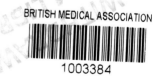

Neonatology Questions and Controversies

ELSEVIER

Neonatology Questions and Controversies

Series Editor

Other Volumes in the Neonatology Questions and Controversies Series

Neonatology Questions and Controversies

Third Edition

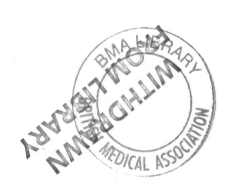

Josef Neu, MD

Professor of Pediatrics
University of Florida College of Medicine
Gainesville, Florida

Brenda Poindexter, MD, MS

Director, Clinical and Translational Research
Perinatal Institute
Cincinnati Children's
Cincinnati, Ohio

Consulting Editor

Richard A. Polin, MD

William T. Speck Professor of Pediatrics
College of Physicians and Surgeons
Columbia University
Director Division of Neonatology
New York Presbyterian
Morgan Stanley Children's Hospital
New York, New York

ELSEVIER

ELSEVIER

1600 John F. Kennedy Blvd.
Ste 1800
Philadelphia, PA 19103-2899

Notices

Knowledge and best practice in this field are constantly changing. As new research and experience broaden our understanding, changes in research methods, professional practices, or medical treatment may become necessary.

Practitioners and researchers must always rely on their own experience and knowledge in evaluating and using any information, methods, compounds, or experiments described herein. In using such information or methods they should be mindful of their own safety and the safety of others, including parties for whom they have a professional responsibility.

With respect to any drug or pharmaceutical products identified, readers are advised to check the most current information provided (i) on procedures featured or (ii) by the manufacturer of each product to be administered, to verify the recommended dose or formula, the method and duration of administration, and contraindications. It is the responsibility of practitioners, relying on their own experience and knowledge of their patients, to make diagnoses, to determine dosages and the best treatment for each individual patient, and to take all appropriate safety precautions.

To the fullest extent of the law, neither the Publisher nor the authors, contributors, or editors, assume any liability for any injury and/or damage to persons or property as a matter of products liability, negligence or otherwise, or from any use or operation of any methods, products, instructions, or ideas contained in the material herein.

Previous editions copyrighted 2012 and 2008.
Library of Congress Cataloging-in-Publication Data

Names: Neu, Josef, editor.
Title: Gastroenterology and nutrition : neonatology questions and
    controversies / [edited by] Josef Neu.
Other titles: Neonatology questions and controversies.
Description: Third edition. | Philadelphia, PA : Elsevier, [2019] | Series:
    Neonatology questions and controversies series | Includes bibliographical
    references and index.
Identifiers: LCCN 2018006369 | ISBN 9780323545020 (alk. paper)
Subjects: | MESH: Gastrointestinal Diseases | Infant, Newborn, Diseases |
    Infant Nutritional Physiological Phenomena | Infant, Newborn
Classification: LCC RJ446 | NLM WS 310 | DDC 616.3/3--dc23 LC record available at
https://lccn.loc.gov/2018006369

Senior Content Strategist: Sarah Barth
Content Development Specialist: Lisa M. Barnes
Book Production Manager: Jeff Patterson
Project Manager: Abigail Bradberry
Design Specialist: Paula Catalano

Printed in China

Last digit is the print number: 9 8 7 6 5 4 3 2 1

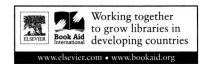

Working together
to grow libraries in
developing countries

www.elsevier.com • www.bookaid.org

Contributors

Kjersti Aagaard-Tillery, MD, PhD, FACOG
Henry and Emma Meyer Chair in Obstetrics & Gynecology
Professor & Vice Chair of Research
Department of Obstetrics & Gynecology, Division of Maternal-Fetal Medicine
Baylor College of Medicine and Texas Children's Hospital
Dallas, Texas
Adult Consequences of Neonatal and Fetal Nutrition: Mechanisms

Lauren Astrug, MD
Neonatal Necrotizing Enterocolitis: Neonatology Questions and Controversies

Cheri Bantilan, MS
Adult Consequences of Neonatal and Fetal Nutrition: Mechanisms

Erika Claud, MD
Professor of Pediatrics and Medicine
Director, Neonatology Research
University of Chicago Medical Center
Chicago, Illinois
Neonatal Necrotizing Enterocolitis: Neonatology Questions and Controversies

Clotilde desRoberts, MD
Adult Consequences of Neonatal and Fetal Nutrition: Mechanisms

Holly J. Engelstad, MD
Fellow
Department of Pediatrics
Washington University in St Louis
St. Louis, Missouri
Nutrition for the Surgical Neonate

Julia B. Ewaschuk
Donor Milk Trials

Steven D. Freedman, MD, PhD
Professor of Medicine
Department of Medicine
Beth Israel Deaconess Medical Center
Boston, Massachusetts
Lipid and Fatty Acid Delivery in the Preterm Infant: Challenges and Lessons Learned from Other Critically Ill Populations

Kathleen M. Gura, BS, PharmD
Clinical Pharmacy Specialist
GI/Nutrition
Pharmacy Department
Clinical Pharmacist
Center for Nutrition;
Clinical Pharmacist
Center for Advanced Intestinal Rehabilitation
Boston Children's Hospital;
Associate Professor
Pharmacy Practice
MCPHS University
Boston, Massachusetts
New Lipid Strategies to Prevent/Treat Neonatal Cholestasis

Anna Maria Hibbs, MD, MSCE
Assistant Professor
Department of Pediatrics
Case Western Reserve University;
Attending Neonatologist
Rainbow Babies and Children's Hospital
Cleveland, Ohio
Maturation of Motor Function in the Preterm Infant and Gastroesophageal Reflux

Sudarshan R. Jadcherla,
MD, FRCPI, DCH, AGAF
Professor
Department of Pediatrics
Sections of Neonatology and Pediatric
Gastroenterology & Nutrition
The Ohio State University College of
Medicine;
Attending Neonatologist
Section of Neonatology;
Director
The Neonatal and Infant Feeding
Disorders Program
Nationwide Children's Hospital;
Principal Investigator
Center for Perinatal Research
The Research Institute at Nationwide
Children's Hospital
Columbus, Ohio
Development of Gastrointestinal Motility
Reflexes

Lisa A. Joss-Moore, PhD
Associate Professor
Pediatrics
University of Utah,
Salt Lake City, Utah
Adult Consequences of Neonatal and Fetal
Nutrition: Mechanisms

Robert H. Lane, MD, MS
Professor and Chair
Department of Pediatrics
Associate Director of Epigenomics
Genomic Science Personalized Medicine
Center
Medical College of Wisconsin
Pediatrician in Chief
The Barri L. and David J. Drury Chair in
Pediatrics
Children's Hospital of Wisconsin
Milwaukee, Wisconsin
Adult Consequences of Neonatal and Fetal
Nutrition: Mechanisms

Mary W. Lenfestey, MD
Postdoctoral Fellow
Pediatric Gastroenterology
University of Florida
Gainesville, Florida
Neonatal Gastrointestinal Tract as a
Conduit to Systemic Inflammation

Camilia R. Martin, MD, MS
Assistant Professor of Pediatrics
Harvard Medical School
Boston, Massachusetts
Lipid and Fatty Acid Delivery in the
Preterm Infant: Challenges and Les-
sons Learned from other Critically Ill
Populations

Nicole Mitchell, MD
Department of Food Science and
Human Nutrition
Michigan State University
Lansing, Michigan
Adult Consequences of Neonatal and Fetal
Nutrition: Mechanisms

Ardythe L. Morrow, PhD, MSc
Professor of Pediatrics, Nutrition &
Environmental Health
University of Cincinnati Colleges of
Medicine & Allied Health
Perinatal Institute
Cincinnati Children's Hospital Medical
Center
Cincinnati, Ohio
Human Milk Oligosaccharides

Josef Neu, MD
Professor
Department of Pediatrics
University of Florida
Gainesville, Florida
Neonatal Gastrointestinal Tract as a
Conduit to Systemic Inflammation
What Are the Controversies, and Where
Will the Field be Moving in the Future?

David S. Newburg, PhD
DSN Medical Consulting
NK Laboratories
Newtonville, Massachusetts
Human Milk Oligosaccharide

Deborah L. O'Connor, PhD, RD
Professor
Department of Nutritional Sciences
University of Toronto,
Senior Associate Scientist
Physiology and Experimental Medicine
The Hospital for Sick Children;
Senior Associate Staff
Pediatrics
Mount Sinai Hospital,
Toronto, Ontario, Canada
Donor Milk Trials

Brenda Poindexter, MD, MS
Director, Clinical and Translational
Research
Professor of Pediatrics
Cincinnati Children's
Cincinnati, Ohio
*What Are the Controversies, and Where
Will the Field be Moving in the Future?*

Sharon L. Unger, MD, FRCP(C)
Neonatologist
Pediatrics
Sinai Health System;
Associate Professor
Medicine
University of Toronto,
Medical Director
Rogers Hixon Ontario Human Milk
Bank;
Clinician Scientist
Lunenfeld-Tanenbaum Research
Institute
Toronto, Ontario, Canada
Donor Milk Trials

Sreekanth Viswanathan, MD, MS
*Development of Gastrointestinal Motility
Reflexes*

Brad W. Warner, MD
Jessie L. Ternberg, MD PhD
Distinguished Professor of Pediatric
Surgery
Surgeon-in-Chief
Washington University School of
Medicine
St. Louis Children's Hospital
Nutrition for the Surgical Neonate

**Jacqueline J. Wessel, Med, RDN,
CNSC, CSP, CLE, LD**
Neonatal Nutritionist
Nutrition Therapy, Intestinal
Rehabilitation
Cincinnati Children's Hospital
Cincinnati, Ohio
Controversies in Short Bowel Syndrome

Series Foreword

Richard A. Polin, MD

"To study the phenomena of disease without books is to sail an uncharted sea, while to study books without patients is not to go to sea at all"

—William Osler

Physicians in training generally rely on the spoken word and clinical experiences to bolster their medical knowledge. There is probably no better way to learn how to care for an infant than to receive teaching at the bedside. Of course, that assumes that the "clinician" doing the teaching is knowledgeable about the disease, wants to teach, and can teach effectively. For a student or intern, this style of learning is efficient because the clinical service demands preclude much time for other reading. Over the course of one's career, it becomes clear that this form of education has limitations because of the fairly-limited number of disease conditions one encounters even in a lifetime of clinical rotations and the diminishing opportunities for teaching moments.

The next educational phase generally includes reading textbooks and qualitative review articles. Unfortunately, both of those sources are often outdated by the time they are published and represent one author's opinions about management. Systematic analyses (meta-analyses) can be more informative, but, more often than not, the conclusion of the systematic analysis is that "more studies are needed" to answer the clinical question. Furthermore, it has been estimated that if a subsequent large randomized clinical trial had not been performed, the meta-analysis would have reached an erroneous conclusion more than one third of the time.

For practicing clinicians, clearly the best way to keep abreast of recent advances in a field is to read the medical literature on a regular basis. However, that approach is problematic given the multitude of journals, unless one reads only the two or three major pediatric journals published in the United States. That approach, however, will miss many of the outstanding articles that appear in more general medical journals (e.g., *Journal of the American Medical Association, New England Journal of Medicine, Lancet,* and the *British Medical Journal*), subspecialty journals, and the many pediatric journals published in other countries.

Although there is no substitute to reading journal articles on a regular basis, the *Questions and Controversies* series of books provides an excellent alternative. This third edition of the series was developed to highlight the clinical problems of most concern to practitioners. The series has been increased from six to seven volumes and includes new sections on genetics and pharmacology. In total, there are 70 new chapters not included previously. The editors of each volume (Drs. Bancalari, Davis, Keszler, Oh, Seri, Ohls, Christensen. Maheshwari, Neu, Benitz, Smith, Poindexter, Cilio, and Perlman) have done an extraordinary job in selecting topics of clinical importance to everyday practice. Unlike traditional review articles, the chapters not only highlight the most significant controversies but also, when possible, incorporate basic science and physiological concepts with a rigorous analysis of the current literature.

As with the first edition, I am indebted to the exceptional group of editors who chose the content and edited each of the volumes. I also wish to thank Lisa Barnes (Content Development Specialist at Elsevier) and Judy Fletcher (Global Content Development Director at Elsevier), who provided incredible assistance in bringing this project to fruition.

Preface

Gastroenterology and Nutrition: Neonatology Questions and Controversies, 3e

As in the previous editions, we address clinically relevant questions and controversies in neonatal nutrition and gastroenterology with up-to-date research in these areas. New information is emerging about the basic developmental physiology of upper intestinal motility as it relates to reflux and feeding tolerance. Immaturities in motility by altering composition of feedings and pharmacologic means is addressed.

The composition of human milk in terms of oligosaccharides and clinical trials that address the efficacy of donor milk in comparison to formula and own mother's milk has been a matter of controversy and is updated in this volume. The developing intestinal tract is known to be much more than a digestive-absorptive organ, and the role of inflammation in systemic diseases in other organs, as well as necrotizing enterocolitis, is addressed.

In this volume, there is also an in-depth analysis of administering lipids to preterm infants, the complications that occur when these are not optimized, and strategies for optimization of providing lipids to infants who are at high risk for complications secondary to suboptimal lipid therapies.

The editors and authors hope to provide continued guidance that will clarify some of the major controversies related to neonatal nutrition and intestinal diseases and help those caring for these vulnerable infants to provide optimal care.

Contents

Neonatology Questions and Controversies

ELSEVIER

CHAPTER 1

Maturation of Motor Function in the Preterm Infant and Gastroesophageal Reflux

Anna Maria Hibbs, MD, MSCE

Gastroesophageal reflux (GER) is defined as the retrograde passage of gastric contents into the esophagus. In term and preterm infants, GER is usually a benign physiologic process, but it meets the definition of gastroesophageal reflux disease (GERD) if it causes clinical symptoms or complications.[1-3] A multitude of gastrointestinal (GI), respiratory, and other symptoms, including apnea, worsening of lung disease, irritability, feeding intolerance, failure to thrive, and stridor, have been attributed to GERD. However, determining whether reflux is the cause of symptoms in an individual patient can be challenging. The approach to an infant with suspected GERD is further complicated by the paucity of available medications demonstrated to be safe or effective in this population.

Upper Gastrointestinal Motility and Physiology

An understanding of GER in infants begins with the physiology of the upper GI tract. Esophageal motor function is well developed in infants as early as 26 weeks' gestational age.[4,5] Swallowing triggers coordinated esophageal peristalsis and lower esophageal sphincter (LES) relaxation, as it does in more mature patients.[4] However, the velocity of propagation is significantly faster in term infants than in preterm infants.[6] Manometry has also documented that spontaneous esophageal activity unrelated to swallowing tends to take the form of incomplete or asynchronous waves; this type of nonperistaltic motor activity occurs more frequently in preterm infants than in adults.[4]

The LES, which blocks GER, is made up of intrinsic esophageal smooth muscle and diaphragmatic skeletal muscle.[7] Although premature infants were once thought to have impaired LES tone, several manometry studies have documented good LES tone, even in extremely low–birth weight infants.[4,8,9] In term and preterm infants, as in older patients, transient LES relaxations (TLESRs) unrelated to swallowing are the major mechanism that allows GER by abruptly dropping lower esophageal pressure below gastric pressure.[4,9,10] These TLESRs may occur several times per hour in preterm infants, although the majority of TLESR events are not associated with GER.[10] Preterm infants with GERD and those without GERD experience a similar frequency of TLESRs, but infants with GERD have a higher percentage of acid GER events during TLESRs.[10] It has been hypothesized that straining or other reasons for increased intra-abdominal pressure may increase the likelihood of a GER event during a TLESR. Although LES relaxations also occur during normal swallowing, these are less often associated with GER events than with isolated TLESR events.[10]

In addition to the anatomic and physiologic factors described that increase the likelihood of the retrograde passage of gastric contents into the esophagus, infants ingest a much higher volume per kilogram of body weight, approximately 180 mL/kg/day, compared with older children and adults.[11] In the neonatal intensive care unit (NICU) population, preterm and term patients with nasogastric or orogastric feeding tubes may experience more reflux episodes as a result of mechanical impairment of the competence of the LES.[12,13]

Gastric emptying is also an important factor in the passage of fluids through the upper GI tract. One small study showed that between 25 and 30 weeks, gastric emptying time seems to be inversely and linearly correlated with gestational age at birth. This study also found that simultaneously decreasing the osmolality and increasing the volume of feeds accelerated gastric emptying, although changes in osmolality or volume alone did not have a significant effect.[14] Emptying also occurs faster with feeding of human milk than of formula. Several small studies suggest that prebiotics, probiotics, and hydrolyzed formulas may speed gastric emptying time in formula-fed infants.[15-17] Fortification of human milk may slow gastric emptying time.[18] The clinical significance of these findings with regard to GER remains uncertain, however. Although it seems logical that slower gastric emptying would be associated with increased GER, a study on the relationship between gastric emptying and GER in preterm infants found no such association.[19]

Diagnosis of Gastroesophageal Reflux and Gastroesophageal Reflux Disease

Although infants have a propensity to experience frequent GER, the majority of GER is physiologic and nonpathologic. GERD is defined as GER that causes complications.[1,2] Unfortunately, in infants, particularly preterm infants, complications of GER are difficult to characterize. Clinicians disagree about which symptoms are caused by GER or GERD.[20] There is mixed evidence in the literature to support or refute most of the proposed complications of GER, including apnea,[21-31] worsening of lung disease,[32-35] and failure to thrive, in infants.[36] An ongoing problem, particularly in the preterm population, is that many of the putative symptoms of GERD also frequently occur for other reasons. For instance, preterm infants without GERD also frequently experience apnea, lung disease, or feeding intolerance.

Physiologic Gastroesophageal Reflux

Nonpathologic GER occurs frequently in both preterm and term infants. Among 509 healthy asymptomatic infants aged 3 to 365 days monitored with an esophageal pH probe, the mean number of acid reflux episodes in 24 hours was 31.28, with a standard deviation of 20.68.[37] The reflux index, the percent of time the esophageal pH was <4, ranged from <1 to 23, with the median and 95th percentile being 4 and 10, respectively. For this reason, a reflux index of 10 is often considered the threshold value for an abnormal study, but it must be remembered that none of the infants in this study were thought to suffer from symptomatic GERD, and clinical correlation with symptoms is required to make the diagnosis of GERD. Among the neonates in this study, the 95th percentile for the reflux index was as high as 13.

In a smaller study of 21 asymptomatic preterm neonates with a median postmenstrual age of 32 weeks, continuous combined esophageal pH and impedance monitoring detected refluxed fluid in the esophagus by impedance for a median of 0.73% (range 0.3%-1.22%) of the recording time, and acid exposure detected by pH monitoring for a median of 5.59% (range 0.04%-20.69%) of the recording time. When using combined pH and multichannel intraluminal impedance (MII) monitoring, detection of acid exposure may exceed volume exposure because the esophageal pH may remain depressed for a time after the majority of the bolus has been cleared, as well as for a variety of other technical reasons.[38] Norms for acid and non–acid reflux are less well defined in preterm than in term infants because of the practical and ethical barriers involved in placing esophageal pH probes in a large number of asymptomatic preterm infants. However, the data from this small study make it clear that GER events occur frequently in asymptomatic infants and that a wide range of reflux measurements may be seen in healthy preterm infants without GERD.

In a study of otherwise healthy infants seen in general pediatric practice, half of all parents reported at least daily regurgitation at 0 to 3 months of age.[39] The peak prevalence occurred at 4 months, with 67% reporting regurgitation, but thereafter it declined rapidly. Thus benign regurgitation was the norm in the first few months of life. Parents reported regurgitation to be a problem when it was associated with increased crying or fussiness, perceived pain, or back arching. The prevalence of regurgitation perceived as a problem peaked at 23% at 6 months but was down to 14% by 7 months. The majority of these children did not receive treatment for GERD from their pediatrician, suggesting that a diagnosis of GERD was only made in a minority of these patients. Infants who did as well as those who did not experience frequent regurgitation between 6 and 12 months of age were subsequently followed-up a year later.[40] At this time, none of the parents described regurgitation as a current problem, and only one child experienced spitting at least daily. That child had not experienced frequent regurgitation at 6 to 12 months of age. Infants who had frequent spitting at 6 to 12 months of age did not experience more ear, sinus, or upper respiratory tract infections or more wheezing. In general, this cohort demonstrated that in the vast majority of infants, regurgitation is a benign process that is outgrown. However, it was noted that in the 1-year follow-up assessment, parents of infants experiencing frequent regurgitation at 6 to 12 months were more likely to report prolonged meal times (8% versus 0%) and frustration about feeding their child (14% versus 4%), even though regurgitation symptoms were no longer present. It is not clear whether this represents a true difference in feeding behavior or parental perception in a group likely to be sensitized to feeding issues.

Gastroesophageal Reflux Disease—Symptoms

Although the definition of GERD hinges on the presence of troublesome symptoms or complications, identifying whether the symptoms in infants are, in fact, caused by reflux can be challenging.[1,2] Symptoms frequently attributed to GERD in infants include regurgitation, Sandifer posturing, worsening of lung disease, food refusal or intolerance, apnea, bradycardia, crying or fussiness, and stridor. Regurgitation may be a symptom of GERD in infants but, in itself, is not a sufficiently sensitive and specific finding to make a diagnosis.[2] In addition, otherwise healthy infants without sequelae from their regurgitation, so-called happy spitters, do not require treatment.[1,3] Clustering regurgitation with other symptoms may increase the accuracy of diagnosis, as demonstrated by the Infant Gastroesophageal Reflux Questionnaire–Revised (I-GERQ-R).[2,41] However, the validity of such questionnaires has not been established in the NICU population, which includes preterm infants and sick term neonates who have multiple competing causes for the symptoms frequently attributed to GERD.

Although GERD and bronchopulmonary dysplasia (BPD) seem to be associated, the presence or direction of causality have not been determined.[2,32-35] Patients with increased work of breathing may generate more negative intrathoracic pressures, thereby promoting the passage of gastric contents into the esophagus. Conversely, aspirated refluxate could injure the lungs. Finally, there may be no causal link in the majority of patients, with immaturity and severity of illness predisposing them to both conditions. In addition, part of the apparent association between BPD and GERD may be caused by an increased index of suspicion for GERD in patients with BPD, leading to increased rates of diagnosis.[34]

A similar issue exists with regard to apnea in premature infants. Although esophageal stimulation may trigger airway protective reflexes in animal models,[42] there is insufficient evidence in human infants to confirm that reflux causes apnea.[2,31] In addition, apnea may itself trigger reflux.[43,44] Finally, it may be that immature infants are simply prone to both apnea and reflux, and there is no causal association.[45] In a cohort of infants referred for overnight esophageal and respiratory monitoring for suspicion of GERD as a cause of apnea, desaturation, or bradycardia, fewer than 3% of all cardiorespiratory events were preceded by a reflux event.[46] The infant with the highest percentage had 4 of 21 cardiorespiratory events preceded by GER. Conversely, 9.1% of reflux events were preceded by a cardiorespiratory event. This study shows that it is more common for a cardiorespiratory event to precede reflux than for reflux to precede a cardiorespiratory event. Cardiorespiratory events preceded by reflux were not more severe than those not preceded by reflux. Furthermore, even in this population referred for suspicion of GER-triggering cardiorespiratory events, only a small minority of cardiorespiratory events were, in fact, preceded by reflux. This suggests that even if all of these temporally related events were also causally related, and even if a treatment were completely efficacious at eliminating GERD, the majority of cardiorespiratory events would not be eliminated by GERD treatment. However, data from small or moderately sized research cohorts cannot rule out the possibility that reflux can trigger the majority of cardiorespiratory events in a small subset of patients. Because bedside recording of apnea events is known to be inaccurate, correlation of apnea with feeding or reflux events in a specific patient requires formal simultaneous respiratory and esophageal monitoring studies.

It is unclear what component of the refluxate triggers complications. Infants experience less acid GER or GERD compared with older children or adults, in large part because of frequent buffering of gastric contents by milk. Although the majority of GER events in infants are nonacid events,[47,48] at least some preterm infants are able to experience significant acid GER, often defined as an esophageal pH <4 for more than 10% of the recording.[23,37] Acid GER predominates preprandially, and nonacid GER postprandially in infants.[45,47] However, it is not clear whether acidity is the mechanism by which reflux causes complications in infants.[2] The other characteristics of the refluxate that have been postulated to be associated with symptoms include the height of the bolus in the esophagus, the volume of the bolus, or the pressure exerted on the esophagus.

Gastroesophageal Reflux Disease—Diagnostic Tests

Numerous tests exist to measure acid and nonacid GER in infants. Esophageal pH probes measure acid reflux, and esophageal MII measures the presence of fluid in the esophagus regardless of pH. Impedance and pH sensors can be combined in one esophageal probe to give the most information about the frequency and timing about both acid and nonacid GER. Many systems have the capacity to be run in conjunction with respiratory monitoring or, for a family member or health care provider to mark the timing of a clinical symptom, to attempt to temporally correlate symptoms and GER events. An upper GI radiographic series is useful for assessing anatomic abnormalities that may contributing to or mimic GER but is a poor measure of the frequency or severity of GER because it only captures a brief window in time. A nuclear medicine scintigraphy study can identify postprandial reflux and aspiration and quantify gastric emptying time. There is no current gold standard diagnostic modality for GERD in infants. Part of the reason is that it is still not clear what component of reflux, such as its frequency, volume, acidity, or height, is most likely to cause complications in infants, and each test measures different parameters. An international consensus statement on GERD described that no single diagnostic test can prove or exclude extraesophageal presentations of GERD in pediatric patients.[2] Furthermore, many NICU patients are too small for endoscopy for direct assessment of esophagitis, so esophageal symptoms can only be inferred from vague symptoms, such as food refusal or fussiness. Finally, because the diagnosis of GERD relies on the presence of clinical complications, no physiologic test that only characterizes the frequency or characteristics of GER events in a patient can, by itself, confirm the diagnosis of GERD (Table 1.1).

Table 1.1 EXAMPLES OF COMMON DIAGNOSTIC TESTS USED TO ASSESS GER IN INFANTS

Test	Strengths	Weakness	Able to Quantify GER Frequency	Able to Diagnose GERD
Upper GI series	Can identify anatomic causes or mimics of GERD, such as a GI obstruction	GER is measured over a brief period, so an assessment of the overall frequency of GER cannot be established Radiation exposure	No	No Correlation with symptoms is necessary
Esophageal pH monitoring	A 12- to 24-hour study allows for a better quantification of the amount of GER experienced by the infant No radiation exposure	It is not clear whether acid or nonacid refluxate triggers certain symptoms Co-monitoring with a probe with both a pH and impedance channel may be a useful option	Yes	No Correlation with symptoms is necessary Many systems may be used in conjunction with cardiorespiratory monitoring or allow for marking of clinical symptoms to try to define the temporal association between symptoms and GER events
Esophageal MII monitoring	Allows for the detection of fluid boluses in the esophagus, regardless of the fluid pH A 12- to 24-hour study allows for a better quantification of the amount of GER experienced by the infant No radiation exposure	Because of technical limitations, some acidic events may not be detected by impedance alone[38]		
Nuclear medicine scintigraphy study (also known as a "milk scan")	Can quantify gastric emptying time Delayed images (usually 12-24 hours) allow for assessment aspirate in the lungs Less radiation than a fluoroscopy-based study	GER is measured over a short total period, even if repeat images are taken, so an assessment of the overall frequency of GER cannot be established Does not distinguish between acid and non-acid GER	No	Yes and no Correlation with symptoms is generally necessary, but a finding of aspiration could result in definitive proof of adverse sequelae

GER, Gastroesophageal reflux; *GERD*, gastroesophageal reflux disease; *GI*, gastrointestinal; *MII*, multichannel intraluminal impedance.

Gastroesophageal Reflux Disease—Treatment

Nonpharmacologic Measures

Nonpharmacologic therapies for GERD include positioning, thickening of feeds, eliminating exposure to cow's milk protein through maternal elimination diets or use of elemental formulas, reducing exposure to environmental tobacco smoke, and decreasing the volume of feeds while increasing the frequency. In a 2013 clinical report, the American Academy of Pediatrics (AAP) Section on Gastroenterology, Hepatology, and Nutrition endorsed these potential lifestyle modifications as potentially beneficial.[49]

The type of milk an infant is consuming may affect GERD symptoms. In the Infant Feeding Practices Study II, direct breastfeeding was protective against reflux compared with formula feeding, but mothers were more likely to wean their babies with reflux.[50] In preterm infants with symptoms of GERD and feeding intolerance, hydrolyzed formula has also been shown to decrease acid reflux measured with an esophageal pH probe, but not regurgitation events measured by impedance.[51] When milk protein allergy is thought to be mimicking or triggering GERD, changing to a more elemental formula may also be appropriate. In the run-in period for a randomized control trial of a pharmacotherapeutic intervention for GERD, the majority of infants seemed to improve over a 2-week period with such a multipronged conservative management strategy, although this effect simply could also be attributed to time and maturation.[52] Thickening of feeds has been shown to decrease episodes of clinical vomiting, although it does not seem to decrease physiologic measures of GER.[53] Thickening can be achieved by adding thickeners or by using commercial GERD formulas that thicken in response to gastric acid. However, thickening of feeds can be challenging for preterm infants as, to date, commercial thickened feeds are nutritionally targeted for term infants and not preterm infants, commercial thickeners may be associated with a risk for necrotizing enterocolitis (NEC), and concerns have been raised about arsenic levels in the infant rice cereals often used for thickening.[49,54-56]

Positioning has also historically been a mainstay of GERD management. Although typical positioning precautions for an infant with a diagnosis of GERD include elevating the head of the bed, there is no advantage to supine-upright positioning versus supine-flat positioning.[53] Prone positioning seems to be associated with fewer GER events compared with supine positioning but is generally contraindicated because of the increased risk of sudden infant death.[53,57] Lateral positioning with the right side down results in more frequent reflux events compared with left lateral positioning, but it is not clear whether this results in more symptoms.[58] In a small study of intubated infants, elevating the head of the bed decreased the detection of gastric pepsin in the airway, presumably indicating a reduction of GER-related aspiration events with positioning.[59]

Pharmacologic Therapy

Medications for the treatment of GERD are among the most common drugs prescribed in the NICU.[60-62] In the United States, pharmacotherapy primarily consists of drugs to decrease gastric acidity, such as the histamine-2 (H_2) receptor antagonists and proton pump inhibitors (PPIs), and prokinetics, such as metoclopramide and erythromycin (Table 1.2). However, an increasing number of studies have questioned the efficacy and safety of these medications in infants. In 2015 the AAP

Table 1.2 COMMON PHARMACOLOGIC THERAPIES FOR GERD IN INFANTS

Drug Type	Mechanisms of Action	Proposed Benefits	Examples of Putative Adverse Effects
H_2 receptor antagonists	Antagonists of the H_2 receptor in acid-producing gastric parietal cells Suppresses basal and meal-induced acid production	Suppression of gastric acidity is thought to mitigate damage to the esophageal mucosa or upper airway caused by the acidity of the refluxate	NEC Late-onset sepsis Respiratory infections Death Intraventricular hemorrhage
Proton pump inhibitors	Irreversibly block the gastric hydrogen/potassium adenosine triphosphatase in parietal cells PPIs are thought to more strongly suppress gastric acidity than H_2 antagonists, leading to the potential for either greater efficacy or more adverse effects	Use of acid suppression is based on the theory that the acidity of the refluxate is the trigger of certain complications, such as fussiness, food refusal, or stridor	Head rubbing or headache Bradycardia Decreased calcium absorption
Metoclopramide	Antagonist of the dopamine-2 receptor subtype	Motility agents are used to promote esophageal clearance of fluids and enhance lower esophageal sphincter tone May also decrease the gastric emptying time	Tarditive dyskinesia Irritability Drowsiness Apnea Emesis Dystonic reaction Oculogyric crisis Gynecomastia and lactation
Erythromycin	Motilin receptor agonist Promotes motility throughout the GI tract by promoting migrating motor complexes		Pyloric stenosis Arrhythmia

GERD, Gastroesophageal reflux disease; *GI*, gastrointestinal; *H_2*, histamine-2; *NEC*, necrotizing enterocolitis.

Section on Perinatal Pediatrics participated in the Choosing Wisely campaign, which charged medical societies with identifying unnecessary tests and treatments that contributed to health care waste. The Section included the following on its list: "Avoid routine use of anti-reflux medications for treatment of symptomatic GERD or for treatment of apnea and desaturation in preterm infants."[63] Nevertheless, because of the wide use of pharmacologic management and its benefit for the exceptional patient, this chapter will review how to gauge response to therapy and the pros and cons of each class of medication. Because both GER and the symptoms commonly linked to GERD, such as feeding intolerance and apnea, change rapidly as functions of time and maturation, valid studies of GERD in infants must account for this effect in their study designs. A study that simply measures symptoms before and after a therapy is likely to find improvement as a result of maturational effects, whether or not the therapy was truly efficacious. In addition, although many studies have demonstrated physiologic changes in response to pharmacotherapy, the gold standard for the treatment of GERD must be improvement in the symptoms that define the disease. Several recent well-conducted studied accounting for maturational changes have raised further questions about the efficacy and safety of common GERD drugs.[64-66]

Because of the difficulties in proving that a possible complication of GER is, indeed, caused by reflux and because of the questionable efficacy of available GERD medications, when treating an individual patient, it must be remembered that treatment failure may stem from either inappropriate application of drugs to treat symptoms not caused by GERD or failure of pharmacotherapy to improve true GERD. Apparent treatment successes may result either from a true treatment effect or from natural maturational changes in GERD or symptoms misclassified as resulting from GERD (Table 1.3). Pharmacotherapy should be stopped if there is no improvement with therapy. If an improvement is seen, trial of cessation of therapy in several weeks should be considered because maturational changes may have been the cause of the initial apparent response or may obviate the need for therapy in the near future.

Table 1.3 POSSIBLE ETIOLOGIES OF APPARENT IMPROVEMENT OR LACK OF IMPROVEMENT AFTER INITIATION OF A GERD THERAPY*

	Symptoms Correctly Attributed to GERD	Symptoms Erroneously Attributed to GERD
Improvement after initiation of therapy	1. The therapeutic intervention was successful. The therapy is efficacious in treating GERD symptoms. -OR- 2. The therapeutic intervention was not successful because of lack of efficacy of the therapy, but improvement in the symptoms due to maturation caused the apparent response to therapy.	1. The therapeutic intervention was not successful because the symptoms were not triggered by GERD, but improvement in the symptoms because of maturation caused the apparent response to therapy. The therapy may or may not be efficacious in treating true GERD.
No improvement after initiation of therapy	1. The therapeutic intervention was not successful due to lack of efficacy of the therapy.	1. The therapeutic intervention was not successful because the symptoms were not triggered by GERD. The therapy may or may not be efficacious in treating true GERD.

*The severity of both GER(D) and the symptoms frequently attributed to GERD, such as apnea, feeding difficulties, or lung disease, rapidly change with time and maturation in infants. Interpretation of a response or lack or response to therapy hinges on understanding that both GERD symptoms and causally unrelated symptoms may change with time, complicating the interpretation of an apparent response to therapy. In addition, many of the symptoms that have been proposed to be triggered by GERD have many other competing causes in preterm infants, and it is difficult to definitively determine whether they are caused by GERD.
GERD, Gastroesophageal reflux disease.

Acid-Blocking Medications

H_2 receptor antagonists and PPIs decrease the acidity of gastric fluid and esophageal refluxate. They act on the H_2 receptors in acid-producing gastric parietal cells, decreasing acid production below normal fasting basal secretion rates as well as suppressing meal-associated acid production. Acid in the esophagus or airway is thought to trigger many of the proposed complications of reflux, such as food refusal, failure to thrive, and pharyngeal or vocal cord edema, in NICU patients. Examples of H_2 receptor antagonists include ranitidine, cimetidine, and famotidine.

Few randomized clinical trials have assessed the impact of H_2 receptor antagonists on GERD symptoms in either neonates or premature infants. In a small but statistically significant crossover trial of combined ranitidine and metoclopramide in preterm infants with bradycardia attributed to GERD, infants experienced significantly more bradycardic events when receiving reflux medications than when receiving placebo.[65] This unexpected finding is biologically plausible; histamine receptors are present in the heart, and ranitidine has been implicated in causing bradyarrhythmias.[67-73] Because most cardiorespiratory events are not associated with GER,[46] the lack of effect found in this study could have been driven either by the misattribution of frequent bradycardia to GERD or by lack of drug efficacy. Bradycardia is likely to have poor specificity for the identification of GERD, given the multiple other triggers for bradycardia in premature infants, including apnea of prematurity and vagal stimulation, and most cardiorespiratory events are not preceded by reflux even among infants suspected of having GERD.[46] Notably, this crossover study of ranitidine and metoclopramide, which appropriately accounted for maturational changes, also demonstrated a clinically and statistically significant decrease in bradycardic events over a 2-week period in both the treatment and placebo groups. This finding underscores the importance of accounting for temporal changes in processes influenced by maturation, such as GER, apnea, and bradycardia.

In a randomized trial of H_2 receptor antagonists, very low–birth weight (VLBW) infants were randomized to cimetidine or placebo.[74] The investigators hypothesized that cimetidine could decrease liver enzyme–mediated oxidative injury in the lung. Although this was not a study of GERD treatment, it is one of the few studies in which VLBW infants were randomized to an H_2 receptor antagonist early in life. Strikingly, it was stopped by the data safety monitoring committee because of increased death and intraventricular hemorrhage in the treatment group. The mechanism of these apparent adverse effects is unknown. The increase in adverse events could have occurred by chance or these events could be true adverse events related to cimetidine and may or may not be generalizable to other H_2 receptor antagonists.

In a small double-blind study, infants aged 1 to 11 months were randomized to a higher or lower dose of famotidine, with a subsequent placebo-controlled withdrawal.[66] Infants receiving famotidine had less frequent emesis compared with those receiving placebo. Infants on the higher famotidine dose also exhibited a decreased crying time and smaller volume of emesis. However, famotidine was also associated with increased agitation and a head-rubbing behavior attributed to headache, raising some concerns about possible side effects in the general infant population.

PPIs irreversibly block the gastric hydrogen/potassium adenosine triphosphatase responsible for secreting hydrogen ions into the gastric lumen. Between 1999 and 2004, PPI prescriptions for infants increased exponentially, with the highest rates of use in infants <4 months of age.[75] Current rates are unknown. Common PPIs include omeprazole, lansoprazole, dexlansoprazole, esomeprazole, pantoprazole, and rabeprazole.

Although physiologic studies have shown that PPIs decrease gastric acidity in infants, PPI trials in infants have generally not shown an improvement in GER symptoms and may have adverse effects. For instance, in a study by Orenstein et al., outpatient infants who had failed a run-in period of nonpharmacologic management were randomized to lansoprazole or placebo.[64] There was no difference in symptoms between the groups, with slightly more than half the infants in each group experiencing improvement over the study period. However, a significant increase in serious adverse events was seen in the lansoprazole group; among these adverse events, a nonsignificant increase in lower respiratory tract infections was noted. In another example, a three-arm trial of delayed release rabeprazole in infants (comparing placebo, 5 mg/day, and 10 mg/day), infants in the 10 mg/day group experienced increased regurgitation.[76] A 2011 systematic review concluded that PPIs should not be prescribed because of insufficient evidence supporting either safety or efficacy.[77] The 2013 AAP clinical report on GER management also cautioned that PPIs have not been shown to be safe or effective in infants.[49]

In addition to drug-specific side effects, such as leukopenia and thrombocytopenia with ranitidine, class effects resulting from the change in gastric pH may be seen with H_2 receptor antagonists and PPIs. For instance, increasing evidence suggests that gastric acidity may play an important role in host immune defense. In an observational study, use of H_2 receptor antagonists was associated with increased NEC.[78] In another cohort study, ranitidine use was associated with late-onset sepsis in NICU patients.[79] In a 2013 meta-analysis, Chung et al. found a significant association between pharmacologic acid suppression and the risk of NEC, sepsis, pneumonia, and GI infections in infants and children.[80] However, in these observational studies, confounding by indication or severity of illness cannot completely be excluded as the cause of this apparent association. Consistent with the findings in the observational studies, in one small interventional study, gastric acidification was shown to decrease NEC.[81] Higher rates of gastric colonization with bacteria or yeast have also been associated with ranitidine, but without a detectable increase in clinical infection.[82] In older patients, a possible association between acid suppression and lower respiratory tract infections, including ventilator associated pneumonia, remains controversial in the literature.[83-91] Acid suppression has also been associated with *Clostridium difficile* infection in some adults. PPIs seem to carry a higher risk compared with H_2 receptor antagonists, presumably because of more effective acid suppression.[92,93] The relationship between PPI use and *C. difficile* colonization or infection has not been reported in infants.

Increasing gastric pH can theoretically also have nutritional consequences. Acid reduction may decrease calcium absorption as a result of decreased ionization of calcium in the stomach. The U.S. Food and Drug Administration (FDA) recently released a class labeling change for PPIs because of concerns that adults on high doses or prolonged courses of PPIs seem to experience more fractures.[94,95] The impact of acid suppression by PPIs or H_2 receptor antagonists on bone health in either healthy neonates or preterm infants with osteopenia of prematurity is unknown. Vitamin B_{12} absorption is also dependent on gastric acidity, but the impact of gastric acid suppression on vitamin B_{12} status in infants has also not been described.

Prokinetics

Drugs to promote GI motility are thought to act by improving esophageal motility and LES tone. Prokinetics are also often used to shorten gastric emptying time, although a relationship between GER and delayed gastric emptying in infants has not been proven.[19]

Metoclopramide and erythromycin are the primary prokinetics currently approved in the United States. Cisapride was removed from the market because of the risk of serious cardiac arrhythmias and QT prolongation.[96] Domperidone is also not approved in the United States because of concerns about QT prolongation in neonates.[97]

Metoclopramide is a dopamine receptor antagonist. The Cochrane systematic review of GERD therapies in children found both therapeutic benefit and increased adverse effects with metoclopramide treatment.[98] However, most of the improvements seen were in physiologic measures of GER and not in the symptoms of GERD. A subsequent systematic review of metoclopramide therapy for GERD in infants found insufficient evidence for either efficacy or safety in this population.[99] Published after these reviews, the previously described placebo-controlled crossover study of ranitidine and metoclopramide demonstrated lack of efficacy and an increase in bradycardia in the treatment group, although this finding could be attributed to ranitidine and not metoclopramide.[65]

Metoclopramide can cause neurologic sequelae because it crosses the blood–brain barrier and acts on central dopamine receptors. Possible neurologic complications of metoclopramide in infants include irritability, drowsiness, oculogyric crisis, dystonic reaction, and apnea.[99] In 2009 the FDA issued a warning about the risk of tarditive dyskinesia with prolonged or high-dose metoclopramide use.[100] Tarditive dyskinesia has no known treatment and consists of involuntary body movements, which may persist after the drug is stopped. It is unknown whether term or preterm infants are at greater or lesser risk of tarditive dyskinesia compared with older patients.

Erythromycin is an analogue of motilin, a hormone normally produced by duodenal and jejunal enterochromaffin cells and which promotes GI migrating motor complexes.[101-103] The prokinetics dose of erythromycin is typically lower than the antimicrobial dose, but a standard promotility dose has not been established in neonates or preterm infants. Infants older than 32 weeks' gestational age may be better able to respond to stimulation of the motilin receptor compared with less mature infants.[104,105]

Most studies of erythromycin in preterm infants have focused on improving feeding intolerance and not specifically on GERD treatment.[104,105] In a masked randomized trial of erythromycin to promote feeding tolerance in 24 preterm infants, GER was measured as a secondary endpoint.[106] Erythromycin did not decrease the time to reach full enteral feeds, and there were no changes in GER measured with an pH probe. GERD symptoms were not reported in this study. A systematic review of erythromycin to promote feeding tolerance in premature infants concluded that erythromycin could promote the establishment of enteral feeding and was not associated with any adverse events.[107] However, the authors cautioned that because long-term adverse events had not been fully studied, erythromycin should be reserved for infants with severe dysmotility.

When used as an antibiotic, erythromycin may promote pyloric stenosis in infants. It is unknown whether a similar effect could occur with the lower doses and longer duration of therapy associated with use as a prokinetic, although pyloric stenosis has not been reported in most of the current trials in preterm infants.[107] Chronic administration of erythromycin has the potential to impact GI colonization, but the impact in the NICU population is unknown.

Erythromycin may increase serum levels of theophylline, digoxin, sildenafil, and some benzodiazepines, and has been implicated in arrhythmias and QT prolongation when co-administered with cisapride. In addition, it also has a direct proarrhythmic effect by itself because of prolongation of the QT interval.[108] In older patients, the risk of sudden death may be increased when erythromycin is used with other inhibitors of the same hepatic enzyme (CYP3A), such as cimetidine and methadone.[108]

Summary

GER is common in both term and preterm infants. The primary mechanism allowing reflux is TLESRs. Although the diagnosis of GERD requires the presence of complication resulting from reflux, ascertaining whether symptoms in a given patient are caused by GERD can be challenging. There is no gold standard diagnostic modality to diagnose GERD in the NICU population. Although esophageal impedance and/or pH measurements are the most commonly reported, linking measured GER with symptoms is still required to diagnose GERD. In the NICU population, few symptoms have been definitively shown to be caused by GERD, and most of the putative symptoms of GERD, such as feeding intolerance or apnea, have many possible etiologies. Furthermore, no pharmacologic interventions have been proven to be safe and effective in this population. Therefore nonpharmacologic expectant management should be the mainstay of treatment for most infants.

REFERENCES

1. Rudolph CD, Mazur LJ, Liptak GS, et al. Guidelines for evaluation and treatment of gastroesophageal reflux in infants and children: recommendations of the North American Society for Pediatric Gastroenterology and Nutrition. *J Pediatr Gastroenterol Nutr*. 2001;32(suppl 2):S1–S31.
2. Sherman PM, Hassall E, Fagundes-Neto U, et al. A global, evidence-based consensus on the definition of gastroesophageal reflux disease in the pediatric population. *Am J Gastroenterol*. 2009;104(5):1278–1295. quiz 96.
3. Vandenplas Y, Rudolph CD, Di Lorenzo C, et al. Pediatric gastroesophageal reflux clinical practice guidelines: joint recommendations of the North American Society for Pediatric Gastroenterology, Hepatology, and Nutrition (NASPGHAN) and the European Society for Pediatric Gastroenterology, Hepatology, and Nutrition (ESPGHAN). *J Pediatr Gastroenterol Nutr*. 2009;49(4):498–547.
4. Omari TI, Benninga MA, Barnett CP, Haslam RR, Davidson GP, Dent J. Characterization of esophageal body and lower esophageal sphincter motor function in the very premature neonate. *J Pediatr*. 1999;135(4):517–521.
5. Omari TI, Barnett C, Snel A, et al. Mechanisms of gastroesophageal reflux in healthy premature infants. *J Pediatr*. 1998;133(5):650–654.
6. Jadcherla SR, Duong HQ, Hofmann C, Hoffmann R, Shaker R. Characteristics of upper oesophageal sphincter and oesophageal body during maturation in healthy human neonates compared with adults. *Neurogastroenterol Motil*. 2005;17(5):663–670.
7. Mittal RK, Balaban DH. The esophagogastric junction. *N Engl J Med*. 1997;336(13):924–932.
8. Omari TI, Miki K, Davidson G, et al. Characterisation of relaxation of the lower oesophageal sphincter in healthy premature infants. *Gut*. 1997;40(3):370–375.
9. Omari TI, Miki K, Fraser R, et al. Esophageal body and lower esophageal sphincter function in healthy premature infants. *Gastroenterology*. 1995;109(6):1757–1764.
10. Davidson G. The role of lower esophageal sphincter function and dysmotility in gastroesophageal reflux in premature infants and in the first year of life. *J Pediatr Gastroenterol Nutr*. 2003;37(suppl 1):S17–S22.
11. Poets CF. Gastroesophageal reflux: a critical review of its role in preterm infants. *Pediatrics*. 2004;113(2):e128–e132.
12. Peter CS, Wiechers C, Bohnhorst B, Silny J, Poets CF. Influence of nasogastric tubes on gastroesophageal reflux in preterm infants: a multiple intraluminal impedance study. *J Pediatr*. 2002;141(2):277–279.
13. Mendes TB, Mezzacappa MA, Toro AA, Ribeiro JD. Risk factors for gastroesophageal reflux disease in very low birth weight infants with bronchopulmonary dysplasia. *J Pediatr (Rio J)*. 2008;84(2):154–159.
14. Ramirez A, Wong WW, Shulman RJ. Factors regulating gastric emptying in preterm infants. *J Pediatr*. 2006;149(4):475–479.
15. Indrio F, Riezzo G, Raimondi F, Bisceglia M, Cavallo L, Francavilla R. The effects of probiotics on feeding tolerance, bowel habits, and gastrointestinal motility in preterm newborns. *J Pediatr*. 2008;152(6):801–806.
16. Indrio F, Riezzo G, Raimondi F, et al. Prebiotics improve gastric motility and gastric electrical activity in preterm newborns. *J Pediatr Gastroenterol Nutr*. 2009;49(2):258–261.
17. Staelens S, Van den Driessche M, Barclay D, et al. Gastric emptying in healthy newborns fed an intact protein formula, a partially and an extensively hydrolysed formula. *Clin Nutr*. 2008;27(2):264–268.
18. Ewer AK, Yu VY. Gastric emptying in pre-term infants: the effect of breast milk fortifier. *Acta Paediatr*. 1996;85(9):1112–1115.
19. Ewer AK, Durbin GM, Morgan ME, Booth IW. Gastric emptying and gastro-oesophageal reflux in preterm infants. *Arch Dis Child Fetal Neonatal Ed*. 1996;75(2):F117–F121.
20. Golski CA, Rome ES, Martin RJ, et al. Pediatric specialists' beliefs about gastroesophageal reflux disease in premature infants. *Pediatrics*. 2010;125(1):96–104.
21. Barrington KJ, Tan K, Rich W. Apnea at discharge and gastro-esophageal reflux in the preterm infant. *J Perinatol*. 2002;22(1):8–11.
22. de Ajuriaguerra M, Radvanyi-Bouvet MF, Huon C, Moriette G. Gastroesophageal reflux and apnea in prematurely born infants during wakefulness and sleep. *Am J Dis Child*. 1991;145(10):1132–1136.
23. Di Fiore JM, Arko M, Whitehouse M, Kimball A, Martin RJ. Apnea is not prolonged by acid gastroesophageal reflux in preterm infants. *Pediatrics*. 2005;116(5):1059–1063.
24. Herbst JJ, Minton SD, Book LS. Gastroesophageal reflux causing respiratory distress and apnea in newborn infants. *J Pediatr*. 1979;95(5 Pt 1):763–768.
25. Molloy EJ, Di Fiore JM, Martin RJ. Does gastroesophageal reflux cause apnea in preterm infants? *Biol Neonate*. 2005;87(4):254–261.
26. Mousa H, Woodley FW, Metheney M, Hayes J. Testing the association between gastroesophageal reflux and apnea in infants. *J Pediatr Gastroenterol Nutr*. 2005;41(2):169–177.
27. Paton JY, Macfadyen U, Williams A, Simpson H. Gastro-oesophageal reflux and apnoeic pauses during sleep in infancy–no direct relation. *Eur J Pediatr*. 1990;149(10):680–686.
28. Peter CS, Sprodowski N, Bohnhorst B, Silny J, Poets CF. Gastroesophageal reflux and apnea of prematurity: no temporal relationship. *Pediatrics*. 2002;109(1):8–11.
29. Spitzer AR, Boyle JT, Tuchman DN, Fox WW. Awake apnea associated with gastroesophageal reflux: a specific clinical syndrome. *J Pediatr*. 1984;104(2):200–205.
30. Corvaglia L, Zama D, Gualdi S, Ferlini M, Aceti A, Faldella G. Gastro-oesophageal reflux increases the number of apnoeas in very preterm infants. *Arch Dis Child Fetal Neonatal Ed*. 2009;94(3):F188–F192.

31. Finer NN, Higgins R, Kattwinkel J, Martin RJ. Summary proceedings from the apnea-of-prematurity group. *Pediatrics*. 2006;117(3 Pt 2):S47–S51.
32. Akinola E, Rosenkrantz TS, Pappagallo M, McKay K, Hussain N. Gastroesophageal reflux in infants < 32 weeks gestational age at birth: lack of relationship to chronic lung disease. *Am J Perinatol*. 2004;21(2):57–62.
33. Farhath S, He Z, Nakhla T, et al. Pepsin, a marker of gastric contents, is increased in tracheal aspirates from preterm infants who develop bronchopulmonary dysplasia. *Pediatrics*. 2008;121(2):e253–e259.
34. Fuloria M, Hiatt D, Dillard RG, O'Shea TM. Gastroesophageal reflux in very low birth weight infants: association with chronic lung disease and outcomes through 1 year of age. *J Perinatol*. 2000;20(4):235–239.
35. Khalaf MN, Porat R, Brodsky NL, Bhandari V. Clinical correlations in infants in the neonatal intensive care unit with varying severity of gastroesophageal reflux. *J Pediatr Gastroenterol Nutr*. 2001;32(1):45–49.
36. Frakaloss G, Burke G, Sanders MR. Impact of gastroesophageal reflux on growth and hospital stay in premature infants. *J Pediatr Gastroenterol Nutr*. 1998;26(2):146–150.
37. Vandenplas Y, Goyvaerts H, Helven R, Sacre L. Gastroesophageal reflux, as measured by 24-hour pH monitoring, in 509 healthy infants screened for risk of sudden infant death syndrome. *Pediatrics*. 1991;88(4):834–840.
38. Di Fiore JM, Arko M, Churbock K, Hibbs AM, Martin RJ. Technical limitations in detection of gastroesophageal reflux in neonates. *J Pediatr Gastroenterol Nutr*. 2009;49(2):177–182.
39. Nelson SP, Chen EH, Syniar GM, Christoffel KK. Prevalence of symptoms of gastroesophageal reflux during infancy. A pediatric practice-based survey. Pediatric Practice Research Group. *Arch Pediatr Adolesc Med*. 1997;151(6):569–572.
40. Nelson SP, Chen EH, Syniar GM, Christoffel KK. One-year follow-up of symptoms of gastroesophageal reflux during infancy. Pediatric Practice Research Group. *Pediatrics*. 1998;102(6):E67.
41. Kleinman L, Rothman M, Strauss R, et al. The infant gastroesophageal reflux questionnaire revised: development and validation as an evaluative instrument. *Clin Gastroenterol Hepatol*. 2006;4(5):588–596.
42. St-Hilaire M, Nsegbe E, Gagnon-Gervais K, et al. Laryngeal chemoreflexes induced by acid, water, and saline in nonsedated newborn lambs during quiet sleep. *J Appl Physiol*. 2005;98(6):2197–2203.
43. Kiatchoosakun P, Dreshaj IA, Abu-Shaweesh JM, Haxhiu MA, Martin RJ. Effects of hypoxia on respiratory neural output and lower esophageal sphincter pressure in piglets. *Pediatr Res*. 2002;52(1):50–55.
44. Omari TI. Apnea-associated reduction in lower esophageal sphincter tone in premature infants. *J Pediatr*. 2009;154(3):374–378.
45. Slocum C, Hibbs AM, Martin RJ, Orenstein SR. Infant apnea and gastroesophageal reflux: a critical review and framework for further investigation. *Curr Gastroenterol Rep*. 2007;9(3):219–224.
46. Di Fiore J, Arko M, Herynk B, Martin R, Hibbs AM. Characterization of cardiorespiratory events following gastroesophageal reflux in preterm infants. *J Perinatol*. 2010;30(10):683–687.
47. Condino AA, Sondheimer J, Pan Z, Gralla J, Perry D, O'Connor JA. Evaluation of infantile acid and nonacid gastroesophageal reflux using combined pH monitoring and impedance measurement. *J Pediatr Gastroenterol Nutr*. 2006;42(1):16–21.
48. Slocum C, Arko M, Di Fiore J, Martin RJ, Hibbs AM. Apnea, bradycardia and desaturation in preterm infants before and after feeding. *J Perinatol*. 2009;29(3):209–212.
49. Lightdale JR, Gremse DA. Section on Gastroenterology H, Nutrition. Gastroesophageal reflux: management guidance for the pediatrician. *Pediatrics*. 2013;131(5):e1684–e1695.
50. Chen PL, Soto-Ramirez N, Zhang H, Karmaus W. Association between infant feeding modes and gastroesophageal reflux. *J Hum Lact*. 2017. https://doi.org/890334416664711.
51. Corvaglia L, Mariani E, Aceti A, Galletti S, Faldella G. Extensively hydrolyzed protein formula reduces acid gastro-esophageal reflux in symptomatic preterm infants. *Early Hum Dev*. 2013;89(7):453–455.
52. Orenstein SR, McGowan JD. Efficacy of conservative therapy as taught in the primary care setting for symptoms suggesting infant gastroesophageal reflux. *J Pediatr*. 2008;152(3):310–314.
53. Carroll AE, Garrison MM, Christakis DA. A systematic review of nonpharmacological and nonsurgical therapies for gastroesophageal reflux in infants. *Arch Pediatr Adolesc Med*. 2002;156(2):109–113.
54. Carignan CC, Punshon T, Karagas MR, Cottingham KL. Potential exposure to arsenic from infant rice cereal. *Ann Glob Health*. 2016;82(1):221–224.
55. Karagas MR, Punshon T, Sayarath V, Jackson BP, Folt CL, Cottingham KL. Association of rice and rice-product consumption with arsenic exposure early in life. *JAMA Pediatrics*. 2016;170(6):609–616.
56. Clarke P, Robinson MJ. Thickening milk feeds may cause necrotising enterocolitis. *Arch Dis Child Fetal Neonatal Ed*. 2004;89(3):F280.
57. American Academy of Pediatrics AAP Task force on infant positioning and SIDS: positioning and SIDS. *Pediatrics*. 1992;89(6 Pt 1):1120–1126.
58. Omari TI, Rommel N, Staunton E, et al. Paradoxical impact of body positioning on gastroesophageal reflux and gastric emptying in the premature neonate. *J Pediatr*. 2004;145(2):194–200.
59. Garland JS, Alex CP, Johnston N, Yan JC, Werlin SL. Association between tracheal pepsin, a reliable marker of gastric aspiration, and head of bed elevation among ventilated neonates. *J Neonatal Perinatal Med*. 2014;7(3):185–192.
60. Clark RH, Bloom BT, Spitzer AR, Gerstmann DR. Reported medication use in the neonatal intensive care unit: data from a large national data set. *Pediatrics*. 2006;117(6):1979–1987.

61. Dhillon AS, Ewer AK. Diagnosis and management of gastro-oesophageal reflux in preterm infants in neonatal intensive care units. *Acta Paediatr*. 2004;93(1):88–93.

62. Malcolm WF, Gantz M, Martin RJ, Goldstein RF, Goldberg RN, Cotten CM. Use of medications for gastroesophageal reflux at discharge among extremely low birth weight infants. *Pediatrics*. 2008;121(1):22–27.

63. Ho T, Dukhovny D, Zupancic JA, Goldmann DA, Horbar JD, Pursley DM. Choosing wisely in newborn medicine: five opportunities to increase value. *Pediatrics*. 2015;136(2):e482–e489.

64. Orenstein SR, Hassall E, Furmaga-Jablonska W, Atkinson S, Raanan M. Multicenter, double-blind, randomized, placebo-controlled trial assessing the efficacy and safety of proton pump inhibitor lansoprazole in infants with symptoms of gastroesophageal reflux disease. *J Pediatr*. 2009;154(4):514–520.e4.

65. Wheatley E, Kennedy KA. Cross-over trial of treatment for bradycardia attributed to gastroesophageal reflux in preterm infants. *J Pediatr*. 2009;155(4):516–521.

66. Orenstein SR, Shalaby TM, Devandry SN, et al. Famotidine for infant gastro-oesophageal reflux: a multi-centre, randomized, placebo-controlled, withdrawal trial. *Aliment Pharmacol Ther*. 2003;17(9):1097–1107.

67. Hu WH, Wang KY, Hwang DS, Ting CT, Wu TC. Histamine 2 receptor blocker-ranitidine and sinus node dysfunction. *Zhonghua Yi Xue Za Zhi (Taipei)*. 1997;60(1):1–5.

68. Alliet P, Devos E. Ranitidine-induced bradycardia in a neonate–secondary to congenital long QT interval syndrome? *Eur J Pediatr*. 1994;153(10):781.

69. Hinrichsen H, Halabi A, Kirch W. Clinical aspects of cardiovascular effects of H2-receptor antagonists. *J Clin Pharmacol*. 1995;35(2):107–116.

70. Nahum E, Reish O, Naor N, Merlob P. Ranitidine-induced bradycardia in a neonate–a first report. *Eur J Pediatr*. 1993;152(11):933–934.

71. Ooie T, Saikawa T, Hara M, Ono H, Seike M, Sakata T. H2-blocker modulates heart rate variability. *Heart Vessels*. 1999;14(3):137–142.

72. Tanner LA, Arrowsmith JB. Bradycardia and H2 antagonists. *Ann Intern Med*. 1988;109(5):434–435.

73. Yang J, Russell DA, Bourdeau JE. Case report: ranitidine-induced bradycardia in a patient with dextrocardia. *Am J Med Sci*. 1996;312(3):133–135.

74. Cotton RB, Hazinski TA, Morrow JD, et al. Cimetidine does not prevent lung injury in newborn premature infants. *Pediatr Res*. 2006;59(6):795–800.

75. Barron JJ, Tan H, Spalding J, Bakst AW, Singer J. Proton pump inhibitor utilization patterns in infants. *J Pediatr Gastroenterol Nutr*. 2007;45(4):421–427.

76. Hussain S, Kierkus J, Hu P, et al. Safety and efficacy of delayed release rabeprazole in 1- to 11-month-old infants with symptomatic GERD. *J Pediatr Gastroenterol Nutr*. 2014;58(2):226–236.

77. van der Pol RJ, Smits MJ, van Wijk MP, Omari TI, Tabbers MM, Benninga MA. Efficacy of proton-pump inhibitors in children with gastroesophageal reflux disease: a systematic review. *Pediatrics*. 2011;127(5):925–935.

78. Guillet R, Stoll BJ, Cotten CM, et al. Association of H2-blocker therapy and higher incidence of necrotizing enterocolitis in very low birth weight infants. *Pediatrics*. 2006;117(2):e137–e142.

79. Bianconi S, Gudavalli M, Sutija VG, Lopez AL, Barillas-Arias L, Ron N. Ranitidine and late-onset sepsis in the neonatal intensive care unit. *J Perinat Med*. 2007;35(2):147–150.

80. Chung EY, Yardley J. Are there risks associated with empiric acid suppression treatment of infants and children suspected of having gastroesophageal reflux disease? *Hospital Pediatrics*. 2013;3(1):16–23.

81. Carrion V, Egan EA. Prevention of neonatal necrotizing enterocolitis. *J Pediatr Gastroenterol Nutr*. 1990;11(3):317–323.

82. Cothran DS, Borowitz SM, Sutphen JL, Dudley SM, Donowitz LG. Alteration of normal gastric flora in neonates receiving ranitidine. *J Perinatol*. 1997;17(5):383–388.

83. Apte NM, Karnad DR, Medhekar TP, Tilve GH, Morye S, Bhave GG. Gastric colonization and pneumonia in intubated critically ill patients receiving stress ulcer prophylaxis: a randomized, controlled trial. *Crit Care Med*. 1992;20(5):590–593.

84. Yildizdas D, Yapicioglu H, Yilmaz HL. Occurrence of ventilator-associated pneumonia in mechanically ventilated pediatric intensive care patients during stress ulcer prophylaxis with sucralfate, ranitidine, and omeprazole. *J Crit Care*. 2002;17(4):240–245.

85. Miano TA, Reichert MG, Houle TT, MacGregor DA, Kincaid EH, Bowton DL. Nosocomial pneumonia risk and stress ulcer prophylaxis: a comparison of pantoprazole vs ranitidine in cardiothoracic surgery patients. *Chest*. 2009;136(2):440–447.

86. Sharma H, Singh D, Pooni P, Mohan U. A study of profile of ventilator-associated pneumonia in children in Punjab. *J Trop Pediatr*. 2009;55(6):393–395.

87. Tablan OC, Anderson LJ, Besser R, Bridges C, Hajjeh R. Guidelines for preventing health-care–associated pneumonia 2003: recommendations of CDC and the healthcare infection control practices advisory committee. *MMWR Recomm Rep*. 2004;53(RR-3):1–36.

88. Beaulieu M, Williamson D, Sirois C, Lachaine J. Do proton-pump inhibitors increase the risk for nosocomial pneumonia in a medical intensive care unit? *J Crit Care*. 2008;23(4):513–518.

89. Kobashi Y, Matsushima T. Clinical analysis of patients requiring long-term mechanical ventilation of over three months: ventilator-associated pneumonia as a primary complication. *Intern Med*. 2003;42(1):25–32.

90. Cook D, Guyatt G, Marshall J, et al. A comparison of sucralfate and ranitidine for the prevention of upper gastrointestinal bleeding in patients requiring mechanical ventilation. Canadian Critical Care Trials Group. *N Engl J Med*. 1998;338(12):791–797.

91. Canani RB, Cirillo P, Roggero P, et al. Therapy with gastric acidity inhibitors increases the risk of acute gastroenteritis and community-acquired pneumonia in children. *Pediatrics*. 2006;117(5):e817–e820.

92. Howell MD, Novack V, Grgurich P, et al. Iatrogenic gastric acid suppression and the risk of nosocomial Clostridium difficile infection. *Arch Intern Med*. 2010;170(9):784–790.

93. Linsky A, Gupta K, Lawler EV, Fonda JR, Hermos JA. Proton pump inhibitors and risk for recurrent Clostridium difficile infection. *Arch Intern Med*. 2010;170(9):772–778.

94. FDA. http://www.fda.gov/Safety/MedWatch/SafetyInformation/SafetyAlertsforHumanMedicalProducts/ucm213321.htm; 2010 [cited 2010 June 24].

95. FDA. http://www.fda.gov/ForConsumers/ConsumerUpdates/ucm213240.htm; 2010 [cited 2010 June 24].

96. FDA. http://www.fda.gov/Safety/MedWatch/SafetyInformation/SafetyAlertsforHumanMedicalProducts/ucm173074.htm; 2000 [cited 2010 June 25].

97. Djeddi D, Kongolo G, Lefaix C, Mounard J, Leke A. Effect of domperidone on QT interval in neonates. *J Pediatr*. 2008;153(5):663–666.

98. Craig WR, Hanlon-Dearman A, Sinclair C, Taback S, Moffatt M. Metoclopramide, thickened feedings, and positioning for gastro-oesophageal reflux in children under two years. *Cochrane Database Syst Rev*. 2004;(4):CD003502.

99. Hibbs AM, Lorch SA. Metoclopramide for the treatment of gastroesophageal reflux disease in infants: a systematic review. *Pediatrics*. 2006;118(2):746–752.

100. FDA. http://www.fda.gov/Safety/MedWatch/SafetyInformation/SafetyAlertsforHumanMedicalProducts/ucm106942.htm; 2009 [cited 2010 June 24].

101. Itoh Z, Nakaya M, Suzuki T, Arai H, Wakabayashi K. Erythromycin mimics exogenous motilin in gastrointestinal contractile activity in the dog. *Am J Physiol*. 1984;247(6 Pt 1):G688–G694.

102. Itoh Z, Suzuki T, Nakaya M, Inoue M, Mitsuhashi S. Gastrointestinal motor-stimulating activity of macrolide antibiotics and analysis of their side effects on the canine gut. *Antimicrob Agents Chemother*. 1984;26(6):863–869.

103. Feighner SD, Tan CP, McKee KK, et al. Receptor for motilin identified in the human gastrointestinal system. *Science*. 1999;284(5423):2184–2188.

104. Ng E, Shah VS. Erythromycin for the prevention and treatment of feeding intolerance in preterm infants. *Cochrane Database Syst Rev*. 2008;(3):CD001815.

105. Patole S, Rao S, Doherty D. Erythromycin as a prokinetic agent in preterm neonates: a systematic review. *Arch Dis Child Fetal Neonatal Ed*. 2005;90(4):F301–F306.

106. Ng SC, Gomez JM, Rajadurai VS, Saw SM, Quak SH. Establishing enteral feeding in preterm infants with feeding intolerance: a randomized controlled study of low-dose erythromycin. *J Pediatr Gastroenterol Nutr*. 2003;37(5):554–558.

107. Ng PC. Use of oral erythromycin for the treatment of gastrointestinal dysmotility in preterm infants. *Neonatology*. 2009;95(2):97–104.

108. Simko J, Csilek A, Karaszi J, Lorincz I. Proarrhythmic potential of antimicrobial agents. *Infection*. 2008;36(3):194–206.

CHAPTER 2

Development of Gastrointestinal Motility Reflexes

Sreekanth Viswanathan, MD, MS, Sudarshan R. Jadcherla, MD, FRCP (Irel), DCH, AGAF

2

Outline

Introduction

Gastrointestinal motility in human infants is a complex function, and the development of the elements to facilitate this is a much more complex process. Briefly, by the 14th week of development, all the cellular components necessary for coordinated neural and muscular activities exist in the fetal gut. However, maturation of neuromuscular functions occurs during mid- and late gestation, and this translates to fully functional coordinated gut motility patterns in the full-term healthy neonate capable of independent feeding, aerodigestive protection, and small and large intestinal peristalsis, besides cyclical regulation of hunger, satiety and feeding. This process continues to mature postnatally and is influenced by the maturational changes in the central and enteric nervous system, gut muscle and interstitial cell of Cajal (ICC), as well as by the diet and rapidly changing anatomy and physiology during infancy. In the vulnerable high-risk preterm infants in neonatal intensive care units (NICUs) the influence of hypoxia, inflammation, sepsis, and other comorbid conditions complicate and alter the postnatal development of gastrointestinal motility. Coordinated movements of gut are crucial for the primary function of the neonatal foregut (to facilitate safe feeding process so as to steer the feedings away from the airway), midgut (gastrointestinal transit of luminal contents to modulate absorption and propulsion), and hindgut (evacuation of excreta to maintain intestinal milieu homeostasis). In this chapter, we will review and summarize the developmental aspects of (1) pharyngo-esophageal motility, (2) gastrointestinal motility, and (3) colonic motility.

Embryologic Aspects of Motility Development

The human gut initially arises as a primitive tube from the endoderm of the trilaminar embryo (week 3) and later receives contributions from all the germ cell layers.[1-3] The endoderm gives rise to the epithelial lining and glands, the ectoderm gives rise to the oral cavity and the anus, and the mesoderm-derived splanchnic mesenchyme gives

A

rise to the smooth muscle and connective tissue. During week 4, the gut differentiates into three distinct regions (foregut, midgut, and hindgut). The foregut later develops into the airway and lung buds, pharynx, esophagus, stomach, and proximal portion of the duodenum; the midgut gives rise to the remainder of the duodenum, small intestine, and portions of the large intestine up to the distal transverse colon; and the hindgut develops into the distal part of the transverse colon, descending colon, rectum, and proximal part of the anal canal.

The smooth muscles are innervated by the intrinsic neurons of the enteric nervous system (ENS), which consists of interconnected ganglia, containing neurons and glial cells.[1-3] The ENS arises from precursor cells derived from the vagal (hindbrain) neural crest that enter the foregut and advance rostrocaudally in the intestine. They colonize the gut through a complex process of migration, proliferation, and differentiation along defined pathways and reach the midgut by week 5 of development and the entire length of the gut by week 7.[2,4-6] A second, more caudal region of the neural crest, that is, the sacral neural crest, also contributes a smaller number of cells that are restricted to the hindgut ENS.[7] The ganglia of the ENS are organized in two plexus layers that span the length of the gut—an outer myenteric plexus, situated between the longitudinal and circular muscle layers, and an inner submucosal plexus lying between the circular muscle and the muscularis mucosae.[8,9] Neurons within the myenteric plexus are primarily involved in the control of gut motility, whereas neurons within the submucosal plexus are mainly involved in controlling mucosal functions, such as electrolyte and hormone secretion.[1,3] The ENS neurons may be classified according to their function as afferent sensory neurons, interneurons, and motor neurons.[1,8,9] Activation of afferent neurons is the first step in the triggering of motor reflexes as they translate stimuli from the intestinal lumen into nerve impulses that are transmitted to interneurons and motor neurons. Interneurons form circuitry chains running both orally and aborally within the myenteric plexus. The orally running interneurons activate excitatory motor neurons, resulting in smooth muscle contraction, and the aborally running interneurons activate inhibitory motor neurons, resulting in smooth muscle relaxation. The excitatory motor neurons release acetylcholine, and the inhibitory motor neurons release nitric oxide or vasoactive intestinal polypeptide. This sequential enteric reflex pattern of ascending contraction and descending relaxation, called *peristalsis*, forms the basis for Starling's Law of the Intestine[10] (Fig. 2.1), which facilitates bolus propulsion in the peristaltic direction. The initiation and regulation of peristalsis is a complex process that involves pacemaker cells (ICCs), in addition to the smooth muscle cells and enteric nerves. ICCs generate spontaneous electrical slow waves, which constitute the basic electrical rhythm in the gut. ICCs develop independent of neural crest–derived enteric neurons or glia and originate mainly from Kit-positive mesenchymal mesodermal precursors.[2]

The ENS is remarkably independent, but its neuronal activity can be modified or modulated by the central nervous system (CNS) via the autonomic nervous system (ANS; parasympathetic and sympathetic nervous systems).[9,11] Much of the parasympathetic innervation to the gut travels via the vagus nerve and the sacral nerves and is primarily excitatory to gut function by promoting secretion and peristalsis. In contrast, sympathetic innervation travels along the mesenteric blood vessels from the prevertebral ganglia and is primarily inhibitory to gut function by decreasing peristalsis and reducing perfusion of the gut.

The human fetal gut, by week 14, has the longitudinal, circular, and muscularis mucosal layers of smooth muscle, submucosal and myenteric plexuses, and ICC networks that are associated with the ENS.[2] However, the first coordinated gut motility patterns do not occur until birth or about that time.[3] By 11 weeks, swallowing ability develops, by 18 to 20 weeks sucking movements appear, and by full-term gestation, the fetus can swallow and circulate nearly 500 mL of amniotic fluid. ENS-mediated contractile activity is prominent in function by full-term birth and is essential for propulsive activity. Variations in gut motility and peristaltic patterns occur in prematurely born neonates and are discussed in the latter part of this chapter.

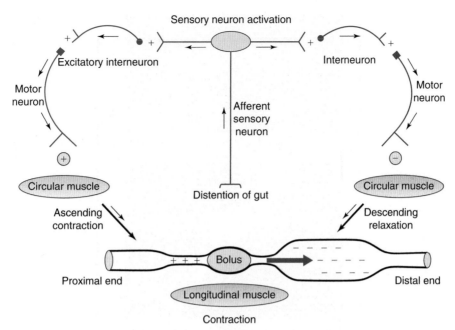

Fig. 2.1 Peristaltic Reflexes: Starling's Law of the Intestine. A schematic representation of the afferent and efferent components of the peristaltic reflex, Starling's Law of the Intestine. When luminal stimulation occurs by mechanoreceptor, chemoreceptor, osmoreceptor, or tension receptor activation, there ensues a cascade of proximal afferent and distal efferent activation. This results in sequential proximal excitatory and distal inhibitory neurotransmission, thus resulting in peristalsis to facilitate gastrointestinal transit. At the level of the esophagus, such sequences also facilitate aerodigestive protection.

Pharyngo-esophageal Motility Reflexes in Human Neonates

Maturation of Esophageal Peristalsis and Upper Esophageal Sphincter and Lower Esophageal Sphincter Functions

Deglutition refers to the whole process of propulsion of a food bolus from the mouth into the stomach and involves the complex coordination of rhythmic sequences of sucking, swallowing, and breathing, followed by well-timed relaxations of the upper and lower esophageal sphincters (UES and LES, respectively) and sequential esophageal contractions.[12] Using micromanometry methods, pharyngeal, UES, esophageal body, and LES functions have been characterized in neonates.[13-15] The UES and the LES maintain a resting tone irrespective of age or activity states, thus protecting the airway from luminal contents. With growth and maturation, the muscle mass and therefore the tone and activity of the UES increase. The average resting UES pressure (mean ± standard deviation) in preterm-born neonates at 33 weeks postmenstrual age (PMA) was 17 ± 7 mm Hg, and in full-term born neonates was 26 ± 14 mm Hg, whereas in adults it was 53 ± 23 mm Hg. Similarly, changes in LES length and tone have been observed with growth.[14,16,17] Additionally, esophageal lengthening occurs in a linear fashion during postnatal growth in both premature and full-term infants.[18]

Maturation of Basal and Adaptive Esophageal Motility

Pharyngeal swallowing and esophageal peristalsis constitute the principal methods used to drive the bolus from the oral cavity to the stomach, at the same time protecting the airways from aspiration or penetration. Pharyngeal swallowing is triggered when a bolus moves from the oral cavity to the pharynx or by direct pharyngeal or esophageal stimulation. Esophageal response to pharyngeal swallowing is termed *primary peristalsis* (triggered by the bolus moving from the oral cavity to the pharynx) or *pharyngeal reflexive swallow* (PRS, by direct pharyngeal stimulation), or

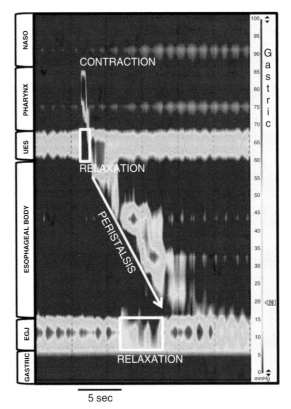

Fig. 2.2 **An Example of Primary Peristalsis.** An example of spontaneous primary esophageal peristalsis in a premature infant evoked upon pharyngeal contraction, upper esophageal sphincter relaxation, forward propagation of esophageal body peristalsis, and lower esophageal sphincter relaxation. Such sequences facilitate swallowing and esophageal clearance.

esophageal deglutition response (EDR, by direct esophageal stimulation) (Fig. 2.2). All three responses are characterized by sequential reflexes that include relaxation of the UES, restoration of UES tone, ordered esophageal body peristalsis, coordinated relaxation of the LES, and restoration of LES tone, all of which ultimately clear the pharynx and propagate the bolus distally into the stomach.[13,19-22] This sequence is normally associated with a respiratory pause called *deglutition apnea* (inspiratory or expiratory) suggesting cross-communications between the pharynx and the airway. This occurs because of the physical closure of the airway by elevation of the soft palate and larynx, by tilting of the epiglottis, and by the neural suppression of respiration in the brain stem.[23] Evaluation of consecutive spontaneous solitary swallows in preterm infants at 33 weeks, preterm infants at 36 weeks, full-term infants, and adults has shown significant age-dependent maturational changes in the sphincter kinetics and in the amplitude and velocity of esophageal peristaltic contractions.[13,19] Importantly, primary esophageal peristalsis exists by 33 weeks PMA; however, it undergoes further maturation and differentiation during postnatal growth and is significantly different from that of adults.[13]

The esophagus is a frequent target for retrograde bolus from the stomach as in gastro-esophageal reflux events, which causes mechanosensitive, chemosensitive, or osmosensitive stimulation of the esophagus. The esophagus clears such luminal contents back into the stomach either by a swallow-dependent EDR or by a more mature, swallow-independent peristaltic sequence response called *secondary peristalsis*.[16,19-21] Secondary peristalsis comprises a coordinated sequence of proximal esophageal contraction and distal esophageal relaxation, coordinated relaxation of the LES, and restoration of LES tone (Fig. 2.3). Similar to the occurrence of secondary peristalsis, esophageal provocation can result in an increase in UES pressure, which increases the pressure barrier against entry of refluxate into the pharynx

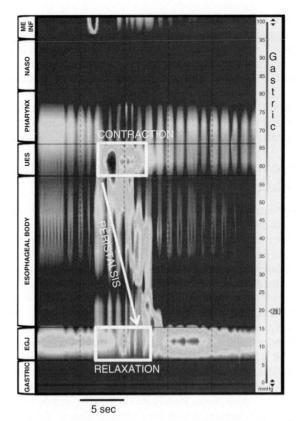

Fig. 2.3 An Example of Secondary Peristalsis. An example of swallow-independent secondary esophageal peristalsis in a premature infant in response to a mid-esophageal infusion. Absence of pharyngeal waveform, presence of propagating esophageal body peristalsis, upper esophageal sphincter contraction, lower esophageal sphincter relaxation, and complete esophageal propagation are also noted. Such sequences are evoked during esophageal provocations and contribute to esophageal and airway protection by facilitating clearance.

(see Fig. 2.3).[19,20] This reflex, referred to as *esophago-UES-contractile reflex*, is mediated by the vagus nerve.[16,19,20] Concurrently, the LES relaxes to facilitate bolus clearance. This is called *LES relaxation reflex response*. These reflexes prevent the ascending spread of the bolus and favor descending propulsion to ensure esophageal clearance.

Although the nature and composition of the bolus within the pharyngeal or esophageal lumen can vary, peristalsis remains the single most important function that must occur to favor luminal clearance away from the airway. These reflexes advance during maturation in premature infants. A study of pharyngeal provocation responses in healthy premature infants at 34 weeks and 39 weeks PMA has shown a higher recruitment frequency of PRS and pharyngeal LES relaxation responses at 39 weeks.[24] Secondary peristalsis upon mid-esophageal provocation has been described as occurring as early as 32 weeks PMA.[12,13,19,20] When premature infants were studied at 33 weeks and 36 weeks PMA for esophageal provocation characteristics, the occurrence of secondary peristalsis and the frequency of completely propagated secondary peristalsis were significantly higher at 36 weeks PMA, with increment in dose volumes of air or liquid esophageal provocation. The occurrence of UES contractile reflex was also volume dependent, and its characteristics showed improvement with advancing maturation. Similarly, the aerodigestive defense mechanisms during the sleep state also mature with time in preterm infants, as evidenced by the greater ability to remain asleep with less cortical arousal, during esophageal provocation.[25] During this maturation process, the peristaltic response becomes faster and more efficient with faster esophageal clearance and greater intraluminal esophageal pressure.[12] These findings are suggestive of the existence of vago-vagal protective reflex mechanisms that facilitate esophageal clearance in healthy premature neonates and indicate that these mechanisms mature with increasing gestational age.

Safe and efficient nutritive sucking in infants requires synchronization of sucking, swallow processing (pharyngeal swallow and esophageal peristalsis), and breathing.[26] Functional immaturity in these components, at either an individual level or an integrated level, is associated with oral feeding difficulties. Many components within each of these levels mature at different times and rates and may explain why infants of similar gestation age demonstrate wide variation in oral feeding skills.[26] A recent study of neonates with significant oral feeding difficulties showed that ability for full oral feeding at NICU discharge was associated with less long-term neurodevelopmental impairment relative to full or partial gastrostomy tube feeding.[27]

Gastrointestinal Motility Reflexes in Human Neonates

Although fetal peristalsis is recognized, local neural transmission and integration of peristalsis mature throughout fetal life and continue to develop during the first postnatal year. These local contractions are coordinated throughout the length of the intestine by neural regulation modulated by the ENS, the ANS, and the CNS. The gut has a network of specialized intrinsic pacemaker muscle cells (ICCs) that also play a role in triggering these coordinated contractions.[28-30] Intestinal myoelectrical activity consists of slow waves and spike bursts. ICCs at the level of the myenteric plexus (ICC-MY) mediate the slow waves whose function is to regulate the maximum rate of muscular contraction.[31] The frequency of slow waves varies along the gut, but each part of the gut has a characteristic frequency. The stomach has the lowest frequency of slow waves, occurring at 3 to 5 times/min, whereas it is fastest in the duodenum (9-11 times/min) and then diminishes distally in the midgut (6-8 times/min).[32-34] The spike bursts are fast action potentials that only appear on the slow-wave plateau when the small intestine contracts and determine the intensity of the intestinal contractions. Finally, motor function can be modulated by gastrointestinal hormones and peptides, which may exert endocrine, paracrine, or neurocrine activity, resulting in inhibitory (e.g., peptide YY, nitrergic, vasoactive intestinal peptide) or excitatory (e.g., cholinergic–muscarinic, cholecystokinin, substance P) modulation.[35] All of the neural and muscular elements are present by 32 weeks' gestation, but full neural and neuroendocrine integration is not achieved until late in infancy.[35,36]

Gastric Motor Functions

Anatomically, the stomach can be divided into the fundus, corpus (body), antrum, and pylorus, whereas, functionally, the proximal stomach (fundus and proximal corpus) acts as a gastric reservoir and the distal stomach (distal corpus and antrum) as a gastric pump where the peristaltic waves occur. The gastric fundus accommodates the ingested nutrients by receptive relaxation reflex. This is largely mediated by the vagus nerve as stimulation of the mechanoreceptors in the mouth and pharynx and of the distal esophagus induces vago-vagal reflexes that cause relaxation of the gastric reservoir by nitrergic pathways.[11,37] Fundus relaxation is a prerequisite for antral contraction and gastric emptying.[11,38] However, receptive relaxation in neonates and infants is not well studied. In contrast to the fundus, the antrum has tonic and phasic activity and is responsible for the churning of nutrients with secretions to initiate early digestion and to empty the stomach contents into the duodenum. Contractile activity in the antrum is coordinated with that in the duodenum to promote emptying of contents into the upper small intestine. Hence, the physical and chemical characteristics of the nutrients entering the duodenum trigger feedback signals to the antrum to hasten or slow emptying. Ultrasonographic studies of the fetal stomach detected gastric emptying occurring as early as 13 weeks of gestation,[39] and the length of gastric emptying cycles in fetuses increases just before birth.[40] The rate of gastric emptying is not influenced by nonnutritive sucking but is influenced by caloric density and osmolality of milk and stress—calorically denser formula accelerates gastric emptying, high milk osmolality, and extreme stress, such as that caused by the presence of systemic illness, delays gastric emptying.[33,41] The administration of drugs for clinical care, such as opioids or mydriatics, may also impair gastrointestinal functioning.[42] Interestingly, bolus feedings appear to delay gastric emptying in some preterm infants, presumably via rapid distention.[43]

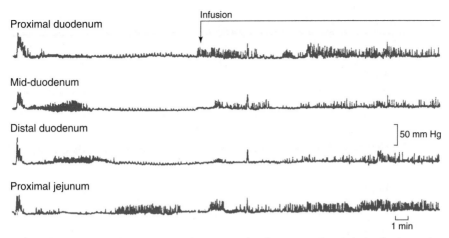

Fig. 2.4 Small intestinal motor activity in term infant (40 weeks of gestational age) during fasting and progressing through initiation of milk infusion. Presence of the migrating motor complex (MMC) is followed by brief period of quiescence before feeding is initiated. Quiescence is replaced by persistent motor activity in all four leads shortly after feeding infusion is begun. Adapted from: Berseth CL. Neonatal small intestinal motility: motor responses to feeding in term and preterm infants. *J Pediatr.* 1990;117:777-782.

Small Intestine Motor Functions

Like in the stomach, there is an ICC network located in the intestinal wall between the internal circular and the external longitudinal muscle layers that initiate the slow waves. Peristaltic waves are far spreading and rapid at the proximal small intestine and become shorter and slower toward the distal gut. The intrinsic contractile rhythm of the stomach, duodenum, and small intestine are present as early as 24 weeks' gestation. Full neural integration is inadequate at birth, and gastric emptying and the overall intestinal transit are slower in the preterm infant than in the full-term infant. Overall gut transit can vary from 7 to 14 days and depends on gestational maturation.

The small intestine exhibits two basic patterns of motor activity: (1) fed response and (2) fasting response. During fed response, the muscle layers contract in a disorganized fashion, resulting in active, continuous mixing and churning of nutrients and secretions resulting in chime (Fig. 2.4). Fed response facilitates transport of nutrients distally to facilitate digestion and absorption. Although an adult-like fed response is seen in most full-term infants in response to bolus feeding, only about 50% of the preterm infants exhibit such a response.[44] In contrast, in the fasting state, the small intestine does not stay quiescent but experiences muscular contractions organized into patterns known as the *interdigestive migrating motor complex* (IMMC) (Fig. 2.5). Depending on the intensity of motor activity, the IMMC cycle can be divided into four periods: phase I, or period of smooth muscle quiescence, during which the intestine is at rest; phase II of random and unorganized motor activity; and phase III (migrating motor complex, MMC), in which bowel contractions occur at maximum frequency and intensity when >90% of slow waves are accompanied by spike bursts. It is usually generated at the duodenum, although it can be generated at any point between the stomach and the ileum.[45] MMCs are responsible for about 50% of the forward movement of nutrients and are considered the "intestinal housekeeper." This robust well-organized pattern is replaced by randomly occurring contractile waveforms that terminate in the reappearance of quiescence (phase IV). The MMC is interrupted by feeding, and the subsequent fed response is characterized by irregular muscle contractions.

Control of the MMC is complex.[46,47] Vagus nerve control of the MMC seems to be restricted to the stomach, as vagotomy abolishes motor activity in the stomach but leaves periodic activity in the small bowel intact.[47] Phase III MMC of antral origin can be induced with intravenous administration of motilin, erythromycin, or ghrelin, whereas administration of serotonin or somatostatin induces phase III MMC of duodenal origin.[47] Preterm infants exhibit comparable fasting levels of motilin to adults,

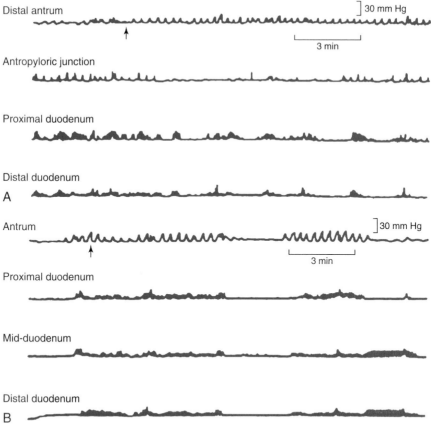

Fig. 2.5 **Nonmigrating and Migrating Gastroduodenal Motility.** An example of (A) nonmigrating and (B) migrating gastroduodenal motility in a human neonate in the fasting state. (A) A representative manometric recording depicting nonmigrating activity in a term infant. Fasting motor activity recorded in the antrum is shown in the top line, activity in the antropyloric junction in the second, and duodenum in the third and fourth. (B) A representative manometric recording in the same infant and three duodenal leads. The *arrow* indicates the presence of migrating motor complex, a phenomenon mediated by motilin, seratoninergic system, or vagal parasympathetic system. Adapted from: Jadcherla SR, Klee G, Berseth CL. Regulation of migrating motor complexes by motilin and pancreatic polypeptide in human infants. *Pediatr Res.* 1997;42:365-369.

but motilin fails to cycle MMC in the preterm infant. Motilin receptor agonists, such as antibiotics (e.g., erythromycin/clarithromycin), can trigger initiation of the MMC in preterm infants whose gestational ages exceed 32 weeks (Fig. 2.6).[36,48,49] The MMC is incompletely developed until 32 weeks of gestation and much uncoordinated in infants at <27 weeks' gestation.[50] Propagating, cyclical MMCs with clearly defined phases develop between 37 weeks and full term.[51] The absence of the MMC in the very premature infant appears to be the result of overall immaturity of the integration of motor pattern, absence of the motilin receptor, and/or the absence of fluctuating levels of motilin.

The method of feeding influences motor patterns during fasting as well as feeding. The provision of small early feedings versus no feeding or nonnutritive feedings (i.e., sterile water) accelerates the maturation of fasting motor patterns,[52-55] which, in turn, are associated with better feeding tolerance. Interestingly, small feedings (i.e., 20 mL/kg/d) induce maturation of motor patterns that is comparable with that induced by larger feedings.[55] This induction of maturation is likely neurally mediated because hormone release is not as robust in response to small feedings as in response to larger feedings.[53] In one animal model, it was shown that the acceleration of maturation of motor patterns is associated with an increase in nitrergic neurons,[56] both of which may regulate motor activity. Additionally, feeding diluted formula slows the onset and intensity of feeding responses.[54,57] Continuous feeds or transpyloric

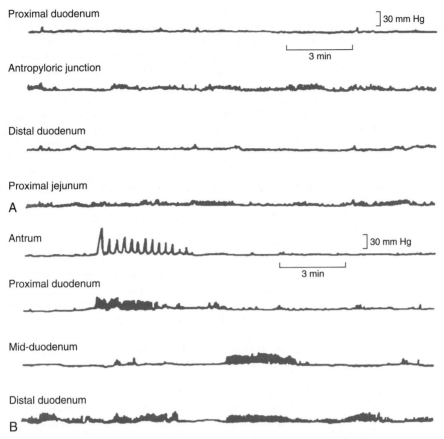

Fig. 2.6 The migrating motor complex (MMC) results from stimulation of motilin receptors after enteral eryth-romycin. (A) Example of motility recording in an infant at 26 weeks' gestation 30 minutes after the enteral eryth-romycin. No evidence of migrating motor activity is seen. (B) Example of motility recording in an infant at 33 weeks' gestation 30 minutes after the administration of intragastric erythromycin. Phasic contractions appear in the antrum and are temporally coordinated with the occurrence of phasic activity in the three duodenal recording ports. Adapted from: Jadcherla SR, Klee G, Berseth CL. Regulation of migrating motor complexes by motilin and pancreatic polypeptide in human infants. *Pediatr Res.* 1997;42:365-369.

feeds may change the intestinal motility pattern by suppressing the fasting periods, thus hampering the intestinal bacterial clearance, and may lead to sepsis.[58] There are reports of the beneficial effects of pre- and probiotics to enhance gastrointestinal motility in preterm infants,[59] but the evidence is not strong enough to recommend its routine use in very premature infants.[60]

Development of Colonic Motility in Human Neonates

The large intestine has two main functions: (1) it is a fermenting chamber in which fiber and indigestible nutrients are hydrolyzed by microbes, and (2) it produces feces by absorption of water. To fulfill these functions, the digesta have to be inten-sively mixed and slowly moved aborally. There is significant lack of data on colonic motility in human preterm infants, and this is largely the result of technical limita-tions, need for invasive approaches, and ethical concerns. Some evidence can be gleaned from animal studies. Colonic motility is quite distinct from small intesti-nal motility, and regionalization of contractions occurs. ICC-mediated slow-wave activity causes colonic contractions when the depolarization is of sufficient ampli-tude. The internal anal sphincter, a specialized thickening of circular muscle, main-tains a state of tonic contraction, thus maintaining continence in association with the external sphincter. Distension of the rectum, typically with feces, results in an

ENS-dependent reflexive relaxation of the sphincter (rectoanal inhibitory reflex).[61] It is not surprising, then, that the passage of meconium is inversely related to gestational age at birth.[62] Although it is highly likely that the propagating contractile activity that occurs before birth contributes to the propulsion of meconium anally before birth, this has yet to be conclusively demonstrated. It may be postulated that colonic distention results in neural feedback, inhibiting motor function in the upper intestine. An observation study in preterm infants undergoing routine glycerin enema to stimulate meconium passage was associated with better feeding tolerance,[63] but a subsequent randomized trial in preterm infants <32 weeks showed no difference in the time to reach full enteral feeds with daily glycerin suppositories.[64] Short-chain fatty acids (SCFAs), such as butyrate, have been proposed as potential therapeutic agents that can modulate neuronal excitability by increasing the cholinergic-mediated colonic contractions, thereby augmenting colonic transit.[65] However, the generation of SCFAs in the colon induces relaxation of the proximal stomach and the LES via release of polypeptide YY hormone, which can slow the gastric emptying.[66]

Summary

In summary, postnatal maturation of the gastrointestinal motility reflexes is dependent on sensory and motor regulation of the intrinsic ENS integrated and modulated by the CNS and the ANS. These reflexes mature in evolution frequency, magnitude, response sensitivity, and associated responses with advanced postnatal maturation.

Implications and Controversies of Gut Motility in Neonatal Gastrointestinal Therapies

- As the relative importance of different neurotransmitters to gastrointestinal contractile activity changes significantly during development, drugs that successfully treat motility disorders in adults will not necessarily have similar effects in infants and children.
- Mechanical gastrointestinal functions, such as suck–swallow processing coordination, UES/LES tone, gastric emptying, and intestinal motility may be immature in preterm infants. As a consequence, they are more prone to oral feeding difficulties, gastroesophageal reflex, gastric residuals, bowel distention, and delayed meconium passage compared with full-term infants.
- Management of gastrointestinal motility issues should be tailed around the functional maturity level in an individual infant, rather than being based on their gestational age or PMA.
- The symptoms and signs of feeding intolerance in preterm infants (gastric residuals, abdominal distention, emesis)—generally an expression of anatomical and functional immaturity of gut—have poor predictive value either for enteral feeding outcomes or pathologic bowel motility in preterm infants. A combination of local and systemic symptoms and signs needs to be considered together while interpreting the clinical and prognostic significance of nonspecific symptoms and signs of feeding intolerance.
- Erythromycin, as a prokinetic agent, may be effective in inducing migrating motor complexes in premature infants >33 weeks PMA. However, its safety and efficacy in preterm infants is not completely defined, so use of oral erythromycin should be limited to rescue treatment of severe persistent feeding intolerance.
- Enteral trophic nutrition is associated with acceleration of gut motility patterns. If feeding intolerance limits the ability to provide full feeding volumes to an infant, smaller feeding volumes may be just as capable of inducing maturation.
- Very premature infants have a small gastric capacity and delayed gastric emptying. An infant who is intolerant to bolus feedings may tolerate feedings that are given as slow intermittent gavage over 1 hour. Similarly, an infant who has large gastric residuals on a 3-hourly feeding regimen may tolerate feeding better with a short-interval (2-hourly) feeding with smaller feeding volume.

REFERENCES

1. Furness JB. Types of neurons in the enteric nervous system. *J Auton Nerv Syst*. 2000;81:87–96.
2. Burns AJ, Hofstra RM. The enteric nervous system: from embryology to therapy. *Dev Biol*. 2016;417(2):127–128.
3. Burns AJ, Roberts RR, Bornstein JC, Young HM. Development of the enteric nervous system and its role in intestinal motility during fetal and early postnatal stages. *Semin Pediatr Surg*. 2009;18(4):196–205.
4. Wallace AS, Burns AJ. Development of the enteric nervous system, smooth muscle and interstitial cells of Cajal in the human gastrointestinal tract. *Cell Tissue Res*. 2005;319(3):367–382.
5. Zhou Y, James I, Besner GE. Heparin-binding epidermal growth factor-like growth factor promotes murine enteric nervous system development and enteric neural crest cell migration. *J Pediatr Surg*. 2012;47(10):1865–1873.
6. Metzger M, Caldwell C, Barlow AJ, Burns AJ, Thapar N. Enteric nervous system stem cells derived from human gut mucosa for the treatment of aganglionic gut disorders. *Gastroenterology*. 2009;136(7):2214–2225. e1–e3.
7. Wang X, Chan AK, Sham MH, Burns AJ, Chan WY. Analysis of the sacral neural crest cell contribution to the hindgut enteric nervous system in the mouse embryo. *Gastroenterology*. 2011;141(3). 992–1002.e1–e6.
8. Costa M, Brookes SJ, Hennig GW. Anatomy and physiology of the enteric nervous system. *Gut*. 2000;47(suppl 4):iv15–iv19. discussion iv26.
9. Gallego D, Malagelada C, Accarino A, et al. Nitrergic and purinergic mechanisms evoke inhibitory neuromuscular transmission in the human small intestine. *Neurogastroenterol Motil*. 2014;26(3):419–429.
10. Goyal RK, Hirano I. The enteric nervous system. *N Engl J Med*. 1996;334:1106–1115.
11. Gallego D, Mañé N, Gil V, Martínez-Cutillas M, Jiménez M. Mechanisms responsible for neuromuscular relaxation in the gastrointestinal tract. *Rev Esp Enferm Dig*. 2016;108(11):721–731.
12. Singendonk MM, Rommel N, Omari TI, Benninga MA, van Wijk MP. Upper gastrointestinal motility: prenatal development and problems in infancy. *Nat Rev Gastroenterol Hepatol*. 2014;11(9):545–555.
13. Jadcherla SR, Duong HQ, Hofmann C, Hoffmann R, Shaker R. Characteristics of upper oesophageal sphincter and oesophageal body during maturation in healthy human neonates compared with adults. *Neurogastroenterol Motil*. 2005;17(5):663–670.
14. Omari TI, Miki K, Fraser R, et al. Esophageal body and lower esophageal sphincter function in healthy premature infants. *Gastroenterology*. 1995;109(6):1757–1764.
15. Staiano A, Boccia G, Salvia G, Zappulli D, Clouse RE. Development of esophageal peristalsis in preterm and term neonates. *Gastroenterology*. 2007;132(5):1718–1725.
16. Gupta A, Gulati P, Kim W, Fernandez S, Shaker R, Jadcherla SR. Effect of postnatal maturation on the mechanisms of esophageal propulsion in preterm human neonates: primary and secondary peristalsis. *Am J Gastroenterol*. 2009;104(2):411–419.
17. Strobel CT, Byrne WJ, Ament ME, Euler AR. Correlation of esophageal lengths in children with height: application to the Tuttle test without prior esophageal manometry. *J Pediatr*. 1979;94(1):81–84.
18. Gupta A, Jadcherla SR. The relationship between somatic growth and in vivo esophageal segmental and sphincteric growth in human neonates. *J Pediatr Gastroenterol Nutr*. 2006;43(1):35–41.
19. Jadcherla SR, Duong HQ, Hoffmann RG, Shaker R. Esophageal body and upper esophageal sphincter motor responses to esophageal provocation during maturation in preterm newborns. *J Pediatr*. 2003;143(1):31–38.
20. Jadcherla SR, Hoffmann RG, Shaker R. Effect of maturation of the magnitude of mechanosensitive and chemosensitive reflexes in the premature human esophagus. *J Pediatr*. 2006;149(1):77–82.
21. Jadcherla SR. Pathophysiology of aerodigestive pulmonary disorders in the neonate. *Clin Perinatol*. 2012;39(3):639–654.
22. Pena EM, Parks VN, Peng J, et al. Lower esophageal sphincter relaxation reflex kinetics: effects of peristaltic reflexes and maturation in human premature neonates. *Am J Physiol Gastrointest Liver Physiol*. 2010;299(6):G1386–G1395.
23. Barlow SM. Central pattern generation involved in oral and respiratory control for feeding in the term infant. *Curr Opin Otolaryngol Head Neck Surg*. 2009;17(3):187–193.
24. Jadcherla SR, Shubert TR, Gulati IK, Jensen PS, Wei L, Shaker R. Upper and lower esophageal sphincter kinetics are modified during maturation: effect of pharyngeal stimulus in premature infants. *Pediatr Res*. 2015;77(1–1):99–106.
25. Jadcherla SR, Chan CY, Fernandez S, Splaingard M. Maturation of upstream and downstream esophageal reflexes in human premature neonates: the role of sleep and awake states. *Am J Physiol Gastrointest Liver Physiol*. 2013;305(9):G649–G658.
26. Lau C. Development of suck and swallow mechanisms in infants. *Ann Nutr Metab*. 2015;66(suppl 5):7–14.
27. Jadcherla SR, Khot T, Moore R, Malkar M, Gulati IK, Slaughter JL. Feeding methods at discharge predict long-term feeding and neurodevelopmental outcomes in preterm infants referred for gastrostomy evaluation. *J Pediatr*. 2017;181:125–130.
28. Miller JL, Sonies BC, Macedonia C. Emergence of oropharyngeal, laryngeal and swallowing activity in the developing fetal upper aerodigestive tract: an ultrasound evaluation. *Early Hum Dev*. 2003;71(1):61–87.

29. Gariepy CE. Intestinal motility disorders and development of the enteric nervous system. *Pediatr Res.* 2001;49(5):605–613.

30. Grundy D, Schemann M. Enteric nervous system. *Curr Opin Gastroenterol.* 2007;23(2):121–126.

31. Hirst GD, Edwards FR. Generation of slow waves in the antral region of guinea-pig stomach–a stochastic process. *J Physiol.* 2001;535(Pt 1):165–180.

32. Berseth CL. Gastrointestinal motility in the neonate. *Clin Perinatol.* 1996;23(2):179–190.

33. Berseth CL. Motor function in the stomach and small intestine in the neonate. *NeoReviews.* 2006;7:e28–e33.

34. Berseth CL. Neonatal small intestinal motility: motor responses to feeding in term and preterm infants. *J Pediatr.* 1990;117:777–782.

35. Jadcherla SR, Klee G, Berseth CL. Regulation of migrating motor complexes by motilin and pancreatic polypeptide in human infants. *Pediatr Res.* 1997;42:365–369.

36. Jadcherla SR, Berseth CL. Effect of erythromycin on gastroduodenal contractile activity in developing neonates. *J Pediatr Gastroenterol Nutr.* 2002;34(1):16–22.

37. Travagli RA, Anselmi L. Vagal neurocircuitry and its influence on gastric motility. *Nat Rev Gastroenterol Hepatol.* 2016;13(7):389–401.

38. Kuiken SD, Tytgat GN, Boeckxstaens GE. Role of endogenous nitric oxide in regulating antropyloroduodenal motility in humans. *Am J Gastroenterol.* 2002;97(7):1661–1667.

39. Sase M, Miwa I, Sumie M, Nakata M, Sugino N, Ross MG. Ontogeny of gastric emptying patterns in the human fetus. *J Matern Fetal Neonatal Med.* 2005;17(3):213–217.

40. Sase M, Miwa I, Sumie M, et al. Gastric emptying cycles in the human fetus. *Am J Obstet Gynecol.* 2005;193(3 Pt 2):1000–1004.

41. Pearson F, Johnson MJ, Leaf AA. Milk osmolality: does it matter? *Arch Dis Child Fetal Neonatal Ed.* 2013;98(2):F166–F169.

42. Bonthala S, Sparks JW, Musgrove KH, Berseth CL. Mydriatics slow gastric emptying in preterm infants. *J Pediatr.* 2000;137(3):327–330.

43. Al Tawil Y, Berseth CL. Gestational and postnatal maturation of duodenal motor responses to intragastric feeding. *J Pediatr.* 1996;129(3):374–381.

44. Al-Tawil Y, Klee G, Berseth CL. Extrinsic neural regulation of antroduodenal motor activity in preterm infants. *Dig Dis Sci.* 2002;47(12):2657–2663.

45. Ye-Lin Y, Garcia-Casado J, Prats-Boluda G, Ponce JL, Martinez-de-Juan JL. Enhancement of the non-invasive electroenterogram to identify intestinal pacemaker activity. *Physiol Meas.* 2009;30(9):885–902.

46. Takahashi T. Interdigestive migrating motor complex—its mechanism and clinical importance. *J Smooth Muscle Res.* 2013;49:99–111.

47. Deloose E, Janssen P, Depoortere I, Tack J. The migrating motor complex: control mechanisms and its role in health and disease. *Nat Rev Gastroenterol Hepatol.* 2012;9(5):271–285.

48. Jones MP, Wessinger S. Small intestinal motility. *Curr Opin Gastroenterol.* 2005;21(2):141–146.

49. Gokmen T, Ozdemir R, Bozdag S, et al. Clarithromycin treatment in preterm infants: a pilot study for prevention of feeding intolerance. *J Matern Fetal Neonatal Med.* 2013;26(15):1528–1531.

50. Berseth CL. Gestational evolution of small intestine motility in preterm and term infants. *J Pediatr.* 1989;115(4):646–651.

51. Bisset WM, Watt JB, Rivers RP, Milla PJ. Ontogeny of fasting small intestinal motor activity in the human infant. *Gut.* 1988;29(4):483–488.

52. Berseth CL, Nordyke C. Enteral nutrients promote postnatal maturation of intestinal motor activity in preterm infants. *Am J Physiol.* 1993;264(6 Pt 1):G1046–G1051.

53. Berseth CL, Nordyke CK, Valdes MG, Furlow BL, Go VL. Responses of gastrointestinal peptides and motor activity to milk and water feedings in preterm and term infants. *Pediatr Res.* 1992;31(6):587–590.

54. Baker JH, Berseth CL. Duodenal motor responses in preterm infants fed formula with varying concentrations and rates of infusion. *Pediatr Res.* 1997;42(5):618–622.

55. Owens L, Burrin DG, Berseth CL. Minimal enteral feeding induces maturation of intestinal motor function but not mucosal growth in neonatal dogs. *J Nutr.* 2002;132(9):2717–2722.

56. Oste M, Van Ginneken CJ, Van Haver ER, Bjornvad CR, Thymann T, Sangild PT. The intestinal trophic response to enteral food is reduced in parenterally fed preterm pigs and is associated with more nitrergic neurons. *J Nutr.* 2005;135(11):2657–2663.

57. Koenig WJ, Amarnath RP, Hench V, Berseth CL. Manometrics for preterm and term infants: a new tool for old questions. *Pediatrics.* 1995;95(2):203–206.

58. Goulet O, Olieman J, Ksiazyk J, et al. Neonatal short bowel syndrome as a model of intestinal failure: physiological background for enteral feeding. *Clin Nutr.* 2013;32(2):162–171.

59. Indrio F, Riezzo G, Raimondi F, Bisceglia M, Cavallo L, Francavilla R. Effects of probiotic and prebiotic on gastrointestinal motility in newborns. *J Physiol Pharmacol.* 2009;60(suppl 6):27–31.

60. Viswanathan S, Lau C, Akbari H, Hoyen C, Walsh MC. Survey and evidence based review of probiotics used in very low birth weight preterm infants within the United States. *J Perinatol.* 2017;37(1):104.

61. Hao MM, Young HM. Development of enteric neuron diversity. *J Cell Mol Med.* 2009;13(7):1193–1210.

62. Weaver LT, Lucas A. Development of bowel habit in preterm infants. *Arch Dis Child.* 1993;68(3 Spec No):317–320.

63. Shim SY, Kim HS, Kim DH, et al. Induction of early meconium evacuation promotes feeding tolerance in very low birth weight infants. *Neonatology.* 2007;92(1):67–72.

64. Khadr SN, Ibhanesebhor SE, Rennix C, et al. Randomized controlled trial: impact of glycerin suppositories on time to full feeds in preterm infants. *Neonatology*. 2011;100(2):169–176.

65. Soret R, Chevalier J, De Coppet P, et al. Short-chain fatty acids regulate the enteric neurons and control gastrointestinal motility in rats. *Gastroenterology*. 2010;138(5):1772–1782.

66. Cherbut C. Motor effects of short-chain fatty acids and lactate in the gastrointestinal tract. *Proc Nutr Soc*. 2003;62(1):95–99.

2

CHAPTER 3

Lipid and Fatty Acid Delivery in the Preterm Infant: Challenges and Lessons Learned from Other Critically Ill Populations

Camilia R. Martin, MD, MS, Steven D. Freedman, MD, PhD

Outline

Introduction

Lipids and fatty acids are critical for optimal cell physiology, organ function, and neurodevelopment. Although these nutrients are delivered to the preterm infant, specific considerations and challenges unique to this population have not been overcome to efficiently extract the physiologic and developmental benefits conferred by these bioactive factors. Some of these factors include understanding the ideal substrate, target dosing, hydrolysis and absorption, and metabolic conversion.

This chapter will discuss the challenges that limit optimal lipid and fatty acid delivery in the preterm infant. Potential strategies to overcome these limitations will be discussed across the spectrum of parenteral to enteral phases of nutrition. Lessons will be drawn from another vulnerable population that share impairments in lipid and fatty acid processing; namely, patients with cystic fibrosis.

Lipids and Fatty Acids Maintaining Function and Health

Thousands of lipid species across six major categories have been detected circulating in the plasma and integrated in cellular membranes.[1] Lipids play critical roles in maintaining function and health throughout an individual's life span and provide an energy-rich source of nutrition supporting normal cellular functions and somatic growth. Lipids form the structure of human cellular and neural membranes vital for cell-to-cell communication and downstream signaling to carry out critical physiologic functions, including organogenesis, immune function, and regulation of inflammation. Fatty acids are a major building block of these lipids and are central to mediating these biologic processes.

To ensure that preterm infants have sufficient nutritional pools of lipids and fatty acids to draw upon and recruit for these critical biologic processes, several key steps must be accomplished: (1) determining the nutritional requirements of lipids and fatty acids to sustain these biologic processes during the postnatal transition after an abrupt discontinuation of maternal supply; (2) employing delivery strategies that span across the parenteral and enteral phases of nutrition; and (3) overcoming the developmental insufficiencies in lipid and fatty acid hydrolysis, absorption, and metabolism. When these steps are unrealized, the accretion of critical lipids and fatty acids is compromised. Equally important, when the metabolism of these nutrients is neither mature nor supported, abnormal generation and accumulation of intermediate metabolites and oxidized byproducts may occur, potentially causing harm.

Several recent reviews have summarized our current understanding of lipid and fatty acid requirements for the preterm infant.[2,3] However, what remains unclear is how to best achieve optimal lipid and fatty acid delivery. How do we best support these requirements during the parenteral and enteral phases of nutrition? This chapter will review each phase of postnatal nutrition and the unique challenges faced by the preterm infant and describe potential strategies that may overcome these obstacles. To address these issues, we will reflect on other populations with fatty acid alterations, largely cystic fibrosis, and draw upon potential parallels in shared physiology that may inform future nutritional strategies in the preterm infant.

Mechanisms and Significance of Fatty Acid Alterations in Cystic Fibrosis

Essential fatty acid deficiency (EFAD), rarely seen in developed countries, is caused by the inadequate consumption in the diet of alpha linolenic acid (18:3, n-3) and gamma linoleic acid (18:2, n-6). These two fatty acids are essential because they cannot be endogenously synthesized and rather must be sourced from the diet. They are also the precursors to the biosynthesis of downstream fatty acids, such as eicosapentaenoic acid (EPA), docosahexaenoic acid (DHA), and arachidonic acid (AA). EFAD can present as dermatitis, thrombocytopenia, and growth failure.[4] The major biochemical changes reflective of EFAD are decreased AA and increased mead acid, the latter being a downstream product of oleic acid, an omega-9 fatty acid. Since cells need to maintain a constant number of double bonds to preserve membrane fluidity and mechanics, EFAD is associated with and diagnosed by a plasma triene/tetraene ratio >0.2.[5,6] The elevated triene/tetraene ratio in patients with cystic fibrosis suggests the presence of a biochemical EFAD and has opened the investigation of altered fatty acid metabolism in this population.[7]

Defects in Fatty Acid Metabolism

Cystic fibrosis (CF) is a multiorgan disease associated with inspissated secretions in the sinuses, lungs, intestine, biliary and pancreatic ducts, and male reproductive tract. Despite identification of the gene responsible for CF as the cystic fibrosis transmembrane conductance regulator (CFTR), a chloride channel, many questions remain as to how this defect leads to the myriad of cellular and host abnormalities seen in CF. This includes the excessive host inflammatory response and viscous secretions with abnormal mucin composition.

The authors' group has been focused on determining whether alterations in fatty acid metabolism may lead to the excessive host inflammatory response in CF, even in the absence of infection. It was first determined that in the pancreas and lung from UNC exon 10 CF knockout mice, compared with wild-type littermates, there was a twofold decrease in membrane-bound DHA and a reciprocal twofold increase in membrane bound AA.[8] Linoleic acid levels were also low. These fatty acid abnormalities were seen only in CF-affected organs and represent the first disease linked to alterations in membrane-bound AA.

Feeding these mice with DHA, 40 mg/day for 7 days, led to normalization of the fatty acid defect and reversal of the CF pathology in the pancreas and ileum.[9] Although there is no spontaneous lung disease in these CF knockout mice, administration of aerosolized *Pseudomonas* lipopolysaccharide once a day for 3 days resulted in an exaggerated host inflammatory response based on bronchoalveolar lavage showing 4 million/mL neutrophils from CF knockout mice compared with 1.5 million/mL in wild-type littermates.[10] Oral DHA, 40 mg/day for 7 days, normalized neutrophil counts in the CF knockout mice to wild-type levels, but DHA had no effect on further reducing neutrophil levels when fed to wild-type mice. The mechanism of action of DHA was through reductions in the downstream eicosanoid metabolites PGF-2α and PGE2, with no effect on tumor necrosis factor and the murine interleukin-8 equivalents MIP2 and KC.[10] The altered fatty acid imbalance was also linked to decreased expression of peroxisome proliferator-activated receptor (PPAR)-[gamma].[11]

Subsequent studies in humans with CF have demonstrated a similar fatty acid abnormality, which is directly correlated with the degree of CFTR dysfunction with progressive alterations seen when progressing from heterozygotes to those with mild CFTR mutations to those with severe CFTR mutations.[12] This was unrelated to age, body mass index, or comorbidities. Furthermore, these fatty acid alterations were not seen in other non-CF inflammatory diseases but, rather, are inherently linked to CFTR dysfunction.

The low linoleic acid levels that have been described in several studies of patients with CF were thought to be reflective of an EFAD despite sufficient linoleic acid in the diet. In airway cells in culture, with or without functional CFTR, by using sense and antisense messenger RNA (mRNA) strategies, it has been observed that the low linoleic acid levels are caused by increased conversion to AA through upregulation of the delta 6 desaturase enzyme.[13-15] Normally this is the rate limiting step in the metabolism of linoleic acid to AA but with loss of normal CFTR function, the "brakes" on this pathway are lost. It remains unknown whether the low DHA levels result from a primary decrease in the biosynthesis of DHA or are secondary to increased AA levels. There are ongoing studies examining whether strategies to increase DHA levels have an impact on CF related disease.

Pancreatic Insufficiency and Lipid Maldigestion

In addition to altered fatty acid metabolism in CF, exocrine pancreatic insufficiency is present in approximately 85% of patients. This inflammatory and fibrosing process begins in utero with full expression of exocrine pancreatic insufficiency typically by the end of the first year of life. Although carbohydrate and protein malabsorption occurs, it is the fat maldigestion that is responsible for most symptoms, including steatorrhea, bloating, and abdominal distention with gas. Typical coefficients of fat absorption, referred to as *coefficient of fat absorption (CFA)*, range from 20% to 70%. Before the advent of pancreatic enzyme replacement therapy, babies with CF died within 1 year as a result of profound protein and fat malnutrition. Institution of pancreatic enzymes has truly been lifesaving in this disease.

Defects in Intestinal Absorption

Not only is there exocrine pancreatic insufficiency resulting in maldigestion in CF, but there is also intestinal malabsorption. Thus whatever hydrolysis of fats occurs as a result of native or exogenous pancreatic enzymes, there is variable impairment in nutrient absorption across the intestinal epithelial cells caused by defective CFTR function. Other mechanisms to explain this malabsorption include thick mucus resulting in a greater unstirred intestinal surface layer; decreased luminal pH affecting pancreatic enzyme function, which has an optimal pH above 6.5, as well as precipitation of bile salts; quantitative and qualitative changes in bile composition; changes in the intestinal microbiome; and alterations in nutrient transporters. Taken together with exocrine pancreatic insufficiency, this combination of maldigestion and malabsorption has a major impact on nutritional status. The importance of nutritional status in CF cannot be overemphasized and is inextricably linked to lung disease. For example, weight-for-age percentile at age 4 years has been shown to be predictive of forced expiratory volume in one second at age 18 years in patients with CF.[16]

Role of Ileal Brake in Feeding Tolerance

Dysmotility is present in at least a third of patients with CF and includes gastroparesis as well as small and large intestinal involvement. The mechanisms are diverse but appear to be a result of altered CFTR function in intestinal ganglia,[17] as well as altered luminal pH and dysbiosis. Diabetes mellitus is present in up to 50% of patients with CF by the time they reach adulthood and can also impact gut function directly by affecting gut innervation and indirectly by altered microbiome and transporters. Furthermore, in the approximately 15% of patients with CF requiring nocturnal enteral tube feeds because of malnutrition, it is not unusual for patients to awaken and display all the signs and symptoms of ileal brake activation due to undigested and/or poorly absorbed full-length triglycerides or free fatty acids.

Each of the mechanisms leading to fatty acid alterations in CF have a potential role in the physiology of lipid digestion and fatty acid balance in the preterm infant—impaired metabolism, pancreatic insufficiency, impaired intestinal absorption, and the ileal brake. Successful strategies to optimize lipid and fatty acid delivery need to consider these facets and within developmental context as the preterm infant transitions from in utero nutrition to receiving parenteral nutrition and finally to the time of full enteral nutrition.

Lipid and Fatty Acids in Preterm Infants

Parenteral Nutrition

With limited time in utero to establish nutritional stores, the preterm infant is highly vulnerable to quickly acquiring postnatal deficits in essential macronutrients as well as their building blocks that serve as important immuno-nutrients for the developing infant. Parenteral nutrition remains the first bridge to minimize these nutritional deficits. The precise postnatal fatty acid requirements of the preterm infant have not been fully established; however, if the goal is to maintain levels that would otherwise be seen in utero, the currently available lipid emulsions fall short of this goal.

Soybean oil lipid emulsions (SOLEs) remain the predominant lipid emulsion used in preterm infants in North America. SOLEs provide the essential fatty acids of linoleic acid (LA, 18:2n6) and alpha-linolenic acid (ALA, 18:3n3) but little to none of the downstream long-chain polyunsaturated fatty acids. Preterm infants exposed to SOLE demonstrate a twofold to threefold reduction in blood levels of DHA (22:6n3) and AA (20:4n6) concomitant with a 2.5-fold increase in LA.[18] Thus the absolute levels of these fatty acids within the first postnatal week, as well as the ratios to one another, are reversed relative to profiles present in utero. Numerous health consequences have been described to be associated with these excesses and deficiencies of systemic fatty acid levels. Clinically, lower DHA levels have been linked to impaired neurodevelopment, retinopathy, and chronic lung disease, whereas low AA has been linked to late-onset sepsis.[18] Preclinical data support the role of fatty acids and their terminal mediators in brain and eye health, pulmonary development, immune function, and intestinal development, including microbial colonization.[19-24] Thus it is critical to understand postnatal fatty acid requirements and how best to deliver these bioactive nutrients before the onset of deficits.

Next-generation lipid emulsions that include various amounts of fish oil, which, compared with SOLE, provide greater concentrations of DHA and EPA (20:4n6), a small amount of AA, and little essential fatty acids (LA and ALA), have been developed. Concentrated fish oil-based lipid emulsions have been shown to alleviate the effects of traumatic brain injury in older children and adults, and this speaks to the potent bioactive properties of these omega-3 polyunsaturated fatty acids.[25] Additionally, in infants, 100% fish oil lipid emulsions (FOLEs) have shown tremendous promise as a therapeutic strategy for parenteral nutrition associated liver disease.[26]

The use of 10% to 15% FOLE has been studied as maintenance therapy in small cohorts of preterm infants with desirable trends in the incidence of bronchopulmonary dysplasia, retinopathy of prematurity, and cholestasis.[27-33] However, of cautionary note, untoward alterations in fatty acid profiles and lipid metabolism are seen with the use of fish oil-based lipid emulsions.[34] As expected, there is an increase in DHA levels when using FOLEs versus SOLEs, but this increase does not eliminate the early postnatal decline in DHA. Additionally, there is a substantial increase in EPA levels. The health effects of an increase in EPA are unknown; however, the well-established role of EPA in inhibiting platelet aggregation is a theoretical concern in the preterm infant. The rise in total omega-3 levels leads to a compensatory reduction in AA even lower than levels observed with SOLEs.[32-34] AA is critical for infant growth and the reduction in systemic AA levels has been linked with an increase in nosocomial sepsis.[18] Thus it is critical to develop a parenteral lipid emulsion that at least minimizes further reductions in AA and preferably maintains birth levels.

The use of FOLE may have other metabolic consequences. An analysis of lipid profiles between two comparable lipid emulsions except for the fish oil content (0% versus 10% fish oil) at a maximum dose of 2.6 to 2.8 g/kg/day revealed reduced lipogenesis in the fish oil group with reduced free cholesterol, cholesterol esters, and phospholipids—all complex lipids essential for organ development.[35] In contrast, preterm infants who received FOLE at a dose of 3.5 g/kg/day versus a SOLE-based product at 2.5 to 3.5 g/kg/day demonstrated increased phospholipid, triglyceride, and free cholesterol levels. The authors suggest that this profile reflects lipid intolerance. However, with the increased need for lipid substrates in organogenesis, it is unclear what the ideal lipid profile is in a rapidly growing preterm infant. In addition, this latter study is confounded by the other compositional differences between the two lipid emulsions.[35] Further studies are needed to understand the precise dose response impact of fatty acid delivery on lipid metabolism. Given the diverse role of complex lipids in human physiology, a sacrifice of one class of lipids for another will unlikely be tolerated well.

In summary, the currently available parenteral SOLEs and FOLEs fail to meet the unique lipid and fatty acid needs of the preterm infant. Ideally, lipid emulsions need to maintain birth levels and mitigate the changes in the systemic fatty acids levels currently observed after delivery. Although FOLEs minimize the postnatal DHA deficit, they induce further declines in AA and considerable increases in EPA. Additionally, as the omega-3 to omega-6 balance changes, it is expected that other complex lipid profiles will be altered as well. In adults, some of these changes, such as decreasing triglyceride levels in hypertriglyceridemia or reducing adipokines, including leptin, are desirable to promote weight loss. However, reduced lipogenesis and alterations of adipokines may not be desirable for preterm infants who rely on these compounds for organ growth and development. The long-term effects of these induced trade-offs with manipulations in the omega-3 to omega-6 balance need to be investigated thoroughly before wide spread adoption in the routine use of FOLEs.

Enteral Nutrition

Preterm infants receive small, steady advancements in enteral nutrition reaching full-volume enteral feedings at an approximate median age of 14 postnatal days. With complete transition from parenteral to enteral nutrition, all lipid and fatty acid requirements must now be met by the enteral diet alone. However, maintaining fatty acid levels close to those seen in utero cannot be achieved enterally using current feeding strategies and available nutritional substrates (human milk, human milk fortifiers, and/or preterm formula). Several factors have led to this conclusion. First, the pace of increasing enteral feeding volumes cannot overcome the deficit in DHA and AA seen within the first postnatal week when the infant is largely dependent on parenteral nutrition. Second, the fatty acid content in human milk, fortifiers, and formula is not sufficient to restore systemic fatty acid levels. Third, preterm infants express a developmentally immature digestive capability for efficient lipid hydrolysis and absorption of fatty acids when fed triglyceride oils. The latter is mediated by developmental exocrine pancreatic insufficiency of the newborn.

Developmental Exocrine Pancreatic Insufficiency

Although not commonly recognized, infants are the largest population of exocrine pancreatic insufficient individuals. In 1980 Lebenthal and Lee conducted a study in which they placed an oral–duodenal tube in healthy term infants and measured amylase, trypsin, and lipase secretion in response to cholecystokinin and secretin stimulation. Up to the first 6 months of life, protease secretion was near adult levels, but there was little amylase and lipase secretion.[36] The lack of the latter two enzymes is compensated for by the presence of amylase and bile salt stimulated lipase in breast milk. However, in formula-fed or donor milk-fed infants, the absence of significant levels of lipase and amylase would be expected to result in fat and carbohydrate malabsorption, respectively.

Fat Maldigestion and Specific Fatty Acid Absorption Coefficients

Humans possess lingual and gastric lipases that assist with fat digestion. Gastric lipase has preference for cleavage at the *sn*-3 position, which favors short- and medium-chain triglycerides, in contrast to pancreatic lipase, which preferentially hydrolyzes at the *sn*-2 position of long-chain triglycerides.[37] Although gastric digestion was initially thought to be higher in preterm infants now it is thought to be similar to adults, where gastric lipase is responsible for 10% to 30% hydrolysis of ingested triglycerides.[38-40] Thus the remainder of fat digestion is largely dependent on pancreatic lipase and the lower gastrointestinal tract.

CFA measurements in term and preterm infants demonstrate the impaired ability of formula-fed infants to digest fat compared with breast milk-fed infants. The authors' group evaluated the coefficients of absorption for specific fatty acids in the diet for a cohort of preterm infant fed with mother's milk or preterm formula.[41] A 3-day collection of feeding and fecal samples allowed for gas chromatography–mass spectrometry quantification of fatty acids entering the body and fatty acids lost in the fecal output and thus not absorbed. An analysis was done at postnatal age 2 and 6 weeks. The authors found that absorption coefficients in preterm infants fed mother's milk were sufficient at >90% for most fatty acids at both time points. In contrast, in formula-fed infants at both time points, a decrease in absorption coefficients was found with saturated and polyunsaturated fatty acids >12 carbons in length. The greatest impairment in fatty acid uptake was seen with DHA, where formula-fed infants were less efficient compared with breast milk-fed infants at postnatal age 2 and 6 weeks (83.4% versus 96.2% and 74.9% versus 97.4%, respectively). Although it has been determined that enteral feeding matures the gut and promotes enzyme maturation and digestive abilities, the fact that at postnatal age 6 weeks, differences were still observed in fatty acid absorption by group, suggests that the dietary substrate is critical to these processes. Additionally, this may also explain why after the initial deficit in AA and DHA in the first postnatal week, enteral diet alone is unlikely to close this deficit. This delayed maturation in lipid digestion must be taken into account when considering approaches to lipid and fatty acid supplementation. It is important to note that deficits in long-chain fatty acid absorption were evident in the authors' study, even though the total fat absorption between these two groups did not differ. Thus future studies in lipid digestion in preterm infants should distinguish between lipid classes and molecules for a more complete assessment of digestive capabilities.

In severe fat maldigestion independent of etiology, impairments in growth and absorption of other nutrients, such as fat-soluble vitamins, are observed. Additionally, pancreatic steatorrhea can present with bloating, abdominal distention, and oily, foul-smelling bulky stools. These symptoms are most evident in adult and pediatric populations with severe pancreatic insufficiency, such as CF, chronic pancreatitis, pancreatic cancer, and Shwachman–Diamond syndrome. Although we rarely ascribe severe fat maldigestion to preterm infants, some of the clinical presentations of feeding intolerance perhaps can be attributed to this impaired process (abdominal distension; loose, foul-smelling stools; and poor growth).

Bioavailability of Other Lipid Classes

Unique to human milk is the delivery of fat as milk fat globules (MFGs). Human MFGs have a triglyceride hydrophobic core surrounded by multiple layers of proteins, enzymes, and other complex lipids, such as phospholipids and cholesterol.

Sphingolipids represent an important class of lipids embedded in these membranes, of which sphingomyelin is the most prevalent at 40% of the total MFG polar lipids. Sphingomyelin and the downstream bioactive metabolites had been shown to have beneficial properties for neonatal gut development as well as immune ontogeny.[42] Interestingly, commensal gut microbiota also produce sphingolipid molecules that have been shown to be critical in the early postnatal period for gut and immune development, further supporting the bioactive role of these compounds.[43]

Lipid digestion of the MFG membrane appears to be independent of pancreatic enzymes (in contrast to the triglycerides present in the core of the fat globule). Sphingomyelin is hydrolyzed from the MFG membrane upon contact with the intestinal brush border by the enzyme alkaline sphingomyelinase, also known as *nucleotide phosphodiesterase pyrophosphatase 7*. Meconium analysis has shown that this enzyme is present at birth for both preterm and term infants.[44] The activity of these enzymes, however, has not been completely defined. Additionally, hydrolysis of sphingomyelin is bile salt dependent, which is limited in the enteral circulation of preterm infants. It would be of interest to further characterize the gestational age dependency of MFG hydrolysis. A parallel concept exists for protein digestion. Although peptidases are present along the preterm intestinal brush border for hydrolysis of small peptide fragments, the pancreatic enzymes that initially hydrolyze the larger intact proteins are deficient. Thus despite the presence of brush border enzymes, the overall efficiency of protein digestion is diminished in preterm infants compared with more mature systems.

Other factors that might dampen the appropriate processing of MFG in the preterm infant are the effects of human milk handling. Takahashi et al.[45] demonstrated that freezing human milk enlarges the diameter of the milk fat globule. In addition, within 12 hours of human milk fortification with a standard human milk fortifier, the milk fat globule size is increased with a decrease in the total surface area per unit of mass. The impact of this on the efficiency of fat digestion is not known.[45]

Complex lipids, such as sphingomyelin, that reside in the membrane of human MFGs are important signaling factors for gut and immune development. To advance the immuno-nutrient potential of the dietary substrates presented to preterm infants, investigation of digestive capabilities and modifiers to this efficiency should be investigated further.

Ileal Brake and Feeding Intolerance

Intestinal digestion, absorption, and motility are tightly controlled to optimize nutrient processing. A feedback loop or network between nutrient presentation, sensing cells, and gut hormone production sets the pace of intestinal motility after a meal. When activated, this feedback system slows gut transit time ("brake") and suppresses appetite to allow appropriate processing time of the meal. Although these "brakes" are in the jejunum and ileum, the most robust feedback system is within the distal ileum. Digested and undigested lipids are the most potent activators of this system, although undigested carbohydrates present in the ileum can also trigger this feedback loop.[46] The greatest inhibition is seen with free fatty acids compared with intact triglycerides. Regarding chain length, long-chain fatty acids are more potent at activating the ileal brake with intermediate responses seen with medium-chain triglycerides. There are multiple signaling pathways that activate the ileal brake. These include glucagon-like peptide 1 (GLP-1) and peptide YY (PYY), which are synthesized and secreted locally within the L cells of the ileum. GLP-1 is also secreted from the pancreatic islets. In addition to inhibition of ileal motility, these two peptides inhibit gastric emptying, and both gastric and pancreatic secretion.[46] Neural pathways, including vagal stimulation, have also been implicated in the ileal brake phenomenon.

In CF, activation of the ileal brake mechanism resulting from the presence of undigested fats and/or malabsorption of free fatty acids or carbohydrates may explain the symptoms of early satiety, bloating, and abdominal distention when continuous nocturnal feedings are delivered through an enteral tube without the benefit of pancreatic enzymes. No formal studies of the ileal brake system have been conducted in the preterm infant. However, not unlike patients with CF, the undigested lipid load reaching the distal ileum can be significant enough to prolong transit time, which can be up to 96 hours. The few studies of gut hormone responses after feeding do suggest an intact GLP-1 and PYY response making it conceivable that the ileal brake in preterm infants may be a factor determining feeding tolerance.

Strategies to Improve Lipid and Fatty Acid Delivery, Digestion, and Absorption

Enzyme-Based Therapies

Infants with CF rarely lived past the first year of life as a result of profound malnutrition secondary to the exocrine pancreatic destruction that began in utero. The advent of pancreatic enzyme replacement therapy containing proteases to digest proteins, amylases to digest carbohydrates, and lipases to digest fats to overcome pancreatic insufficiency has been lifesaving for patients with CF and was the first pharmaceutical to significantly extend survival in these patients. Pancreatic enzyme replacement therapies are also used for other conditions of pancreatic insufficiency, such as chronic pancreatitis and pancreatic cancer.

As discussed previously, there has been a long-standing acceptance that preterm and term infants are born with pancreatic insufficiency. Although many patents exist for enzyme supplementation in formula, this strategy has not been successfully implemented to date, presumably because of the challenges in enzyme stability in a liquid formulation as well as stability of hydrolyzed triglycerides.

The authors' group and others have studied the potential impact of enzyme-based therapies to optimize hydrolysis and absorption. Most recently, Casper et al.[47] published the results of a double-blind, placebo-controlled study in which they used a recombinant bile salt stimulated lipase (rhBSSL; Swedish Orphan Biovitrum) with pasteurized human milk and infant formula in preterm infants <32 weeks' gestation.[47] Fifteen milligrams of rhBSSL was reconstituted in 1 mL of sterile water (8700 units of lipase) and was added to 100 mL of feeding. Enzyme therapy was started once enteral feedings reached 100 mL/kg/day. For the entire cohort, the addition of rhBSSL did not improve growth, which was the primary outcome of the study. In a subanalysis of small-for-gestational-age infants, the mean growth velocity in the recombinant group was higher than that of the placebo group (17.1 versus 15.15 g/kg/day, respectfully). Interestingly, the infants in the recombinant group had more reported adverse events compared with the infants in the placebo group. These events included an increase in gastrointestinal signs and symptoms, including necrotizing enterocolitis. The physiologic basis for these increased events could not be determined. One consideration is that 8700 lipase units per 100 mL of feeding (unit/g of fat) exceeds the recommended dose given to infants and children with other disorders of pancreatic insufficiency, such as cystic fibrosis. The current recommended dose is 2000 to 4000 lipase units/120 mL according to the U.S. Food and Drug Administration (FDA) guidelines (https://www.fda.gov/downloads/Drugs/DevelopmentApprovalProcess/DevelopmentResources/UCM323253.pdf).

To counteract the potential undesirable consequences of recombinant or exogenous lipase contact with an immature gut epithelium, the authors' team has been investigating a strategy of ex vivo lipolysis, where enteral feedings are passed through an in-line cartridge of lipase immobilized to beads for prehydrolysis before entering the body (Alcresta Pharmaceuticals). Two clinical trials have been registered with clinicaltrials.gov for patients with CF to determine safety and tolerability (NCT02750501, NCT02598128). These studies have been completed; however, the final results have not been published so far.

Although there is sufficient evidence that providing mother's milk is the best nutrition for the preterm infant often demonstrating total fat absorption of >90%, multiple factors remain, propelling the need to consider additional nutritional strategies to optimize lipid and fatty acid delivery. These factors include (1) delayed milk delivery; (2) lipid and fatty acid composition insufficient to meet the needs of the rapidly developing preterm infant; and (3) potential alterations in human milk as a result of storage and fortification strategies.

Supplementation

Because of the complexity of providing stable enzymes in formula products, strategies to improve lipid and fatty acid delivery mainly comprised adding these nutrients largely in their native triglyceride form. A review of the literature on fatty acid supplementation for preterm infants, mostly DHA alone, will reveal mixed results and few have long-term follow-up. Meta-analyses of fatty acid supplementation in preterm and term infants have concluded that no benefit has been proven with enteral supplementation of long-chain polyunsaturated fatty acids.[48,49] Inconsistent outcomes with fatty acid supplementation support the premise that until the developmental limitations in lipid metabolism, such as pancreatic insufficiency, are overcome, supplementation of triglyceride oils alone will unlikely achieve the goals of increasing lipid and fatty acid delivery, absorption, tissue utilization, and ultimately health benefit.

Limitations that need to be addressed include suboptimal emulsification caused by decreased bile acids at the site of action; decreased hydrolysis caused by immature production of pancreatic lipase; and dose-finding to achieve an optimal balance of fatty acids to minimize counterregulatory reductions in critical omega-6 fatty acids levels (e.g., AA) with increasing levels of omega-3 fatty acids.[50]

One approach to overcome these physiologic limitations is to more directly provide the downstream bioactive metabolites of the parent fatty acids. Metabolite derivatives of DHA, EPA, and AA have been shown to regulate inflammation, cellular differentiation, and immune function.[51,52] In adult animal models of lung injury, Duvall et al. have shown that these specialized resolving mediators, such as resolvins, can attenuate the inflammatory response, and await studies in humans.[53] In a neonatal model of hyperoxia-induced lung injury, the authors' group demonstrated that the intraperitoneal injection of resolvin D1 (a derivative of DHA) and lipoxin A4 (a derivative of AA) alleviated the inflammatory changes and alveolar simplification observed in the hyperoxia-alone group.[22] These results demonstrate that these moieties not only have antiinflammatory properties but also play a major role in organogenesis.

Structured Lipids

Structured lipids are designed to mimic specific lipid and fatty acid composition and structure found in human milk. Examples of structured lipids include biochemical engineering (1) to force a specific fatty acid to reside in a specific *sn* position along the glycerol backbone of a triglyceride molecule (stereospecific positioning); (2) to enhance specific fatty acid delivery by increasing their presence on the glycerol backbone; and (3) to bind the lipid or fatty acid to a carrier or molecule that facilitates hydrolysis and/or absorption. The first example represents the most prolific investigation of structured lipids in neonatal health primarily involving the fatty acid palmitic acid (PA; 16-0). PA is the second most abundant fatty acid in human milk and is naturally found in the *sn*-2 position in human milk. After hydrolysis during which cleavage of covalent ester bonds preferentially occurs at the *sn*-1 and *sn*-3 position, PA as an *sn*-2 monoglyceride is generated. This configuration is optimally absorbed and confers multiple host physiologic benefits, including functions related to intestinal health and fat and calcium absorption (improving bone health).[54] In contrast, vegetable oils used in infant formulas have the PA in the *sn*-1 or *sn*-3 position. After hydrolysis at the outer positions, the resultant free PA binds to calcium, forming calcium soaps, and any host benefits conferred in intestinal health are lost. Formula-fed term infants with PA in the *sn*-2 position, compared with infants with the standard PA configuration that is found in vegetable oils, demonstrated softer stools, improved calcium and fat absorption, improved bone health, and intestinal microbial patterns with greater abundance of lactobacilli and bifidobacteria.[55-57] The benefits in absorption and mineral balance conferred by adding structured PA in the *sn*-2 position to infant formula have also been shown for preterm infants.[58,59]

The second example of structured lipids is the manipulation of the fatty acid composition bound to the glycerol backbone. This strategy is mostly utilized to increase the amount of omega-3 fatty acids in the diet, such as DHA and EPA. Additionally, similar to the PA experience, efforts have been made to preferentially place DHA in the *sn*-2 position for optimal delivery. Kenler et al. investigated the tolerance and potential benefit of a structured lipid formula containing fish oil and medium-chain triglycerides in adult patients recovering from major abdominal surgery.[60] In a small cohort of 50 adult patients, compared with a standard formula, patients demonstrated tolerance of the fish oil structured lipid formula, increased absorption and incorporation of EPA in plasma and red blood cell phospholipids, and fewer gastrointestinal complications and infections. In a 12-week hamster study, diets enriched with structured lipids containing DHA in the *sn*-2 position demonstrated higher tissue incorporation in DHA, including brain tissue, compared with diets containing natural fish oil configurations.[61] Current technology allows for multiple configurations of structured lipids, including stereospecific combinations of omega-3 fatty acids and beta (*sn*-2) PA on the glycerol backbone of the triglyceride molecule.[62,63] To date, no infant trials seem to have been conducted or are being conducted utilizing these newer generation structured lipids with stereospecific polyunsaturated fatty acids aimed at increasing their amounts in formula while optimizing absorption and tissue incorporation.

The third example of structured lipids is to take advantage of carrier molecules that optimize absorption and tissue incorporation. Unique to the brain, delivery efficiency of DHA is increased when it is bound to phosphatidylcholine in the *sn*-2 position (a molecule also known as *lysoPC-DHA*). Hachem et al. reported equal efficacy in DHA delivery to the brain using a synthesized phospholipid mimicking the lysoPC-DHA structure[64] and that this molecule maintained regional specificity in brain tissue, concentrating in the cortex, hippocampus, and cerebellum.

Milk Fat Globule Membrane Fragments

The concept of structured lipids can be extended to include engineering formula fats in a structure similar to the human MFGs. Gallier et al. described a novel infant milk formula with processed fats to mimic human milk fats in droplet size distribution, membrane structure, and outer membrane composition.[65] Like human milk, these artificially processed fats were encased in a membrane with other lipid classes, including phospholipids and cholesterol. A clinical trial involving healthy term infants is currently registered with clinicaltrials.gov (NCT01609634). The study is registered as "ongoing, but not recruiting participants"; no results are currently available.

In term piglets, the addition of milk fat and MFG membrane fragments to formula accelerated intestinal morphology, primed mucosal immunity from a Th2-Treg profile to a Th1 profile, and altered the microbiota approximating the status found in a control group of piglets solely sow fed.[66] Similarly, in a neonatal rat model, formula supplemented with MFG membrane fragments accelerated intestinal development and fostered the expression of tight junction proteins and microbial patterns comparable with dam-fed animals.[67]

Other Strategies

Bile salts are a necessary component to aid in the emulsification of lipids. Preterm infants possess a decreased pool of circulating bile salts that partly contributes to an inadequate or incomplete fat digestion. Although it would seem reasonable to restore levels of enteral bile salts to improve fat digestion, specific interventions to accomplish this are largely unexplored.

Summary

During infancy, especially in the preweaning phase, 40% to 60% of nutritional energy comes from lipids.[68] These diverse, complex lipids and fatty acids facilitate critical biologic functions vital for healthy survival. Although human milk is the most natural source of the lipid molecules, the altered environment and immature development of the preterm infant preclude efficient and optimal delivery of lipids and their bioactive metabolites. Inadequate delivery, hydrolysis and absorption of dietary fat limit their bioactive potential and may potentially lead to metabolic consequences that are harmful to health. Strategies to overcome these limitations and restore lipid and fatty acid delivery are critical to foster optimal health in the developing preterm infant. In doing so, concomitant evaluation of other lipid-mediated metabolic pathways needs to be undertaken to monitor for potential trade-offs of improved long-chain polyunsaturated fatty acid delivery.

REFERENCES

1. Quehenberger O, Armando AM, Brown AH, et al. Lipidomics reveals a remarkable diversity of lipids in human plasma. *J Lipid Res*. 2010;51:3299–3305.
2. Robinson DT, Martin CR. Fatty acid requirements for the preterm infant. *Semin Fetal Neonatal Med*. 2017;22:8–14.
3. Delplanque B, Gibson R, Koletzko B, Lapillonne A, Strandvik B. Lipid quality in infant nutrition: current knowledge and future opportunities. *J Pediatr Gastroenterol Nutr*. 2015.
4. Yamanaka WK, Clemans GW, Hutchinson ML. Essential fatty acids deficiency in humans. *Prog Lipid Res*. 1980;19:187–215.
5. Holman RT, Smythe L, Johnson S. Effect of sex and age on fatty acid composition of human serum lipids. *Am J Clin Nutr*. 1979;32:2390–2399.
6. Holman RT. The ratio of trienoic: tetraenoic acids in tissue lipids as a measure of essential fatty acid requirement. *J Nutr*. 1960;70:405–410.
7. Rosenlund ML, Kim HK, Kritchevsky D. Essential fatty acids in cystic fibrosis. *Nature*. 1974;251:719.
8. Freedman SD, Katz MH, Parker EM, Laposata M, Urman MY, Alvarez JG. A membrane lipid imbalance plays a role in the phenotypic expression of cystic fibrosis in cftr(-/-) mice. *Proc Natl Acad Sci U S A*. 1999;96:13995–14000.
9. Beharry S, Ackerley C, Corey M, et al. Long-term docosahexaenoic acid therapy in a congenic murine model of cystic fibrosis. *Am J Physiol Gastrointest Liver Physiol*. 2007;292:G839–G848.
10. Freedman SD, Weinstein D, Blanco PG, et al. Characterization of LPS-induced lung inflammation in cftr-/- mice and the effect of docosahexaenoic acid. *J Appl Physiol*. 2002;92:2169–2176.
11. Ollero M, Junaidi O, Zaman MM, et al. Decreased expression of peroxisome proliferator activated receptor gamma in cftr-/- mice. *J Cell Physiol*. 2004;200:235–244.
12. Freedman SD, Blanco PG, Zaman MM, et al. Association of cystic fibrosis with abnormalities in fatty acid metabolism. *N Engl J Med*. 2004;350:560–569.
13. Andersson C, Al-Turkmani MR, Savaille JE, et al. Cell culture models demonstrate that CFTR dysfunction leads to defective fatty acid composition and metabolism. *J Lipid Res*. 2008;49:1692–1700.
14. Zaman MM, Martin CR, Andersson C, et al. Linoleic acid supplementation results in increased arachidonic acid and eicosanoid production in CF airway cells and in cftr-/- transgenic mice. *Am J Physiol Lung Cell Mol Physiol*. 2010;299:L599–L606.
15. Al-Turkmani MR, Andersson C, Alturkmani R, et al. A mechanism accounting for the low cellular level of linoleic acid in cystic fibrosis and its reversal by DHA. *J Lipid Res*. 2008;49:1946–1954.
16. Yen EH, Quinton H, Borowitz D. Better nutritional status in early childhood is associated with improved clinical outcomes and survival in patients with cystic fibrosis. *J Pediatr*. 2013;162:530–535.e1.
17. Xue R, Gu H, Qiu Y, et al. Expression of cystic fibrosis transmembrane conductance regulator in ganglia of human gastrointestinal tract. *Sci Rep*. 2016;6:30926.
18. Martin CR, Dasilva DA, Cluette-Brown JE, et al. Decreased postnatal docosahexaenoic and arachidonic acid blood levels in premature infants are associated with neonatal morbidities. *J. Pediatr*. 2011;159:743–749.e1-2.
19. Robertson RC, Seira Oriach C, Murphy K, et al. Omega-3 polyunsaturated fatty acids critically regulate behaviour and gut microbiota development in adolescence and adulthood. *Brain Behav Immun*. 2017;59:21–37.
20. Lu J, Jilling T, Li D, Caplan MS. Polyunsaturated fatty acid supplementation alters proinflammatory gene expression and reduces the incidence of necrotizing enterocolitis in a neonatal rat model. *Pediatr Res*. 2007;61:427–432.
21. Calder PC. The relationship between the fatty acid composition of immune cells and their function. *Prostaglandins Leukot Essent Fatty Acids*. 2008;79:101–108.
22. Martin CR, Zaman MM, Gilkey C, et al. Resolvin D1 and lipoxin A4 improve alveolarization and normalize septal wall thickness in a neonatal murine model of hyperoxia-induced lung injury. *PloS one*. 2014;9:e98773.
23. Connor KM, SanGiovanni JP, Lofqvist C, et al. Increased dietary intake of omega-3-polyunsaturated fatty acids reduces pathological retinal angiogenesis. *Nat Med*. 2007;13:868–873.
24. Bhatia HS, Agrawal R, Sharma S, Huo YX, Ying Z, Gomez-Pinilla F. Omega-3 fatty acid deficiency during brain maturation reduces neuronal and behavioral plasticity in adulthood. *PloS one*. 2011;6:e28451.
25. Barrett EC, McBurney MI, Ciappio ED. Omega-3 fatty acid supplementation as a potential therapeutic aid for the recovery from mild traumatic brain injury/concussion. *Adv Nutr*. 2014;5:268–277.
26. Gura KM, Duggan CP, Collier SB, et al. Reversal of parenteral nutrition-associated liver disease in two infants with short bowel syndrome using parenteral fish oil: implications for future management. *Pediatrics*. 2006;118:e197–e201.
27. Tomsits E, Pataki M, Tolgyesi A, Fekete G, Rischak K, Szollar L. Safety and efficacy of a lipid emulsion containing a mixture of soybean oil, medium-chain triglycerides, olive oil, and fish oil: a randomised, double-blind clinical trial in premature infants requiring parenteral nutrition. *J Pediatr Gastroenterol Nutr*. 2010;51:514–521.

28. Pawlik D, Lauterbach R, Walczak M, Hurkala J, Sherman MP. Fish-oil fat emulsion supplementation reduces the risk of retinopathy in very low birth weight infants: a prospective, randomized study. *J Parenter Enteral Nutr*. 2013.

29. Pawlik D, Lauterbach R, Turyk E. Fish-oil fat emulsion supplementation may reduce the risk of severe retinopathy in VLBW infants. *Pediatrics*. 2011;127:223–228.

30. Le HD, de Meijer VE, Robinson EM, et al. Parenteral fish-oil-based lipid emulsion improves fatty acid profiles and lipids in parenteral nutrition-dependent children. *Am J Clin Nutr*. 2011;94:749–758.

31. Skouroliakou M, Konstantinou D, Agakidis C, et al. Cholestasis, bronchopulmonary dysplasia, and lipid profile in preterm infants receiving MCT/omega-3-PUFA-containing or soybean-based lipid emulsions. *Nutr Clin Pract*. 2012;27:817–824.

32. D'Ascenzo R, Savini S, Biagetti C, et al. Higher Docosahexaenoic acid, lower Arachidonic acid and reduced lipid tolerance with high doses of a lipid emulsion containing 15% fish oil: a randomized clinical trial. *Clin Nutr*. 2014;33:1002–9.

33. D'Ascenzo R, D'Egidio S, Angelini L, et al. Parenteral nutrition of preterm infants with a lipid emulsion containing 10% fish oil: effect on plasma lipids and long-chain polyunsaturated fatty acids. *J Pediatr*. 2011;159:33–38.e1.

34. Zhao Y, Wu Y, Pei J, Chen Z, Wang Q, Xiang B. Safety and efficacy of parenteral fish oil-containing lipid emulsions in premature neonates. *J Pediatr Gastroenterol Nutr*. 2015;60:708–716.

35. Biagetti C, Vedovelli L, Savini S, et al. Double blind exploratory study on de novo lipogenesis in preterm infants on parenteral nutrition with a lipid emulsion containing 10% fish oil. *Clin Nutr*. 2015.

36. Lebenthal E, Lee PC. Development of functional responses in human exocrine pancreas. *Pediatrics*. 1980;66:556–560.

37. Rogalska E, Ransac S, Verger R. Stereoselectivity of lipases. II. Stereoselective hydrolysis of triglycerides by gastric and pancreatic lipases. *J Biol Chem*. 1990;265:20271–20276.

38. Roman C, Carriere F, Villeneuve P, et al. Quantitative and qualitative study of gastric lipolysis in premature infants: do MCT-enriched infant formulas improve fat digestion? *Pediatr Res*. 2007;61:83–88.

39. Hamosh M, Bitman J, Liao TH, et al. Gastric lipolysis and fat absorption in preterm infants: effect of medium-chain triglyceride or long-chain triglyceride-containing formulas. *Pediatrics*. 1989;83:86–92.

40. Carriere F, Barrowman JA, Verger R, Laugier R. Secretion and contribution to lipolysis of gastric and pancreatic lipases during a test meal in humans. *Gastroenterology*. 1993;105:876–888.

41. Martin CR, Cheesman A, Brown J, et al. Factors determining optimal fatty acid absorption in preterm infants. *J Pediatr Gastroenterol Nutr*. 2016;62:130–136.

42. Nilsson A. Role of sphingolipids in infant gut health and immunity. *J Pediatr*. 2016;173(suppl):S53–S59.

43. An D, Oh SF, Olszak T, et al. Sphingolipids from a symbiotic microbe regulate homeostasis of host intestinal natural killer T cells. *Cell*. 2014;156:123–133.

44. Nilsson A, Duan R-D. Absorption and lipoprotein transport of sphingomyelin. *J Lipid Res*. 2006;47:154–171.

45. Takahashi K, Mizuno K, Itabashi K. The freeze-thaw process and long intervals after fortification denature human milk fat globules. *Am J Perinatol*. 2012;29:283–288.

46. Shin HS, Ingram JR, McGill A-T, Poppitt SD. Lipids, CHOs, proteins: can all macronutrients put a 'brake' on eating? *Physiol Behav*. 2013;120:114–123.

47. Casper C, Carnielli VP, Hascoet JM, et al. rhBSSL improves growth and LCPUFA absorption in preterm infants fed formula or pasteurized breast milk. *J Pediatr Gastroenterol Nutr*. 2014;59:61–69.

48. Schulzke SM, Patole SK, Simmer K. Long-chain polyunsaturated fatty acid supplementation in preterm infants. *Cochrane Database Syst Rev*. 2011;(2):CD000375.

49. Jasani B, Simmer K, Patole SK, Rao SC. Long chain polyunsaturated fatty acid supplementation in infants born at term. *Cochrane Database Syst Rev*. 2017;3:CD000376.

50. Levy BD, Serhan CN. Resolution of acute inflammation in the lung. *Annu Rev Physiol*. 2013.

51. Serhan CN. Discovery of specialized pro-resolving mediators marks the dawn of resolution physiology and pharmacology. *Mol Aspects Med*. 2017;58:1–11.

52. Chiang N, Serhan CN. Structural elucidation and physiologic functions of specialized pro-resolving mediators and their receptors. *Mol Aspects Med*. 2017;58:114–29.

53. Duvall MG, Bruggemann TR, Levy BD. Bronchoprotective mechanisms for specialized pro-resolving mediators in the resolution of lung inflammation. *Mol Aspects Med*. 2017;58:44–56.

54. Bar-Yoseph F, Lifshitz Y, Cohen T. Review of sn-2 palmitate oil implications for infant health. *Prostaglandins Leukot Essent Fatty Acids*. 2013;89:139–143.

55. Yaron S, Shachar D, Abramas L, et al. Effect of high beta-palmitate content in infant formula on the intestinal microbiota of term infants. *J Pediatr Gastroenterol Nutr*. 2013;56:376–381.

56. Kennedy K, Fewtrell MS, Morley R, et al. Double-blind, randomized trial of a synthetic triacylglycerol in formula-fed term infants: effects on stool biochemistry, stool characteristics, and bone mineralization. *Am J Clin Nutr*. 1999;70:920–927.

57. Carnielli VP, Luijendijk IH, van Goudoever JB, et al. Structural position and amount of palmitic acid in infant formulas: effects on fat, fatty acid, and mineral balance. *J Pediatr Gastroenterol Nutr*. 1996;23:553–560.

58. Carnielli VP, Luijendijk IH, van Goudoever JB, et al. Feeding premature newborn infants palmitic acid in amounts and stereoisomeric position similar to that of human milk: effects on fat and mineral balance. *Am J Clin Nutr*. 1995;61:1037–1042.

59. Carnielli VP, Luijendijk IH, van Beek RH, Boerma GJ, Degenhart HJ, Sauer PJ. Effect of dietary triacylglycerol fatty acid positional distribution on plasma lipid classes and their fatty acid composition in preterm infants. *Am J Clin Nutr*. 1995;62:776–781.

60. Kenler AS, Swails WS, Driscoll DF, et al. Early enteral feeding in postsurgical cancer patients. Fish oil structured lipid-based polymeric formula versus a standard polymeric formula. *Ann Surg.* 1996;223:316–333.

61. Bandarra NM, Lopes PA, Martins SV, et al. Docosahexaenoic acid at the sn-2 position of structured triacylglycerols improved n-3 polyunsaturated fatty acid assimilation in tissues of hamsters. *Nutr Res.* 2016;36:452–463.

62. Liu Y, Guo Y, Sun Z, et al. Production of structured triacylglycerols containing palmitic acids at sn-2 position and docosahexaenoic acids at sn-1, 3 positions. *J Oleo Sci.* 2015;64:1227–1234.

63. Li R, Sabir JSM, Baeshen NA, Akoh CC. Enzymatic synthesis of refined olive oil-based structured lipid containing omega -3 and -6 fatty acids for potential application in infant formula. *J Food Sci.* 2015;80:H2578–H2584.

64. Hachem M, Geloen A, Lo Van A, et al. Efficient docosahexaenoic acid uptake by the brain from a structured phospholipid. *Mol Neurobiol.* 2016;53:3205–3215.

65. Gallier S, Vocking K, Post JA, et al. A novel infant milk formula concept: mimicking the human milk fat globule structure. *Colloids Surf B Biointerfaces.* 2015;136:329–339.

66. Le Huërou-Luron I, Bouzerzour K, Ferret-Bernard S, et al. A mixture of milk and vegetable lipids in infant formula changes gut digestion, mucosal immunity and microbiota composition in neonatal piglets. *Eur J Nutr.* 2016:1–14.

67. Bhinder G, Allaire JM, Garcia C, et al. Milk fat globule membrane supplementation in formula modulates the neonatal gut microbiome and normalizes intestinal development. *Sci Rep.* 2017;7:45274.

68. Abrahamse E, Minekus M, van Aken GA, et al. Development of the digestive system–experimental challenges and approaches of infant lipid digestion. *Food Dig.* 2012;3:63–77.

CHAPTER 4

Human Milk Oligosaccharide

Ardythe L. Morrow, PhD, MSc, David S. Newburg, PhD

- Human milk oligosaccharide (hMOS) is a major component of human milk, similar in quantity to protein.

- The structure of hMOS is distinct from other commercially available oligosaccharide or prebiotics. hMOSs are structural homologues to oligosaccharide components of glycoproteins in the infant gut and contain fucose and sialic acid.

- Bovine milk (and most infant formulas) contains sparse quantities of acidic oligosaccharide that lack fucose.

- There is variation in the hMOS content of human milk among mothers and over the course of lactation.

- Infants do not directly digest hMOS, but some of the hMOS consumed is absorbed into the circulation, and some of it is metabolized by mutualist bacteria, which produces beneficial metabolites.

- The functions of hMOS include prebiotic effects, inhibition of pathogen binding, neurodevelopment, and immunomodulation. After intestinal challenge, hMOS reduces gut inflammation while enhancing infant immunity, intestinal adaptation, and growth recovery.

- Major hMOSs of human milk are being tested as additives to infant formula. Preclinical studies and clinical trials have established their safety, with no effects on normal growth. Consumption of hMOS through infant formula confers immune and metabolic benefits.

Introduction

Human milk oligosaccharide (hMOS) is a major fraction of human milk. This fraction is composed of carbohydrate chains ranging in size from 3 to 32 sugars that use lactose as a core molecule.[1] hMOS in nutrition was overlooked for many years, but the number

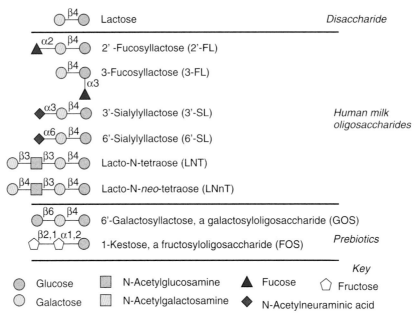

Fig. 4.1 Structural comparison of carbohydrates found in human milk or formula. *Upper row,* The disaccharide lactose, which is the most abundant carbohydrate found in human milk, and the core for human milk oligosaccharides. *Rows 2 through 7,* Selected examples of simple human milk oligosaccharide (hMOS) structures. Shown are two fucosylated structures (2'-FL and 3'-FL), two sialylated (acidic) structures (3'-SL and 6'-SL), and two precursor molecules without fucose or sialic acid. Rows 8 and 9: Two commercially available prebiotic carbohydrates are shown (fructo-oligosaccharide [FOS] and galacto-oligosaccharide [GOS]).

of publications indexed on hMOS in PubMed per year nearly tripled between 2009 and 2016, indicating that hMOS has emerged as a major focus of investigation. Heightened attention to hMOS is likely the result of the emerging evidence of its effects on health and development, as well as the distinctive composition of the oligosaccharides of human milk and their homology to gut glycans.[2] Technical developments have now led to commercial biosynthesis of major individual hMOS molecules, enabling preclinical and clinical studies. Several companies have obtained U.S. Food and Drug Administration approval of synthetically produced hMOS, 2'-fucosyllactose (2'-FL) and lacto-*N*-neotretraose (LNnT), as "generally recognized as safe". Initial human trials have demonstrated safety and potential health benefits of 2'-FL in combination with other oligosaccharides in infant formula.[3-5] In this chapter, we examine the structure and composition of human milk, the effects of hMOS on the infant gut microbial community, and other probable health effects of hMOS.

Structure and Composition

Human milk oligosaccharides are distinct in structure from commercially available oligosaccharides—fructo-oligosaccharide and galacto-oligosaccharide (GOS)—that were synthesized and first added to formula as substitutes for hMOS more than 10 years ago (Fig. 4.1). Remarkably, the oligosaccharide is more abundant and complex in human milk compared with the milk of most other mammalian species and comprises more than 150 individual molecules.[6-14] The absolute quantity of hMOS in mature milk may be as high as 5 to 20 g/L, with higher levels in early milk; the quantity of hMOS declines about 30% over the course of lactation.[7] The quantity of hMOS in early preterm milk is about 10% higher than that in term milk within the first 14 days after delivery.[8] The reported quantity of hMOS in mother's milk is generally similar to that of protein. However, there is significant variation in the hMOS content of milk among mothers, over the course of lactation, and by maternal genetics. Measurement of hMOS content is also influenced by differences in methods, including milk collection, hMOS isolation, and analytic techniques.[7,12,14,15]

Table 4.1 HIGHLY ABUNDANT HMOS IN HUMAN MILK

Oligosaccharide (abbreviation)	Structure	Type and size
2'-fucosyllactose (2'-FL)	Fucose $\alpha_{1,2}$ γαλαχτοσε$\beta_{1,4}$ glucose	Fucosylated, neutral, triose
Lacto-*N*-fucopentaose I (LNFPI)	Fucose $\alpha_{1,2}$-Gal $\beta_{1,3}$-GlcNAc $\beta_{1,3}$-Gal $\beta_{1,4}$-Glc,	Fucosylated, neutral, tetraose
Lacto-*N*-difucohexose I (LNDFHI)	Fucose $\alpha_{1,2}$-Gal $\beta_{1,3}$-(Fuc-$\alpha_{1,4}$)- GlcNAc $\beta_{1,3}$-Gal $\beta_{1,4}$-Glc	Difucosylated, neutral, hexaose
Lacto-*N*-fucopentose II (LNFPII)	Gal $\beta_{1,3}$-(Fuc $\alpha_{1,4}$)-GlcNAc $\beta_{1,3}$-Gal $\beta_{1,4}$-Glc	Fucosylated, neutral, pentaose
3-Fucosyllactose (3-FL)	Fuc $\alpha_{1,3}$-(Gal $\beta_{1,4}$)-Glc	Fucosylated, neutral
Lactodifucotetraose (LDFT)	Fuc$\alpha_{1,2}$Gal$\beta_{1,4}$(Fuc$\alpha_{1,3}$)Glc	Difucosylated, neutral, tetraose
Disialyllacto-*N*-tetraose (DSLNT)	Neu5Ac $\alpha_{2,3}$-Gal $\beta_{1,3}$-(Neu5Ac $\alpha_{2,6}$)-GlcNAc $\beta_{1,3}$-Gal $\beta_{1,4}$-Glc	Disialylated, acidic, hexaose
3'- sialyllactose (3'-SL)	Neu5Ac $\alpha_{2,3}$-Gal $\beta_{1,4}$-Glc	Sialyl, acidic, triose
6'- sialyllactose (6'-SL)	Neu5Ac $\alpha_{2,6}$-Gal $\beta_{1,4}$-Glc	Sialylated, acidic, triose
Monofucosylmonosialyllacto-*N*-hexaose (MFMSLNH)	Neu5Ac $\alpha_{2,6}$-(Gal $\beta_{1,3}$)-GlcNAc $\beta_{1,3}$-(Gal $\beta_{1,4}$-[Fuc $\alpha_{1,3}$-] GlcNAc $\beta_{1,6}$-)Gal $\beta_{1,4}$-Glc	Sialylated and fucosylated, acidic octaose
Lacto-*N*-tetraose (LNT)	Gal $\beta_{1,3}$-GlcNAc $\beta_{1,3}$-Gal $\beta_{1,4}$-Glc	Nonfucosylated, neutral, tetraose
Lacto-*N*-neotetraose (LNnT)	Gal $\beta_{1,4}$-GlcNAc $\beta_{1,3}$-Gal $\beta_{1,4}$-Glc	Nonfucosylated, neutral, tetraose

From two thirds to three quarters of total hMOS are neutral.[6,7,12,13,15] The majority of the neutral oligosaccharides comprises molecules containing one or more fucose moieties. A minority of the neutral oligosaccharide fraction consists of precursor molecules (e.g., lacto-*N*-tetraose [LNT], LNnT, and lacto-*N*-hexaose [LNH]) that lack fucose. Maternal ability to synthesize fucosylated hMOS depends on encoded enzymes made by specific fucosyltransferase (*FUT*) genes. Synthesis of hMOS containing the Fuc-α1,2-Gal linkage requires the *FUT2* ("secretor") enzyme. This class of hMOS may constitute half of the hMOS fraction when the mother is *FUT2*$^+$ ("secretor"). Individual oligosaccharides containing this linkage include 2'-FL and lacto-*N*-fucopentaose I (LNFP I). However, nearly 25% of the U.S. population and many other populations worldwide are homozygous recessive for the *FUT2* gene and therefore are incapable of synthesizing this class of hMOS. Mothers who are secretors have significantly higher hMOS content of milk compared with mothers who are nonsecretors.[6,12]

Another strong genetic influence on neutral hMOS phenotype is the *FUT3* ("Lewis") enzyme, which is required for synthesis of Fuc-α1,4-Gal linkages. Some major hMOSs containing this linkage include lacto-*N*-difucohexaose I (LNDFH I) and LNFP II. But the *FUT3* gene can also have inactivating mutations. As a result, about 10% of mothers cannot make Lewis hMOS. About two thirds of the population are both *FUT2*+ and *FUT3*+ and are thus capable of synthesizing all hMOSs. However, the remaining third of the population is nonsecretors, Lewis negative, or both and therefore lack the corresponding hMOS. Mothers with polymorphisms in *FUT2* and *FUT3* genes ("nonsecretor" and Lewis negative) typically have lower total hMOS concentrations, despite compensatory increase in acidic or precursor hMOS that do not require the *FUT2* or *FUT3* encoded enzymes.[6,12,16]

Sialic-acid containing hMOSs range from about 25% to 40% of the hMOS fraction. The highest proportions are found in early lactation, with the percentage declining rapidly over the first few months of lactation. Synthesis of sialylated hMOS requires sialyltransferase (ST)3Gal enzymes to produce sialic acid–containing α2,3 linkages (which includes 3'-sialyllactose [3'-SL]) and ST6Gal gene enzymes to produce sialic acid-containing α2,6 linkages (which includes 6'-sialyllactose [6'-SL]).

Although human milk contains hundreds of distinct hMOSs, as much as 75% of the hMOS fraction of human milk consists of 12 individual hMOSs (Table 4.1 and Fig. 4.2), including six fucosylated neutral hMOSs, two precursor nonfucosylated hMOSs, and four sialylated (acidic) hMOSs. As shown in Fig. 4.2, the relative abundance of these different hMOS shifts over the course of lactation. The most abundant neutral

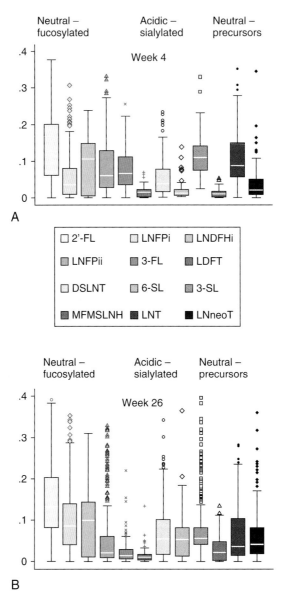

Fig. 4.2 Box plots of 12 highly abundant human milk oligosaccharide (hMOS) across three global urban populations (Cincinnati, OH, USA; Shanghai, China; Mexico City, Mexico), including samples collected at week 4 (A) and
week 26 (B). Data are from the Global Exploration of Human Milk (GEHM) study. This longitudinal study includes
360 mothers (120 per site). Analysis was performed in the Newburg laboratory by using mass spectrometry. The
Y-axis is relative abundance and indicates the percentage of total hMOS that the specific individual oligosaccharide constitutes at that time point. In the box plots, the upper line of the box represents the 75th percentile, the
middle line represents the median, and the lower line of the box represents the 25th percentile. The vertical lines
of the box represent adjacent values; points above or below the vertical lines represent outlier values. Upper panel,
Week 4 milk samples, box plot of the most abundant hMOS, grouped by type of structure: 6 neutral fucosylated;
4 acidic (sialylated); 2 neutral precursors. Within each group, ordered by relative abundance. Lower panel, Week
26 milk samples, box plot of the most abundant hMOS, grouped by type of structures, same hMOS as above.
Ordered by relative abundance shown in upper panel. For both graphs, From left to right the first 6 hMOS are
neutral fucosylated: 2'-fucosyllactose (2'-FL), Lacto-N-fucopentaose I (LNFP-I), lacto-N-difucohexaose I (LNDFH-I),
LNFP-II, 3-fucosyllactose (3-FL), lacto-difucotetraose (LDFT) (top row). From left to right, the second six hMOSs are
acidic: disialyl lacto-N-tetraose (DSLNT), 6-SL, 3-SL, monofucosylmonosialylacto-N-hexaose (MFMSLNH) (the latter
contains one fucose and one sialic acid), followed by the neutral precursor oligosaccharides: lacto-N-tetraose (LNT)
and lacto-N-neotetraose (LNnT).

Box 4.1   HEALTH FUNCTIONS OF hMOS

- Inhibition of pathogen binding—provide soluble receptor analog to competitively inhibit pathogen binding to infant gut receptors
- Prebiotic effects—guiding ontogeny of early gut colonization and restitution of microbiota homeostasis
- Immunomodulation through signal control:
  - Attenuate inflammatory response to pathogens and irritation
  - Enhance mutualist interkingdom signaling
  - Preserve and restore homeostasis
  - Support normal gut ontogeny
- Reduce overall risk of infectious and inflammatory diseases:
  - Diarrhea, necrotizing enterocolitis, respiratory, and urinary tract
- Neurodevelopment—enhance development and function of brain through gut microbiota-brain axis

---

oligosaccharide over the course of lactation is typically 2'-FL, but depending on maternal genetics and the timing of lactation, there are other major abundant neutral hMOSs, including the neutral precursor molecules LNT, and LNnT and the fucose-containing molecules LNFP I, LNDFH I, LNFP II, 3-fucosyllactose (3-FL), and lacto-difucotetraose. Among the many acidic oligosaccharides found in milk, the most abundant are disialyl lacto-*N*-tetraose (DSLNT), the two trisaccharide molecules 6'-SL and 3'-SL, and monofucosylmonosialylacto-*N*-hexaose, a molecule that contains both fucose and sialic acid.

The relative abundance of different hMOSs shifts over the course of lactation. For example, the total quantity of hMOSs reduces over the course of lactation, and the quantity of sialic acid-containing hMOSs declines more rapidly than neutral hMOS.[6,7,16] The biologic significance of these shifts in hMOS composition is not known.

Digestion and Absorption

Infants lack the enzymes necessary to hydrolyze or digest hMOS, and thus in a strict sense, hMOS is not a human nutrient, but a form of dietary fiber. Some hMOSs are absorbed in the small intestine, found intact in the infant's circulation, and excreted in urine.[4,17] More of the hMOSs are fermented by bifidobacteria and other mutualist bacteria in the colon; this fermentation produces short-chain fatty acids and small organic acids. However, a large proportion of the hMOS fraction is found intact in the infant's stool.[17] These findings are consistent with the multiple functions that have been identified for hMOSs, as described later.

Functions

Oligosaccharides are among the most abundant bioactive molecules of human milk and have multiple functions, including metabolic, antiinfective, and immunomodulatory functions. The individual hMOS molecules appear to have some common, or redundant, functions, but there is increasing evidence that individual hMOS molecules also have distinct effects (see Box 4.1).

Prebiotic Functions

In infancy, human milk feeding shapes the composition of microbiota, favoring colonization by bifidobacteria. The bifidogenic impact of human milk was first observed by the eminent Dr. Paul Gyorgy, whose pioneering work on human milk led to his discovery of a "bifidus factor" in human milk,[18] that is, hMOS and hMOS bound to glycoprotein. Indeed, the predominance of bifidobacteria in the microbiota of exclusively breastfed infants is largely shaped by the hMOS fraction of human milk.[19]

The hMOS fraction and the individual hMOS molecules are effective prebiotics, defined as dietary carbohydrates that are indigestible by humans but utilized by gut bacteria for anaerobic fermentation. hMOS is avidly utilized by the mutualist microbes *Bifidobacterium longum infantis* and *Bacteroides* spp., but not by the nonmutualists *Campylobacter jejuni*, *Clostridium perfringens*, or *Escherichia coli*. Mutualist bacteria ferment hMOS into small organic acids and short-chain fatty acids that acidify the gut and inhibit pathogens. However, even in this general function, specific bacteria differ in their ability to hydrolyze and metabolize specific hMOS molecules, depending on their genomic capacities, resulting in distinct patterns of bacterial growth and metabolic products with different combinations of hMOS.[20-22]

Antiinfective Functions

Human milk oligosaccharides protect infants against enteric, urinary, and respiratory pathogens through several different protective mechanisms. The most highly studied are the hMOSs that protect against enteric pathogens. The protection that hMOSs offer against enteric infection may be attributed to multiple mechanisms, including their prebiotic effects. However, the primary mechanism of protection may be through competitive inhibition of pathogen binding to homologous gut receptors. The intestinal tract displays an abundant quantity of oligosaccharides lining the mucosal surface. The oligosaccharides located on terminal end of membrane-bound gut glycans can be used as binding sites by enteric pathogens, which then infect gut enterocytes.[15] Competitive inhibition of this binding by hMOS is thought to depend on the degree of homology between milk and gut oligosaccharide structures. Nevertheless, the specificity of pathogen binding varies, allowing some hMOSs to inhibit multiple pathogens through competitive binding.

The fucose of fucosylated glycans, and the sialic acid (*N*-acetylneuraminic acid) of acidic glycans, are common components of bacterial and viral mucosal receptors. Human milk acidic glycans include mucins, glycoproteins, and the gangliosides GM1, GD3, and GM3. MUC1 and MUC4 are the principal mucins of human milk. These human milk mucins (MUCs) are heavily glycosylated (i.e., contain copious oligosaccharides) and contain serine, threonine, and proline repeats and terminal cysteine-rich domains as part of their structures. Protection of mucosa through competitive binding of mucin to pathogens may often depend on the relative quantity of fucosylated and sialylated moieties available to bind the pathogen, thereby inhibiting binding to the infant's mucosal glycan receptor. MUC1 and MUC4 are able to inhibit infection by *Salmonella typhimurium*. MUC1 also inhibits infection by rotavirus, and binding by norovirus, *E. coli*, and human immunodeficiency virus (HIV).[23]

Acidic human milk glycans include the glycolipid gangliosides GM1 and GM3, which also bind to pathogens. The ganglioside GM1 limits the adhesion of enterotoxigenic *E. coli* to Caco-2 cells to less than 20% of the positive control. GM3 depresses adhesion of enterotoxigenic *E. coli* and enteropathogenic *E. coli* in vitro. The most prevalent acidic hMOSs are the sialyllactoses, which inhibit *E. coli*, *Pseudomonas aeruginosa*, *Aspergillus fumigatus conidia*, and *Helicobacter pylori*.[1]

Human milk secretory immunoglobulin A (sIgA) was recognized early as a milk component that protects infants against human pathogens. When sIgA binds an antigen, it renders the pathogen less infective. Oligosaccharides on the surface of sIgA play general structural and functional roles and appear to increase the binding of sIgA.[24,25] Human milk bile salt–stimulated lipase (BSSL) binds to dendritic cell–specific intercellular adhesion molecule-3-grabbing nonintegrin (DC-SIGN), a nonenzymatic function, and inhibits HIV type 1 transfer to the CD4+ class of T cells.[26] Human milk lactoferrin is a multifunctional glycoprotein that displays innate antibacterial, antivirus, antifungal, and antiprotozoan activity and can block cell–virus interaction and disrupt bacterial cell membranes.[1]

Many enteric pathogens use $\alpha_{1,2}$-fucosylated gut glycan structures for binding—this includes *C. jejuni*, *Vibrio cholerae*, enteropathogenic *E. coli*, human rotaviruses, and most major noroviruses, including GII.4, GII.17 and GII.10 strains. This predilection for pathogen binding to $\alpha_{1,2}$-fucosylated glycans explains the finding that acute diarrheal disease was more prevalent in *FUT2+* secretors than in nonsecretors in population-based studies, including a recent genome wide association study (GWAS).[27,28] Consistent with that finding, norovirus is inhibited by the large milk glycoproteins, mucin and BSSL, only when their source is milk from a secretor mother.[29] Among "secretor-binding pathogens," however, there are differences in the ability of simple oligosaccharide structures or large glycans of human milk to effectively inhibit binding to the gut receptor.[15,30,31]

Some simple hMOSs bind to specific pathogens, competing with the ability of the pathogen to bind its homologous carbohydrate moiety on the host cell surface receptor. For example, *C. jejuni* is the most common agent of bacterial diarrhea worldwide. The receptor of *C. jejuni* contains an H-2-fucosylated critical determinant: *C. jejuni* has high avidity for the fucosylated antigen H-2 (Fucα1,2-Galβ1,4-GlcNAc); monoclonal antibodies against the H-2 epitope inhibit *C. jejuni* binding. Conversely, overexpression of H-2- fucosylated antigen on Chinese hamster ovary cells transforms these cells from *C. jejuni* nonbinding cells to *C. jejuni* binding cells. Ligands that bind to H-2 epitope, such as *Ulex europaeus* agglutinin and *Lotus tetragonolobus* lectins, inhibit *C. jejuni* adhesion. 2'-FL, the most prevalent of the milk oligosaccharides, is a major source of H-2 epitope in human milk. 2'-FL competes with H-2 epitopes of the host cell surface receptors for binding to *C. jejuni*. Thus 2'-FL inhibits *C. jejuni* binding to fucosylated H-2 epitopes on the apical surface of epithelial cells of the intestinal mucosa, thereby preventing *C. jejuni* adhesion to the host.[32]

The clinical relevance of these in vitro and in vivo laboratory results was tested in a cohort of 93 breastfeeding mother–infant pairs. *C. jejuni* diarrhea occurred significantly less in infants consuming milk that contained high levels of 2'-FL but was unrelated to levels of other hMOSs, strongly supporting clinical relevance of protection by 2'-FL consumption. Similarly, the hMOS LDFH-I binds to Norwalk virus in vitro and specifically inhibits the ability of the virus to infect cells. In the aforementioned clinical study, only LDFH-I levels in milk consumed by the infants was inversely related to the risk of norovirus-associated diarrhea; levels of other hMOSs were not related. More recently, mice infected with a human cutivar of virulent *Campylobacter* exhibited the pathobiology, morbidity, and mortality of the human disease. Feeding physiologic human milk levels of 2'FL during the campylobacter infection reduced the pathobiology to the extent that the sick but treated mice resembled uninfected controls.[33]

Thus the hMOSs and glycoproteins are strongly implicated as responsible for a major portion of the protection of human milk against infant diarrhea.[15]

Immune Regulation

Human milk oligosaccharides regulate immune processes in the intestinal epithelium and in the central circulation. For example, in vitro, hMOSs reduce platelet-neutrophil complex formation, which decreases neutrophil β_2-integrin expression. At physiologically plausible concentrations, an acidic hMOS fraction reduced platelet–neutrophil complex formation up to 20%, and neutrophils showed a dose-dependent decrease in β_2-integrin expression.[34] The neutral hMOS fraction had no effect.

In a variety of inflammatory diseases, excessive leukocyte infiltration causes severe tissue damage. This initial step of leukocyte extravasation is mediated by selectin binding to the glycan moiety of glycoconjugate ligands. Monocytes, lymphocytes, and neutrophils isolated from human peripheral blood, when passed over activated human umbilical vein endothelial cells under hemodynamic shear stress, adhere to the endothelial cells. Within physiologic concentrations, the acidic hMOS fraction significantly inhibited leukocyte rolling and adhesion. Individual hMOSs may serve as antiinflammatory components that contribute to the lower incidence of inflammatory diseases in human milk–fed infants.[35]

Relative to the mature intestinal mucosa, that of the immature intestine overexpresses inflammatory genes and underexpresses feedback regulatory genes, making neonatal epithelial cells prone to exaggerated responses to proinflammatory stimuli. Moreover, the T helper cell 2 (Th2) bias that remains from prenatal immune regulation renders the neonatal mucosa hyperresponsive to bacterial infection and susceptible to food allergy. The oligosaccharides of human colostrum curb inflammatory genes and cytokine expression in the neonatal intestine. These genes are involved in the major immunologic signal pathways: immune cell trafficking, hematologic system development, promotion of Th1 cell activation and function, and suppression of Th2 cell activation and function.[36] Colostrum hMOS modulates Toll-like receptor 3 (TLR3), TLR5 and interleukin-1 (IL-1β)–dependent pathogen-associated molecular pattern signaling pathways, depressing acute phase inflammatory cytokine protein expression. 3'-galactosyllactose, an oligosaccharide found in especially high concentrations in colostrum relative to mature milk, specifically quenches polyinosine–polycytidylic acid (the TLR3 ligand)–induced IL-8 levels.[36]

The human milk oligosaccharide 2'-FL modulates CD14 expression through decreasing CD14 messenger RNA (mRNA) transcription and decreases the amount of CD14 bound to membrane. Modulation of CD14 expression and binding quenches inflammation elicited by type I pili *E. coli* infection in human enterocytes.[37] Feeding 2'-FL to mice modified their gene expression, changed microbiota species, and increased survival during dysbiosis (DSN, personal communication). Other examples of modulating the neonatal immune system through hMOS have also been reported.[38] LNFP III, a human milk oligosaccharide containing the Lewis X (Lex) epitope, strongly promotes a Th2 response in vivo. LNFP III induces recruitment of suppressor macrophages and accelerates maturation of dendritic cells. Sialyl $\alpha_{2,3}$-lactose (3'-SL) arouses mesenteric lymph node CD11c+ dendritic cells and causes release of cytokines that expand Th1 and Th17 T lymphocytes. Although the precise mechanism of many other antiinflammatory effects of hMOS in diverse inflammatory disease conditions has not been elucidated, such putative antiinflammatory functions of hMOS could contribute to the lower incidence of inflammatory diseases in breastfed versus formula-fed infants.

Somatic Growth

A number of studies in diverse populations have examined the relationship between administration of hMOS and infant growth. Before reviewing these studies, we first consider biologic plausibility. In the "as consumed" form, hMOSs are not directly a human nutrient, given that human infants (and adults) lack the enzymatic repertoire to digest hMOS. Given this, what is the potential mechanism by which hMOS could influence infant growth? One possibility, as previously noted, is the potential for hMOS to reduce infections and gut inflammation, which could, in turn, improve growth by making the nutrient content of human milk more bioavailable to the infant. Another potential explanation pertains to the prebiotic role of hMOS. Providing hMOS can shift the microbiota beneficially, supporting the growth of mutualist bacteria and reducing the burden of potentially pathogenic bacteria. The fermentation of hMOS by bacteria in the small intestine and colon can produce metabolites, including small-chain fatty acids and small organic acids, that can beneficially influence bacterial metabolism in the gut and the metabolites found in the infant's circulation.[5] Furthermore, provision of hMOS can restore gut architecture[39,40] after intestinal insult. These several putative mechanisms provide ample justification for studying the role of hMOS in infant growth.

Because hMOS composition varies significantly among mothers, it is possible to examine the association between varied composition and infant health outcomes using epidemiology. Several longitudinal studies of mother-infant pairs have reported that variation in hMOS composition affects infant growth, but the findings appear inconsistent. In a longitudinal study of 25 term infants in Oklahoma, the growth of breastfed infants was measured at 1 and 6 months of postnatal life. Higher diversity and evenness of hMOSs measured in mothers' milk was associated with lower infant fat mass. Individual hMOSs showed varying relationships to growth: LNFP I was associated with lower infant weight and lower lean mass, whereas LNnT was associated with lower body fat. Other individual hMOS molecules—DSLNT and LNFP II—were associated with greater fat mass. A longitudinal study of 33 Gambian mother–infant pairs at 4, 16, and 20 weeks postpartum also reported that the relative abundance of other hMOSs in mothers' milk was associated with growth. But the pattern differed from that reported in infants in Arizona. The Gambian study found that infant weight-for-age

Z-score growth was positively associated with the abundance of 3'-SL, whereas there was a negative association with LSTc abundance in mother's milk. Several other hMOSs—LNFP I/III and DFLNHa—were positively associated with infant height-for-age Z-scores. The findings of a third longitudinal study of 50 infants in Singapore measured hMOSs at a single time point, and examined growth at 30, 60, and 120 days of postnatal life. In the Singapore infants, no significant differences were found in body weight, body length, or body mass index in relation to hMOS concentrations.[41]

In addition to these observational studies in breastfed term infants, two randomized, controlled trials (RCTs) were conducted in the United States and Europe, and these studies compared the growth of infants given standard formula with those given formula with hMOS. Neither trial found a significant difference in the growth of hMOS-fed and non–hMOS-fed control infants.[3,4]

Taken together, the results of these studies do not support a consistent association between total or relative intake of specific hMOSs and growth in healthy, term infants. The two observational studies that reported growth effects related to individual hMOSs were conducted in distinct populations and environments and could potentially have been influenced by particular microbe–hMOS interactions found within each study population. Alternatively, the findings in those two studies might have been influenced by chance, given the multiple comparisons made within each study.

However, several preclinical studies support a role for hMOS in growth recovery after infection, malnutrition, or gut insult. Mouse models of growth recovery after intestinal resection,[40] after dextran sulfate sodium (DSS)–induced colitis,[42] and in mice recovering from necrotizing enterocolitis (NEC)[39] all showed that 2'-FL was associated with significantly greater growth recovery. These studies are reviewed in greater depth in the following sections.

Reduced Severity of Necrotizing Enterocolitis

Nearly 7% of very low–birth weight preterm infants (infants born <33 weeks gestational age) are affected by NEC.[43] NEC, which is a major gastrointestinal emergency in preterm infants, results in significant mortality. Although the exact cause of NEC is not known, the condition has a sudden onset and represents an immature, hyperinflammatory response to intestinal stimuli, resulting in necrosis and ischemia. Dysbiosis appears to be a major contributing factor, with evidence of a surge in microbes of the family Enterobacteriaceae, although other forms of dysbiosis have also been reported.

Feeding human milk is one of the best-evidenced clinical interventions to reduce the risk and severity of NEC. The epidemiology of NEC and the results of human milk feeding trials have raised the possibility that the oligosaccharide fraction of human milk may explain some of this protective effect.

Several studies using a rat model of NEC have demonstrated that hMOSs prevent morbidity and mortality caused by NEC. These preclinical studies found that the strongest and most consistent protective effect occurs with the disialylated (acidic) oligosaccharide DSLNT but that the neutral hMOS fraction of milk, and 2'-FL specifically, also protects against NEC. In a multisite epidemiologic study of NEC in preterm infants, it was found that human milk lacking DSLNT was significantly predictive of NEC in human milk–fed infants.

Several other preclinical studies suggest the potential for 2'-FL to reduce risk or severity of NEC. He et al tested 2'-FL in T84 and H4 cells and found that exposure to 2'-FL attenuates inflammatory response to uropathogenic *E. coli* (UPEC) and other pathogenic *E. coli*.[38] The relevance of this to the neonatal gut was supported by the finding of Ward et al.[44] that UPEC is a major contributor to NEC in some populations. In a neonatal mouse model of NEC, Good et al.[39] tested 2'-FL and found that it significantly reduced the severity of NEC, helped preserved intestinal mucosal architecture, and modestly enhanced growth in mice with NEC. The mechanism thought to be responsible for these effects were that 2'-FL upregulated the vasodilatory molecule endothelial nitric oxide synthase (eNOS) and thereby restored intestinal perfusion. Administration of 2'-FL to eNOS-deficient mice or to mice that received eNOS inhibitors did not protect against NEC. Although 16S analysis indicated that 2'-FL also shifted the microbiota of the neonatal mouse gut, these changes did not seem to explain the observed reduction in NEC severity. In cultured endothelial cells, 2'-FL treatment induced eNOS, linking eNOS and hMOS in the endothelium. Thus 2'-FL protects against NEC, in part through maintaining mesenteric perfusion via increased eNOS expression. This suggests that 2'-FL found in human milk may mediate some of the protective benefits of breast milk against more severe NEC or recovery from NEC.[39]

However, providing 2'-FL has not shown effectiveness in all preclinical models. Cilieborg et al.[45] tested 5 g/L of 2'-FL in a neonatal preterm pig model of NEC. They found no significant difference in NEC lesion scores between pigs given 2'-FL-fortified formula versus regular formula. Although the 2'-FL–fed pigs tended to have less anaerobic bacteria in cecal contents, no significant difference between groups was found in gut microbiota, as measured by fluorescence in situ hybridization and 454 pyrosequencing.

Taken as a whole, the evidence for hMOS protection against NEC is compelling. Human milk trials indicate protection by human milk feeding against NEC, and preclinical studies and one epidemiologic study have indicated protection by one or more hMOSs. To date, DSLNT appears to be the strongest candidate oligosaccharide for reduction of NEC risk in animal models, with some evidence that 2'-FL could contribute to reducing NEC severity through restoration of intestinal perfusion and potentially other mechanisms. Although additional clinical epidemiology of DSLNT as a predictor of NEC risk should be conducted, the depth of evidence to date is such that testing DSLNT as a protective molecule in clinical trials may be warranted. However, few hMOSs are currently available for clinical testing, as noted at the end of this chapter. Thus additional effort is needed toward the synthesis and commercial manufacturing of a larger repertoire of hMOSs for clinical testing and use.

Intestinal Adaptation

Normal intestinal adaptation occurs between intrauterine life and extrauterine life, and is related to gut glycosylation. hMOS may support intestinal adaptation under circumstances of intestinal failure and reduce the burden of extrauterine growth retardation associated with intestinal failure.

At birth, the gut mucosa of mice is heavily sialylated but becomes heavily fucosylated at weaning, with a decrease in sialylation. Germ-free mice do not develop highly fucosylated mucosa, but fucosylation is rapidly induced by bacterial colonization.[46] Likewise, minimizing the colonization of conventional mice by treatment with a cocktail of antibiotics reduces gut fucosylation while depleting the microbiota restores gut fucosylation, fut2 mRNA, and fucosyl transferase enzyme. TLR4 is essential for transcellular signaling that leads to fucosylation. TLR4 and MyD88 knockout mice are unable to induce fut2 upon colonization. Extracellular signal-regulated kinase (ERK) and Jun kinase (JNK) signal transduction pathways downstream from TLR4 and MyG88 are activated by restitution of bacterial colonization. Drugs that specifically inhibit ERK and JNK activation strongly inhibit colonization-dependent fut2 induction, confirming the direct involvement of these pathways in signaling. The nuclear transcription factors activated by the ERK and JNK pathways, activating transcriptor factor-2 and c-jun, together activate genetic control element AP1 domains, two of which are contained in the control region of the fut2 gene. Goto et al. demonstrated that fucosylation is induced by type 3 innate lymphoid cells via IL-22 signaling in a bacteria-dependent manner.[47] The ability of microbes to induce fucosylation in their host to create a more favorable niche without inducing an inflammatory response is a clear form of mutualism: The bacteria benefit from fucosylation, and the host benefits from the presence of mutualist bacteria.

The benefit of gut glycosylation to the host was tested in a mouse model of DSS-induced colitis. Conventionally colonized mice with highly fucosylated mucosa successfully recovered from mucosal injury, but with minimally fucosylated mucosa as a result of bacterial depletion by antibiotics, recovery was impaired. Replacement of the bacterial community, or just monocolonization with fucose-utilizing *Bacteriodes fragilis*, induced mucosal fucosylation and supported recovery from injury. In contrast, colonization by a mutant *B. fragilis* unable to utilize fucose did not promote recovery. Thus colonization, signaling, and fucosylation central to this type of mutualism are intrinsic to resilience and return to homeostasis by the gut.[46]

The previous data suggest that through the provision of hMOS, feeding human milk could enhance the availability of oligosaccharides to the growing infant gut, and augment the capacity of the gut to adapt and recover from insult. This view is supported by three preclinical studies conducted by different teams studying different forms of enteric insult or injury. In a mouse model of NEC, described previously, Good et al.[39] demonstrated that mouse pups that developed NEC grew better and had less severe disease if concurrently fed 2'-FL. The effect was attributed to upregulation of eNOS and restoration of intestinal perfusion. In a mouse model of DSS-induced colitis, Weiss et al.[42] tested two hMOSs–2'-FL and 3-FL. In mice fed 2'-FL, recovery from DSS challenge was faster compared with controls: mice fed 2'-FL recovered weight more quickly, had lower postchallenge fecal calprotectin levels, and had a more diverse microbial community with increased abundance of *Barnesiella* organisms that can metabolize 2'-FL.[42] In a mouse model of intestinal adaptation following ileocecal resection (ICR), Mezoff et al. tested 2'-FL in half the mice, which were supplemented postoperatively compared with mice given their regular feeds.[40] All ICR mice steadily increased weight gain over the postoperative study period of 56 days. But the 2'-FL-supplemented mice had a significantly greater weight recovery after 21 days, a greater crypt depth at 56 days compared with control ICR mice, increased microbial alpha diversity measured from small bowel luminal content following resection, and a bloom in organisms of the genus *Parabacteroides* (this organism is crypt-dwelling and can metabolize 2'-FL). Transcriptional analysis of the intestine revealed enriched ontologies and pathways related to antimicrobial peptides, metabolism, and energy processing.[40] Thus 2'-FL supplementation assisted recovery and intestinal adaptation after several different forms of gut injury or insult.

Neurodevelopment

The gut microbiota–brain axis has become a major scientific focus because of the recent observations that the gut microbiota influence neurobehavior, including anxiety, depression, and aggressive behavior. Gut microbes may influence neurodevelopment by several different mechanisms: by modifying inflammation or the immune system, via gut metabolites absorbed into circulation, or via the enteric nervous system.

An increasingly compelling body of evidence links human milk feeding to improved neurodevelopment. Much of the effect of human milk on neurodevelopment may be attributable to hMOS. Historically, most studies of hMOS and neurodevelopment have focused on the impact of sialylated hMOS for enrichment of sialic acid in gangliosides, which constitute a critical component of the nervous system. Several recent in vivo studies have tested two dominant forms of sialyllactose, 6'-SL and 3'-SL, for their impact on neurobehavior. Mice fed for 2 weeks were then exposed to a social disruption stressor. Exposure to the stressor significantly changed gut microbial composition and resulted in anxiety-like behavior under controlled conditions. But in mice fed hMOS, the stressor exposure did not significantly change microbial community structure. Further, 3'SL and 6'SL helped maintain normal behavior on tests of anxiety. In another study, the two sialyllactose isomers were studied to determine the impact of ingestion of these hMOS on brain sialic acid content, and on modulation of the microbiome of neonatal piglets, which were randomly allocated to the following diets for 21 days: control, 2 or 4 g 3'-SL/L, 2 or 4 g 6'-SL/L, or 2 g polydextrose and 2 g GOS/L. Dietary sialyllactose did not affect feed intake, growth, or fecal consistency. Ganglioside-bound sialic acid in the corpus callosum of pigs fed 2 g 3'-SL or 6'-SL/L increased by 15% in comparison with control pigs. Similarly, ganglioside-bound SA in the cerebellum of pigs fed 4 g 3'-SL/L increased by 10% in comparison with control pigs. Significant microbiome differences were observed in the proximal and distal colons of piglets fed control formula compared with those fed sialyllactose. Thus supplementation of formula with 3'-SL or 6'-SL can enrich ganglioside sialic acid in the brain and modulate gut-associated microbiota in neonatal pigs.

In addition, recent studies of 2'-FL have indicated that this hMOS may have a distinct role in neurodevelopment. In a rodent model, Vazquez et al.[48] showed that ingested 2'-FL enhances learning, memory, and hippocampal long-term potentiation and impacts a variety of brain molecular markers. A subsequent study using the same model aimed to determine whether oral 2'-FL has an effect on the development of newborn brain and cognitive skills later in life. Rat pups received an oral supplementation of 2'-FL or water during the lactation period. 2'-FL fed rats performed significantly better in learning tasks compared with controls. Long-term potentiation was more intense and longer lasting in the rats supplemented with 2'-FL than in control animals, both in young and adult animals. Oral administration of 2'-FL exclusively during lactation also enhanced cognitive abilities in adulthood.[49] These findings indicate the impact of 2'-FL on brain development. The influence of 2'-FL on neurobehavior could be direct or through indirect mechanisms, such as via gut microbial composition and metabolism.

2'-FL can also affect neuronally dependent gut motor function. Using a standard ex vivo colonic preparation, Bienenstock et al.[50] examined the acute effects of a variety of fucosylated and sialylated hMOSs, and determined that only 2'-FL and a related oligosaccharide, 3-FL, decreased colonic smooth muscle contractions. Specifically, 2'-FL and 3-FL reduced the amplitude, velocity and frequency of migrating motor complexes within 10 to 15 minutes after administration, whereas other hMOS molecules, GOS, and lactose elicited no response. These data suggest that 2'-FL and 3-FL contribute to functional regulation of gut motility, which may be especially important to the healthy gut maturation and function of preterm infants.

Randomized Controlled Trials in Healthy, Term Infants

Human milk contains a higher concentration and a greater structural diversity of oligosaccharides than are found in the milk of many other species.[51] Bovine milk is the source from which most infant formulas are produced. Bovine colostrum contains low levels of acidic oligosaccharides, and bovine milk is particularly lacking in fucosylated oligosaccharide. Thus manufacturers of formula milk have considerable interest in advancing infant feeding through the addition of hMOS to infant formula.

To date, several RCTs have reported on hMOS added to infant formula. The first such trial was a growth and tolerance study conducted in 424 formula-fed healthy, singleton infants born at term in the United States.[4] Infants were enrolled by day 5 of life and followed up for 4 months. All were fed a standard formula containing a total oligosaccharide quantity of 2.4 g/L. The three formula study groups each tested a specific combination of 2'-FL and GOS, respectively: group 1—0 g/L and 2.4 g/L; group 2—0.2 g/L and 2.2 g/L; and group 3—1.0 g/L and 1.4 g/L. The trial also included a human milk–fed reference group. In the formula groups, each study dose combination was well tolerated over the 4-month study period. Study groups did not differ in weight, length, head circumference growth, average stool consistency, number of stools per day, or the occurrence of reflux. In formula-fed infants, similar to breastfed infants, 2'-FL was detected in plasma and urine samples. A substudy was conducted for analysis of blood samples drawn at 6 weeks of age.[5] In the plasma samples analyzed, breastfed infants and infants fed one of the formulas with 2'-FL did not differ from one another, but they had significantly lower concentrations of inflammatory cytokines compared with the control group fed regular formula. In ex vivo respiratory syncytial virus-stimulated peripheral blood mononuclear cell cultures, breastfed infants and infants fed one of the formulas with 2'-FL again did not differ from one another but had lower concentrations of inflammatory cytokines compared with infants fed the control formula.

A separate RCT was conducted in 175 formula-fed European infants to compare the effects of infant formula supplemented with two different hMOSs on infant growth, tolerance, and morbidity.[3] Healthy infants, 0 to 14 days old, were randomized to an intact-protein, cow's milk–based infant formula or the same formula with addition of 1.0 g/L 2'-FL and 0.5g/L LNnT, which were fed for the first 6 months of life. All study infants received standard formula without hMOS from 6 to 12 months of life. Weight gain did not differ between study groups. Digestive symptoms and behavioral patterns were also typically similar between groups, but the intervention groups had softer stool ($P = .021$) and fewer nighttime wake-ups at 2 months. Infants receiving test (versus control) had significantly fewer parental reports of bronchitis, lower rates of respiratory tract infections, and less antibiotic use through 12 months of age (42% versus 60.9%).

These trials of hMOS added to infant formula represent a promising step in narrowing the compositional gap between human milk and infant formula. But it is unclear whether the addition of only one or two hMOSs found in breast milk will recapitulate the complexity of actions exerted by the complex mixture of hMOS ingested by breastfed infants. Thus as more individual hMOS molecules become commercially available, we anticipate that more oligosaccharides will be added to infant formula as mixtures, either hMOS alone or in combination with other prebiotics.

Summary

Although human milk contains many bioactive molecules, the oligosaccharide fraction is the most abundant. Increasing evidence suggests that many of the protective effects of breastfeeding may be attributed, at least in part, to hMOS functions, including prebiotic effects, pathogen inhibition, antiinflammatory effects, immune modulation, and enhanced neurodevelopment. The oligosaccharide fraction is a major component of human milk that differs qualitatively and quantitatively from that of other mammals. The molecular structures of hMOSs are also distinct from other commercially available oligosaccharides; hMOS is more similar in structure to the oligosaccharide moieties found lining the infant gut. However, the composition of hMOS differs among mothers and changes over the course of lactation. Most infant formula presently contains no hMOS, and donor milk from late lactation may typically provide lower levels of oligosaccharide than that found in mother's milk early in lactation. A few studies indicate that compositional variation in mother's milk can modify infant outcomes. More studies are needed of the biologic impact of the compositional variation of hMOS on outcomes in high-risk infants. The few available epidemiologic data suggest that variability in hMOS composition can influence risk of diarrhea[14] and respiratory infection in term infants[3,52,53] and the risk of NEC in preterm infants.[54]

Pure hMOS molecules are now being commercially synthesized and tested as supplements to infant formulas. Although human milk naturally contains many different hMOSs, the initial formulations brought to market with hMOS added are likely to contain 2'-FL and possibly one or two other oligosaccharide structures. The addition of one or two hMOSs to infant formula represents a major advance at this time, and there is evidence of safety and immune benefits from preclinical studies and two clinical trials to date.[3,4] Additional studies on the health effects of hMOS when provided in infant formula are underway to address the long-term goal of bringing the qualities of infant formula as close as possible to that of human milk. Because of its complexity, however, the full range of hMOSs cannot be replicated by commercial formulas, so human milk remains the "gold standard" for infant nutrition, including the oligosaccharide fraction.

REFERENCES

1. Newburg DS, He Y. Neonatal gut microbiota and human milk glycans cooperate to attenuate infection and inflammation. *Clin Obstet Gynecol.* 2015;58(4):814–826.
2. Marcobal A, Southwick AM, Earle KA, Sonnenburg JL. A refined palate: bacterial consumption of host glycans in the gut. *Glycobiology.* 2013;23(9):1038–1046.
3. Puccio G, Alliet P, Cajozzo C, et al. Effects of infant formula with human milk oligosaccharides on growth and morbidity: a randomized multicenter trial. *J Pediatr Gastroenterol Nutr.* 2017;64(4):624–631.
4. Marriage BJ, Buck RH, Goehring KC, Oliver JS, Williams JA. Infants fed a lower calorie formula with 2'-fucosyllactose (2'FL) show growth and 2'FL uptake like breast-fed infants. *J Pediatr Gastroenterol Nutr.* 2015;61(6):649–658.
5. Goehring KC, Marriage BJ, Oliver JS, Wilder JA, Barrett EG, Buck RH. Similar to those who are breastfed, infants fed a formula containing 2'-fucosyllactose have lower inflammatory cytokines in a randomized controlled trial. *J Nutr.* 2016;146(12):2559–2566.
6. Thurl S, Munzert M, Henker J, et al. Variation of human milk oligosaccharides in relation to milk groups and lactational periods. *Br J Nutr.* 2010;104(9):1261–1271.

7. Chaturvedi P, Warren CD, Altaye M, et al. Fucosylated human milk oligosaccharides vary between individuals and over the course of lactation. *Glycobiology*. 2001;11(5):365–372.

8. Gidrewicz DA, Fenton TR. A systematic review and meta-analysis of the nutrient content of preterm and term breast milk. *BMC Pediatr*. 2014;14:216.

9. Coppa GV, Gabrielli O, Pierani P, Catassi C, Carlucci A, Giorgi PL. Changes in carbohydrate composition in human milk over 4 months of lactation. *Pediatrics*. 1993;91(3):637–641.

10. Viverge D, Grimmonprez L, Cassanas G, Bardet L, Solere M. Variations in oligosaccharides and lactose in human milk during the first week of lactation. *J Pediatr Gastroenterol Nutr*. 1990;11(3):361–364.

11. Polonowski M, Lespagnol A. Sur la nature glucidique de la substance lévogyre du lait de femme. *Bull Soc Biol*. 1929;101:61–63.

12. McGuire MK, Meehan CL, McGuire MA, et al. What's normal? Oligosaccharide concentrations and profiles in milk produced by healthy women vary geographically. *Am J Clin Nutr*. 2017;105(5):1086–1100.

13. Alderete TL, Autran C, Brekke BE, et al. Associations between human milk oligosaccharides and infant body composition in the first 6 mo of life. *Am J Clin Nutr*. 2015;102(6):1381–1388.

14. Morrow AL, Ruiz-Palacios GM, Altaye M, et al. Human milk oligosaccharides are associated with protection against diarrhea in breast-fed infants. *J Pediatr*. 2004;145(3):297–303.

15. Newburg DS, Ruiz-Palacios GM, Morrow AL. Human milk glycans protect infants against enteric pathogens. *Annu Rev Nutr*. 2005;25:37–58.

16. Newburg DS, Ruiz-Palacios GM, Altaye M, et al. Innate protection conferred by fucosylated oligosaccharides of human milk against diarrhea in breastfed infants. *Glycobiology*. 2004;14(3):253–263.

17. Chaturvedi P, Warren CD, Buescher CR, Pickering LK, Newburg DS. Survival of human milk oligosaccharides in the intestine of infants. *Adv Exp Med Biol*. 2001;501:315–323.

18. Gyorgy P, Jeanloz RW, von Nicolai H, Zilliken F. Undialyzable growth factors for Lactobacillus bifidus var. pennsylvanicus. Protective effect of sialic acid bound to glycoproteins and oligosaccharides against bacterial degradation. *Eur J Biochem*. 1974;43(1):29–33.

19. Wang J, Chen C, Yu Z, He Y, Yong Q, Newburg DS. Relative fermentation of oligosaccharides from human milk and plants by gut microbes. *Eur Food Res Technol*. 2017;243(1):133–146.

20. Yu ZT, Chen C, Newburg DS. Utilization of major fucosylated and sialylated human milk oligosaccharides by isolated human gut microbes. *Glycobiology*. 2013;23(11):1281–1292.

21. Sela DA, Mills DA. The marriage of nutrigenomics with the microbiome: the case of infant-associated bifidobacteria and milk. *Am J Clin Nutr*. 2014;99(3):S697–S703.

22. Zivkovic AM, German JB, Lebrilla CB, Mills DA. Human milk glycobiome and its impact on the infant gastrointestinal microbiota. *Proc Natl Acad Sci U S A*. 2011;108(suppl 1):4653–4658.

23. Liu B, Yu Z, Chen C, Kling DE, Newburg DS. Human milk mucin 1 and mucin 4 inhibit Salmonella enterica serovar Typhimurium invasion of human intestinal epithelial cells in vitro. *J Nutr*. 2012;142(8):1504–1509.

24. Liu B, Newburg DS. Human milk glycoproteins protect infants against human pathogens. *Breastfeed Med*. 2013;8(4):354–362.

25. Mantis NJ, Rol N, Corthesy B. Secretory IgA's complex roles in immunity and mucosal homeostasis in the gut. *Mucosal Immunol*. 2011;4(6):603–611.

26. Naarding MA, Dirac AM, Ludwig IS, et al. Bile salt-stimulated lipase from human milk binds DC-SIGN and inhibits human immunodeficiency virus type 1 transfer to CD4+ T cells. *Antimicrob Agents Chemother*. 2006;50(10):3367–3374.

27. Bustamante M, Standl M, Bassat Q, et al. A genome-wide association meta-analysis of diarrhoeal disease in young children identifies FUT2 locus and provides plausible biological pathways. *Hum Mol Genet*. 2016;25(18):4127–4142.

28. Currier RL, Payne DC, Staat MA, et al. Innate susceptibility to norovirus infections influenced by FUT2 genotype in a United States pediatric population. *Clin Infect Dis*. 2015;60(11):1631–1638.

29. Ruvoen-Clouet N, Mas E, Marionneau S, Guillon P, Lombardo D, Le Pendu J. Bile-salt-stimulated lipase and mucins from milk of 'secretor' mothers inhibit the binding of Norwalk virus capsids to their carbohydrate ligands. *Biochem J*. 2006;393(Pt 3):627–634.

30. Hansman GS, Shahzad-Ul-Hussan S, McLellan JS, et al. Structural basis for norovirus inhibition and fucose mimicry by citrate. *J Virol*. 2012;86(1):284–292.

31. Nasir W, Frank M, Koppisetty CA, Larson G, Nyholm PG. Lewis histo-blood group alpha1,3/alpha1,4 fucose residues may both mediate binding to GII.4 noroviruses. *Glycobiology*. 2012;22(9):1163–1172.

32. Ruiz-Palacios GM, Cervantes LE, Ramos P, Chavez-Munguia B, Newburg DS. Campylobacter jejuni binds intestinal H(O) antigen (Fuc alpha 1, 2Gal beta 1, 4GlcNAc), and fucosyloligosaccharides of human milk inhibit its binding and infection. *J Biol Chem*. 2003;278(16):14112–14120.

33. Yu ZT, Nanthakumar NN, Newburg DS. The human milk oligosaccharide 2'-fucosyllactose quenches campylobacter jejuni-induced inflammation in human epithelial cells HEp-2 and HT-29 and in mouse intestinal mucosa. *J Nutr*. 2016;146(10):1980–1990.

34. Bode L, Rudloff S, Kunz C, Strobel S, Klein N. Human milk oligosaccharides reduce platelet-neutrophil complex formation leading to a decrease in neutrophil beta 2 integrin expression. *J Leukoc Biol*. 2004;76(4):820–826.

35. Bode L, Kunz C, Muhly-Reinholz M, Mayer K, Seeger W, Rudloff S. Inhibition of monocyte, lymphocyte, and neutrophil adhesion to endothelial cells by human milk oligosaccharides. *Thromb Haemost*. 2004;92(6):1402–1410.

36. He Y, Liu S, Leone S, Newburg DS. Human colostrum oligosaccharides modulate major immunologic pathways of immature human intestine. *Mucosal Immunol*. 2014;7(6):1326–1339.

37. He Y, Liu S, Kling DE, et al. The human milk oligosaccharide 2'-fucosyllactose modulates CD14 expression in human enterocytes, thereby attenuating LPS-induced inflammation. *Gut*. 2014;65(1):33–46.

38. He Y, Lawlor NT, Newburg DS. Human milk components modulate toll-like receptor-mediated inflammation. *Adv Nutr.* 2016;7(1):102–111.
39. Good M, Sodhi CP, Yamaguchi Y, et al. The human milk oligosaccharide 2'-fucosyllactose attenuates the severity of experimental necrotising enterocolitis by enhancing mesenteric perfusion in the neonatal intestine. *Br J Nutr.* 2016;116(7):1175–1187.
40. Mezoff EA, Hawkins JA, Ollberding NJ, Karns R, Morrow AL, Helmrath MA. The human milk oligosaccharide 2'-fucosyllactose augments the adaptive response to extensive intestinal. *Am J Physiol Gastrointest Liver Physiol.* 2016;310(6):G427–G438.
41. Sprenger N, Lee LY, De Castro CA, Steenhout P, Thakkar SK. Longitudinal change of selected human milk oligosaccharides and association to infants' growth, an observatory, single center, longitudinal cohort study. *PloS one.* 2017;12(2):e0171814.
42. Weiss GA, Chassard C, Hennet T. Selective proliferation of intestinal Barnesiella under fucosyllactose supplementation in mice. *Br J Nutr.* 2014;111(9):1602–1610.
43. Neu J, Walker WA. Necrotizing enterocolitis. *N Engl J Med.* 2011;364(3):255–264.
44. Ward DV, Scholz M, Zolfo M, et al. Metagenomic sequencing with strain-level resolution implicates uropathogenic E. coli in necrotizing enterocolitis and mortality in preterm infants. *Cell Rep.* 2016;14(12):2912–2924.
45. Cilieborg MS, Bering SB, Ostergaard MV, et al. Minimal short-term effect of dietary 2'-fucosyllactose on bacterial colonisation, intestinal function and necrotising enterocolitis in preterm pigs. *Br J Nutr.* 2016;116(5):834–841.
46. Meng D, Newburg DS, Young C, et al. Bacterial symbionts induce a FUT2-dependent fucosylated niche on colonic epithelium via ERK and JNK signaling. *Am J Physiol Gastrointest Liver Physiol.* 2007;293(4):G780–G787.
47. Goto Y, Obata T, Kunisawa J, et al. Innate lymphoid cells regulate intestinal epithelial cell glycosylation. *Science (New York, NY.* 2014;345(6202).
48. Vazquez E, Barranco A, Ramirez M, et al. Effects of a human milk oligosaccharide, 2'-fucosyllactose, on hippocampal long-term potentiation and learning capabilities in rodents. *J Nutr Biochem.* 2015;26(5):455–465.
49. Oliveros E, Ramirez M, Vazquez E, et al. Oral supplementation of 2'-fucosyllactose during lactation improves memory and learning in rats. *J Nutr Biochem.* 2016;31:20–27.
50. Bienenstock J, Buck RH, Linke H, Forsythe P, Stanisz AM, Kunze WA. Fucosylated but not sialylated milk oligosaccharides diminish colon motor contractions. *PloS one.* 2013;8(10):e76236.
51. Warren CD, Chaturvedi P, Newburg AR, Oftedal OT, Tilden CD, Newburg DS. Comparison of oligosaccharides in milk specimens from humans and twelve other species. *Adv Exp Med Biol.* 2001;501:325–332.
52. Weichert S, Jennewein S, Hufner E, et al. Bioengineered 2'-fucosyllactose and 3-fucosyllactose inhibit the adhesion of Pseudomonas aeruginosa and enteric pathogens to human intestinal and respiratory cell lines. *Nutr Res.* 2013;33(10):831–838.
53. Stepans MB, Wilhelm SL, Hertzog M, et al. Early consumption of human milk oligosaccharides is inversely related to subsequent risk of respiratory and enteric disease in infants. *Breastfeed Med.* 2006;1(4):207–215.
54. Autran CA, Kellman BP, Kim JH, et al. Human milk oligosaccharide composition predicts risk of necrotising enterocolitis in preterm infants. *Gut.* 2017;67(6):1064–1070.

CHAPTER 5

Donor Milk Trials

Sharon L. Unger, MD, FRCP(C), Julia B. Ewaschuk, PhD, Deborah L. O'Connor, PhD, RD

5

Introduction

Care of the preterm infant has undergone several major transformations over the past 120 years, and an integral part of this has been nutrition. This was outlined in an excellent review by Greer, in which he points out that from the turn of the 20th century, feeding human milk has been recognized as a priority in the care of the preterm infant or "weakling".[1] In a publication from 1922, mother's milk or donor milk was the "gold standard" practice initiated at 140 mL/kg/d and increased to 200 mL/kg/d over the first 3 weeks of life, with gavage feeding provided to infants unable to nurse.[2] If no human milk was available, a buttermilk and skim milk mixture or boiled milk with water and sugar added was recommended.[2] The 1940s and 1950s brought two major changes to the nutritional care of preterm infants. First, withholding of feedings for the first 12 to 72 hours of life became common practice, as it was believed that delaying oral intake would reduce the incidence of aspiration pneumonia and prevent retention of extracellular fluid.[3] Second, investigators began studying the effects of feeding cow's milk formulations to preterm infants. Various diets, including evaporated milk, skimmed or partially skimmed milk, diluted milk, and with various additives, such as dextran-maltose, sugar, and olive oil, were studied.[1] Feeding some of these preparations was demonstrated to result in accelerated growth compared with human milk feeding,[4] leading to a change in clinical practice to a predominance of artificial formula feeding.[5] Artificial formula feeding of preterm infants was widespread in the 1950s and 1960s.

Beginning in the 1970s, a body of research began to challenge the artificial formula feeding practices of the mid-20th century, bringing about a resurgence in the interest in human milk feeding. Indeed, it is now increasingly standard practice to feed very low birth weight (VLBW; <1500 g) infants donor milk when mother's milk is unavailable. The World Health Organization (WHO) recently published a recommendation that low birth weight babies (<2500 g) who cannot be fed mother's milk should be fed donor human milk and advocated for the establishment of safe and affordable milk-banking facilities.[6] In 2012 the American Academy of Pediatrics (AAP) Breastfeeding Policy Statement recommended that preterm infants be given human milk and that donor milk be used if mother's milk is unavailable.[7] A clinical report on donor milk from the AAP in 2016 recommended that priority should be given to providing donor human milk to infants born weighing <1500 g.[8] In a recently reaffirmed Position Statement of the Canadian Paediatric Society, it is similarly recommended that mother's milk be the preferred nutrition for newborn infants and that pasteurized donor milk be the recommended alternative for hospitalized neonates when availability of mother's milk is limited.[9] Even in the settings of the authors' home institutions with high rates of use of mother's milk, for a variety of reasons, about two thirds of mothers are unable to provide a sufficient volume of their own milk; these findings are similar to those in other reports in the literature.[10,11] Although a growing body of evidence indicates that use of mother's milk increases when mothers are offered lactation support, it is clear that a supplement is frequently required.[12,13]

This chapter will describe the history of the use of donor milk and review the randomized clinical trials (RCTs) that have been conducted over the past 40 years informing modern recommendations for the feeding of the preterm infant (Table 5.1).

History of Donor Milk

From the once-common practice of "wet nursing," to the current rapid expansion of not-for-profit and commercial donor milk banks, donated human milk has long been a crucial aspect of feeding sick and vulnerable infants. From as early as 2000 BC until the early 20th century, mothers who were unable to breastfeed their infants employed the services of "wet nurses."[14] There are ancient depictions of wet nursing in many areas of the world, including Egypt, India, China, and Israel, among others. Eventually, advances in technology and hygiene permitted the collection and storage of donated human milk, and facilities to bank and distribute donor milk became feasible. This is detailed by Frances Jones in her paper entitled "History of north american donor milk banking: one hundred years of progress."[15] Briefly, the first documented human milk bank opened in 1909 in Vienna, Austria,[16] followed by milk banks in the United States (1910)[17] and Germany (1919).[18] These early banks were established primarily in response to the diminishing number of available wet nurses. Donor mothers were initially compensated for their contribution of their milk,[19] but concerns regarding the possibility of mothers denying their own babies milk or tampering with milk volumes led to the cessation of this practice which had continued until recently.

Preservation of milk in the absence of refrigeration presented a significant challenge, and many strategies were attempted in those first decades of milk banking, including chemical preservation with peroxides, boiling, autoclaving, and spray drying.[15] All of these methods posed substantial problems, either with maintenance of bacteriologic safety or with extensive destruction of nutritional and bioactive components.[15] In spite of these challenges, milk banking was widespread in the 1930s and 1940s, with more than 12 North American milk banks existing in 1939.[15]

A decline in the use of donor milk occurred in the 1950s and 1960s as artificial formula feeding became more common. Once the shortcomings of artificial formula feeding were recognized, milk banking once again increased in popularity, peaking in the 1980s with 53 operational donor milk banks existing in North America.[20,21] The human immunodeficiency virus/acquired immunodeficiency syndrome (HIV/AIDS) crisis of the mid-1980s and awareness that the virus could be secreted into human milk subsequently resulted in the closure of the majority of these banks and a cessation in donor milk research. A resurgence in milk banking began in the early 2000s with the ability to thoroughly screen donor mothers and the safety of donor milk being further ensured through standardized donor milk processing and pasteurization techniques. In this current era of neonatal care and feeding the preterm infant, there has been an unprecedented growth in donor milk banking.

Table 5.1   RANDOMIZED CONTROLLED TRIALS INVESTIGATING THE IMPACT OF FEEDING DONOR MILK TO PRETERM INFANTS

Author, Year	Country	Participants	Intervention Groups	Outcomes Measured	Results
O'Connor, 2016[10]	Canada	VLBW infants (<1500 g)	Double blind RCT MM, DM, BBF (n = 181) MM, PF, BBF (n = 182) Intervention: 90 days or hospital discharge	Primary: Neurodevelopment (18 month BSID III) Secondary: BSID III language and motor scores, growth, mortality and morbidity index	No difference in cognitive score (BSID III) DM 92.9; PF 94.5 Mean difference −2.0 (95% CI −5.8 to 1.8) No difference in language, motor (BSID III) No difference in growth No difference in morbidity and mortality index Lower incidence of NEC stage ≥II in DM group (1.7%) compared with PF group (6.6%), P = .02
Corpeleijn, 2016[70]	The Netherlands	VLBW infants (<1500 g)	Double blind RCT MM, DM (n = 183) MM, PF (n = 190) Intervention: 10 days	Primary: Serious infection or NEC within first 60 days	No difference in composite outcome (serious infection or NEC to 60 days): DM 42.1%; PF 44.7% Hazard ratio 0.87 (0.63-1.19), P = .37
Hair, 2014[36]	USA	Preterm infants (750-1250 g)	Unmasked RCT MM, DM, HBF (n = 39) MM, DM, HBF, with human-based cream when human milk <67 kcal/dL (n = 39) Intervention: to 36 weeks corrected age	Primary: Growth velocity	Faster weight (14.0 ± 2.5 vs. 12.4 ± 3.9 g/kg/d, P = .03) and length (1.03 ± 0.33 vs. 0.83 ± 0.41 cm/wk, P = .02) growth in cream-fortified group No difference in head growth No difference in rate of sepsis No occurrences of NEC or death
Cristofalo, 2013[35]	USA, Austria	Preterm infants (500-1250 g)	Double blind RCT PF (n = 24) DM, HBF (n = 29) Intervention: 91 days, hospital discharge or attainment of 50% oral feeds	Primary: Duration of parenteral nutrition Secondary: Growth, respiratory support, NEC	Fewer parenteral nutrition days in DM group (27 vs. 36 days, P = .04) Reduced incidence of NEC in DM group (3% vs. 21%, P = .08) No difference in duration of mechanical ventilation or oxygen, ROP or death
Sullivan, 2010[37]	USA, Austria	Preterm infants (500-1250 g)	RCT MM, DM, HBF at 100 mL/kg/d (n = 67) MM, DM, HBF at 40 mL/kg/d (n = 71) MM, PF, BBF (n = 69) Intervention: 91 days, hospital discharge or attainment of 50% oral feeds	Primary: Duration of parenteral nutrition Secondary: Select morbidities and growth	No differences in duration of parenteral nutrition No difference in sepsis, ROP, BPD or growth Significant difference between groups in rate of NEC (1.7% HBF at 100 mL/kg/d, 3.2% HBF 40 mL/kg/d, 15.3% PF; P = .006)

Continued

5

Table 5.1 RANDOMIZED CONTROLLED TRIALS INVESTIGATING THE IMPACT OF FEEDING DONOR MILK TO PRETERM INFANTS—cont'd

Author, Year	Country	Participants	Intervention Groups	Outcomes Measured	Results
Schanler, 2005[11]	USA	Preterm infants (<30 weeks)	Double blind RCT MM, BBF (n = 70) MM, DM, BBF (n = 81) MM, PF, BBF (n = 92) Intervention: 90 days or hospital discharge	Primary: Infection related events (sepsis, NEC, meningitis, UTI) Secondary: Milk intake, growth, duration of hospital stay	No difference in infection related events between DM (77 ± 103 death or infection related event per 100 infants) and PF (85 ± 111) but fewer in MM only (47 ± 70); P = .012 21% of DM group switched to PF for poor weight gain Greater enteral intake but lower weight gain in DM group but no difference in length or head circumference gains Shorter duration of stay for MM group
Morley, 2000[53]	UK	Preterm infants (<1850 g) Patients from Lucas, 1990[47]	Long-term follow-up n = 781	Primary: Late growth (7.5-8 y)	No differences in weight, height, head circumference, skinfold thickness or BMI between groups, at age 7.5-8 y
Lucas, 1994[49]	UK	Preterm infants (<1850 g) Overlap of patients with Lucas, 1990[47]	RCT with blinded outcome assessor DM (sole or supplement) (n = 212) PF (sole or supplement) (n = 210) Intervention: to 2000 g or discharge, transfer to nonparticipating center or death	Primary: Neurodevelopment (18 month BSID)	No differences in neurodevelopmental indices between groups at 18 months DM: MDI 98.6 ± 1.3 PTF: MDI 100.1 ± 1.5 Advantage for PF: 1.5 (95% CI −2.4 to 5.4) DM: PDI 92.2 ± 1.2 PTF: PDI 90.9 ± 1.3 Advantage for PF: −1.3 (95% CI −4.8 to 2.3)
Lucas, 1990[47]	UK	Preterm infants (<1850 g) Overlap of patients with Lucas, 1989[50]	RCT Formula only: PF or TF (n = 236) MM, PF, or TF (n = 437) Human milk only: MM or DM (n = 253)	Primary: NEC	Significant difference in the incidence of NEC: PF or TF: 7.2% MM, PF, or TF: 2.5% MM, DM: 1.2% OR of formula only compared with human milk only 6.5 (95% CI 1.9-22; P < .001)

Continued

5

Lucas, 1989[50]	UK	Preterm infants (<1850 g) Overlap of patients with Lucas, 1984[48]	RCT with blinded outcome assessor DM (sole or supplement) (n = 195) PF (sole or supplement) (n = 174) Intervention: to 2000 g or discharge, transfer to nonparticipating center or death	Primary: Neurodevelopment at 9 months corrected age (Knobloch et al. developmental screening inventory) Secondary: Neurologic examination at 9 and 18 months corrected age	Significantly better overall developmental quotient in PF group: PF: 100.4 ± 10.7 DM: 97.9 ± 9.6 (95% CI 0.4-4.6; $P < .025$) Difference greater for subgroup where supplement was >50% of intake: PF: 101.4 ± 10.5 DM: 96.5 ± 9.9 (95% CI 1.3-8.5; $P \le .01$) No difference between groups for diagnosis of neurologic impairment at 9 or 18 months
Lucas, 1984[48]	UK	Preterm infants (<1850 g)	RCT DM (n = 29) PF (n = 33) MM, DM (n = 67) MM, PF (n = 65) Intervention: to 2000 g or discharge, transfer to nonparticipating center or death	Primary: Days to regain birth weight Weight, length, and head circumference gains while in hospital	More days to regain birth weight for DM fed as sole diet or as supplement Slower weight, length gains for DM fed as sole diet or as supplement Slower head circumference gain for DM as sole diet
Tyson, 1983[41]	USA	VLBW infants (<1500 g)	Unblinded RCT DM (n = 34) PF (n = 42) Intervention commenced at day 10 to exclude babies receiving MM	Primary: Early growth (10-30 postnatal days) Secondary: milk intake, biochemical indices, neonatal responsiveness (Brazelton Neonatal Behavioural Assessment Scale at 37 weeks corrected age), maternal interaction	Slower growth in DM group compared with PF group (weight gain 15 vs. 30 g/d; length gain 0.7 vs. 1.1 cm/wk; head circumference gain 0.8 vs. 1.2 cm/wk) Greater milk intake in DM group No clinically significant differences between groups in biochemical indices (serum chemistry, amino acids) Increased responsiveness in PF infants compared with DM Brazelton orientation scale: PF: 3.4 ± 1.4 vs. DM: 2.6 ± 1.0; $P < .10$ Brazelton inanimate stimuli: PF: 7.5 ± 3.0 vs. DM: 5.0 ± 2.1; $P < .02$ No reported differences in mother–infant interaction

Table 5.1 RANDOMIZED CONTROLLED TRIALS INVESTIGATING THE IMPACT OF FEEDING DONOR MILK TO PRETERM INFANTS—cont'd

Author, Year	Country	Participants	Intervention Groups	Outcomes Measured	Results
Gross, 1983[39]	USA	Preterm infants (<1600 g and 27-33 weeks)	RCT TF (n = 20) Preterm DM (n = 20) Term DM (n = 20) Intervention until weight of 1800 g	Primary: Early growth	Mean time to regain birth weight was significantly longer in the mature DM (18.8 ± 1.7) group compared with preterm DM (11.4 ± 0.8) or TF (10.3 ± 0.8), P < .001 All growth parameters significantly better in TF and preterm DM compared with term DM Weight gain: TF 27.0 ± 0.8, preterm DM 23.7 ± 1.1, term DM 15.8 ± 0.8 g/d, P < 0.001 4 cases of NEC all withdrawn from the study, 3 in TF group and 1 in mature DM group
Svenningsen, 1982[46]	Sweden	Preterm infants (<2000 g)	RCT MM (n = 12) DM (n = 6) PF1 (2.3 g/100 kcal) (n = 14) PF2 (3.0 g/100 kcal) (n = 16) Intervention: weeks 2-15	Primary: Growth until 2 years Secondary: Metabolic responses at 3, 5, and 7 weeks, Neurodevelopment examination at 2 years	No differences between groups in early growth Higher weight gain between 15 and 20 weeks in PF2 No differences in growth at 2 years Higher BUN and metabolic acidosis in PF1, PF2, compared with MM ± DM No differences in neurodevelopment
Schultz, 1980[40]	Hungary	Preterm infants (<2000 g)	RCT DM (n = 10) PF (n = 10) Intervention: 4 weeks	Primary: Metabolic indices at 4 weeks Secondary: Growth	PF group had lower fasting blood glucose compared with DM PF group had significantly higher BUN, higher plasma free amino acids and metabolic acidosis compared with DM group No difference in weight gain
Davies, 1977[38]	Wales	Preterm infants (<36 weeks)	RCT 28-32 weeks DM (n = 14) PF (n = 14) 33-36 weeks: DM (n = 20) PF (n = 20) Intervention: 2 months	Primary: Growth (birth to 1 month, 1 month to 2 months)	Slower linear growth and head growth in group born at 28-32 weeks fed DM compared with PF in the first month of life with similar growth in second month No difference in growth for either period for babies born at 33-36 weeks

| Raiha, 1976[34] | Finland | LBW infants (<2100 g) | RCT
DM (n = 22)
PF1 (60:40 whey/casein ratio, 1.5 g/dL protein) (n = 21)
PF2 (60:40, 3.0 g/dL) (n = 20)
PF3 (18:82, 1.5 g/dL) (n = 22)
PF4 (18:82, 3.0 g/dL) (n = 21)
Intervention: to 2400 g | <u>Primary:</u> Early growth (up to 2400 g)
<u>Secondary:</u> Metabolic responses | No differences among groups in growth parameters with exception of longer time to regain birth weight and longer time to reach 2400 g in those born 34-36 weeks and fed DM
BUN significantly higher in infants fed 3.0 g/dL protein formula compared with DM
Blood ammonia significantly higher in casein predominant and 3.0 g/dL whey predominant formula compared with DM group
Total protein higher in 3.0 g/dL groups compared with DM or 1.5g/dL
Late acidosis (5 weeks) observed with 3.0 g/dL casein predominant formula |

BBF, Bovine-based fortifier; BPD, bronchopulmonary dysplasia; BMI, body mass index; BSID, Bayley Scales of Infant Development; BUN, blood urea nitrogen; CI, confidence interval; DM, donor milk; HBF, human-based fortifier; LBW, low birth weight; MM, mother's milk; MDI, mental development Index; NEC, necrotizing enterocolitis; OR, odds ratio; PDI, psychomotor development index; PF, preterm formula; RCT, randomized controlled trial; ROP, retinopathy of prematurity; TF, term formula; UK, United Kingdom; USA, United States of America; UTI, urinary tract infection; VLBW, very low birth weight.

Current State of Milk Banking

There are two large international groups that are at the forefront of publishing guidelines for human milk banking: the European Milk Bank Association and the Human Milk Banking Association of North America (HMBANA). Member banks are nonprofit and follow their respective organization's established guidelines and protocols to ensure the consistent quality and safety of donor milk. The Program for Appropriate Technology in Health, funded by the Gates Foundation, also provides guidance, with an international perspective, on the core requirements and quality principles for human milk banks.[22] Last, for-profit suppliers of donor milk are now established in the United States and operate as food manufacturers under regulations that vary by state.

Both nonprofit and for-profit banks, according to the applicable guideline and/or regulatory requirements, conduct medical screening and blood testing of potential donors to reduce the risk of disease transmission. Pooling of milk from several mothers is generally recommended to ensure uniformity in nutritional content, and then the milk is pasteurized to remove known pathogens. Donor milk is cultured after pasteurization, and these cultures must show negative results before distribution. Typical donor milk processing is depicted in Fig. 5.1.

Nutrient and Bioactive Composition of Donor Milk

Most donor milk used in the hospital setting globally is pasteurized using the Holder Method (30 minutes at 62.5° C; see Fig. 5.1). Heat treatment, per se, does not substantially compromise the macronutrient composition of donor milk,[23] although transferring milk from container to container does result in loss of lipid content. Pasteurization partially inactivates some of the bioactive components found in human milk (Table 5.2).[24] Obliteration of all cellular activity (T cells, B cells, macrophages, neutrophils) occurs,[25] along with a reduction in antibody (immunoglobulin A reduced by 0%-48%), lactoferrin (reduced by 57%-80%), lysozyme (reduced by 0%-60%), erythropoietin, growth factor, and cytokine concentrations (interferon-γ, tumor necrosis factor-α, interleukin [IL]-1β, IL-10).[26] Despite these heat-induced alterations to the bioactive components of human milk, pasteurized milk maintains a degree of bacteriostatic[27] and immune-stimulating[28] properties.

Human milk, whether mother's own milk or donor milk, does not contain adequate protein to meet the elevated needs of the very preterm infant.[29] To address this deficiency, fortifiers are added to donor milk, either by using ready-made multinutrient fortifiers, or by adding modular components of each macronutrient. Three fortification strategies are currently being used in neonatal intensive care units (NICUs) in North America.[30]

- Standard fortification is a fixed-dose approach that assumes the uniform macronutrient composition of all donor milk.
- Adjustable fortification uses the infant's blood urea nitrogen (BUN) as an indicator of protein requirement; fortifier strength is adjusted to maintain BUN within a target range.
- Target fortification involves the regular assessment of macronutrient composition of milk samples and adjustment to target levels.

Most HMBANA milk banks do not provide a nutritional analysis for their donor milk and normal concentrations must be assumed from the literature. Typical estimates for protein are 0.9 g/dL[31] compared with 1.2 g/dL for mature mother's milk. Further, most NICUs utilize the standard fortification approach and target protein intakes based on these references ranges for human milk.

There are numerous fortification products on the market, currently available in liquid or powder form. The majority are concentrated bovine products, although a human milk-based fortifier now exists. Carbohydrates, fat, electrolytes, calcium, phosphate, vitamins, and minerals, in addition to protein, are usually present in fortifier formulations.

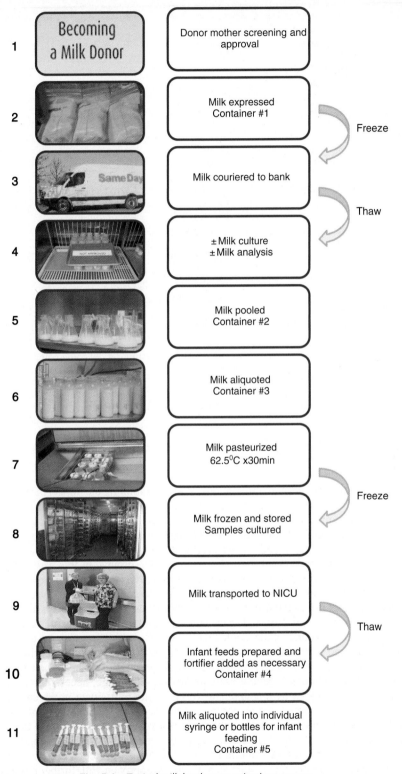

Fig. 5.1 Typical milk bank pasteurization process.

Table 5.2 EFFECTS OF PASTEURIZATION ON HUMAN MILK MACRO- AND MICRONUTRIENTS

Component	Maintained (>90%)	Maintained (50%–90%)	Maintained (10%–50%)	Abolished (<10%)
Macronutrients	Carbohydrate (lactose, oligosaccharides)	Protein Total fat		
Micronutrients	Calcium Copper Magnesium Phosphorus Potassium Sodium Zinc	Iron		
Vitamins	Vitamin A	Folate Vitamin B$_6$ Vitamin C		
Biologically active (immune)	IL-8, IL-12p70, IL-13 TGF-α	IgA, sIgA IgG IGF-1, IGF-2, IGF-BP2,3 IFN-γ IL-1β, IL-4, IL-5, IL-10 TGF-β Gangliosides	CD14 (soluble) IL-2 Lactoferrin-iron-binding capacity Lysozyme	IgM Lymphocytes
Biologically active (metabolism)	Epidermal growth factor Heparin binding growth factor	Adiponectin Amylase Insulin	Erythropoietin Hepatocyte growth factor	Bile salt–dependent lipase Lipoprotein lipase

Bioactive components are impacted to varying degrees by Holder pasteurization; some components remain intact, whereas cellular components are completely abolished.
Ig, Immunoglobulins; *IGF*, insulin-like growth factor; *IFN-γ*, Interferon-γ; *IL*, interleukin; *TGF*, transforming growth factor.
Copyright cleared by Wolters Kluwer Health, Inc. License Number 4035491086494.

Strengths and Challenges of Conducting and Comparing Donor Milk Trials

The potential for bias in open-label and observational studies examining the impact of supplemental donor milk versus infant formula is well known. Views on which is the superior form of nutrition may influence, for example, how long clinicians wait until mother's milk is available before feeding a supplement and/ or advancement of enteral feeds. A blinded RCT with random allocation of infants between supplement groups should address these biases and ensure even distribution of known and unknown confounding variables (e.g., birth weight, early acuity, etc.) between the two groups. In this way, differences in outcomes can reasonably be ascribed to the intervention. Feeding RCTs in neonates are subject to a host of unique challenges. Foremost are ethical considerations for randomizing infants to various feeding protocols. If NICUs are already using donor milk as a supplement, the health care team may not feel there is sufficient clinical equipoise to ethically randomize infants. Given the recent data, this could be an issue for future research in this area. Second, clinical outcomes of interest, such as necrotizing enterocolitis (NEC), have a low prevalence and recruiting a sufficient sample size to yield meaningful interpretation may be difficult and time consuming, particularly for the VLBW baby (1.4% of births in the United States[32]).

The blinding of supplemental feeding assignments is a challenge, necessitating preparation in a designated milk preparation area by a technician who does not participate in the care of the neonate. Feeds must be placed in individual opaque syringes because those caring for the neonate can discern differences in color, smell, and appearance between various feed types. A strategy needs to be developed to ensure provision of vitamin and mineral drops that meets the needs of infants in both arms of the study as a differential approach may unblind the study. Not unexpectedly, these trials are very costly to run, especially so if the sample size requires a multicenter approach with further costs accruing if the outcome of interest requires long-term follow-up.

Quigley and McGuire [33] published a Cochrane review in 2014 on the use of donor milk for feeding preterm infants. Examination of the studies included emphasizes the challenges of comparing the results of different RCTs now available.[33] This meta-analysis includes nine trials, of which seven were conducted before 1985, reflecting a different era in the care and feeding of preterm infants. Only the two most recent trials used nutrient fortified donor milk. The authors highlighted weaknesses in the included studies, particularly the lack of blinding in many and the lack of long-term follow-up in most studies.[33] Differences in subject inclusion criteria alone can heavily impact outcomes as the possible benefit, or risk, of using a supplement will likely be affected by the vulnerability of the sample studied. For example, some studies have included infants with a birth weight as high as 2100 g,[34] where recent trials have more intensively studied higher-risk infants in the 500 to 1250 g range.[35-37] The timeline for inclusion of infants in the study may substantially influence findings, with some studies enrolling infants immediately after birth and other protocols including infants only after a predetermined feeding tolerance has been achieved. This results in a "healthier" and more homogeneous study population through the exclusion of very ill infants.

Feeding protocols differed substantially among the trials included in the Cochrane meta-analysis. Early study protocols usually included a group that received strictly cow's milk formula, with no mother's milk provided.[34,38-41] Once it became clear that mother's milk exerted beneficial effects, it became unethical to randomize infants to receive no mother's milk. In light of this, many recent studies employ a pragmatic approach that includes mother's milk, whenever available, in all feeding groups.[10,11,36,37] Others selected infants of mothers who did not intend to breast-feed,[35] which may reflect a different demographic of infants. Donor milk fortification strategies varied significantly among trials.

Finally, no data on using donor milk in term infants are available; all studies, to date, have investigated health outcomes of feeding donor milk to preterm infants.

Outcomes of Randomized Controlled Clinical Trials of Donor Milk

Since the late 1970s, several trials have been conducted investigating the clinical impact of various strategies for feeding preterm infants human donor milk, initially with a focus on growth and metabolic outcomes; later trials investigated infection-related outcomes, NEC, and neurodevelopment. Trials in this review were identified by searching the Medline database by using the search terms "donor milk" or "pasteurized donor milk." RCTs that compared feeding of donor milk (with or without fortification) to preterm infants with other feeding strategies (formula, mother's milk, or a combination of these) are reviewed in this section and in Table 5.1. Trials that did not randomize subjects are discussed in section 5, Nonrandomized Studies of Donor Milk.

Growth

Early Growth

Although a subject of debate, the goal of providing nutrition for preterm infants is to facilitate growth that mimics intrauterine fetal growth rates and body composition changes.[42,43] There are multiple health concerns related to intrauterine and postnatal growth restriction, including both short- and long-term neurodevelopmental delays.[44,45] Early studies that prompted the widespread feeding of cow's milk-based formulas to preterm infants did so by demonstrating improved growth parameters for various formulas over human milk.[4,5] One of the first trials that began to challenge the growth advantages of formula over donor milk was conducted by Raiha et al. between 1972 and 1975.[34] This randomized controlled study investigated not only the quantity but the quality of protein provided. This study of 106 low birth weight babies (<2100 g) randomized infants to one of five feeding regimens: (1) 1.5 g/dL protein with a whey/casein ratio of 60:40; (2) 3 g/dL protein with whey/casein ratio of 60:40; (3) 1.5 g/dL protein with whey/casein ratio of 18:82; and (4) 3 g/dL protein with whey/casein ratio of 18:82, with all these four formulas containing the same quantities of minerals and vitamins; and (5) pooled donor human milk, supplemented with vitamins A, D, and C, and iron. No infants were fed mother's milk. Subjects were also divided into three groups based on gestation: (1) 28 to 30 weeks; (2) 31 to 33 weeks; and (3) 34 to 36 weeks. This strategy yielded a final number of six to eight subjects per group. Feeding was initiated within the first 24 hours (typically 6-9 hours), and increased to 150 mL/kg/d within the first week of life. Protein intakes were 2.25 g/d for the 1.5 g/dL protein formula groups, 4.5 g/d for the 3 g/dL protein formula groups, and 1.63 g/d for the human milk group. No differences were observed among groups for initial weight loss, but in the group of infants born at 34 to 36-weeks' gestation, all formula-fed infants regained birth weight more rapidly compared with donor milk-fed infants. Once birth weight was achieved, there were no differences among groups in attaining a body weight of 2400 g. No differences were observed in any groups in linear growth (measured by crown–rump length), head circumference, skinfold thickness, or hematocrit. BUN was significantly higher in infants fed the 3 g/dL protein formula, compared with those fed donor milk. Blood ammonia was higher in all formula groups compared with the donor milk group, except for the 1.5 g/dL whey-predominant formula. Feeding the casein-predominant 3 g/dL protein formula resulted in a late (5 weeks) acidosis. Overall no growth advantage was observed over the range and type of bovine protein fed to preterm infants, compared with donor milk. The authors identified the importance of the quality of the protein in infant formulas for preventing the development of metabolic acidosis arising from feeding large amounts of casein. An alternative explanation is that the sample size (n = 6-8 infants/group) was insufficient to detect a difference in growth. In planning a five-group study, 26 infants per group would be required to detect a 1 standard deviation (SD) difference in growth with 80% power an alpha-level of 0.05.

This study was quickly followed by a growth study of Welsh preterm infants (28-32 weeks, n = 28; 33-36 weeks, n = 40).[38] Subjects were randomized to be fed either mature pooled, pasteurized donor milk (protein 1.1 g/dL), as assessed in a prior study, or a cow's milk-based formula (protein 2.7 g/dL). Feeding was initiated at 50 mL/kg/d and increased by 15 mL/kg/d daily until a daily oral intake of 200 mL/kg/d was achieved. All infants received vitamin and iron supplementation. In infants born at 28 to 32 weeks' gestation, there were no significant differences in the rate of weight gain over the first 2 months of life; however, linear growth and head circumference were higher in the formula-fed group from birth to 1 month, but not from 1 to 2 months. No differences in any growth parameter were observed between the two feeding groups in the infants born at 33 to 36 weeks' gestation. The authors concluded that the slower growth of the head and length of the donor milk-fed infants in the lower gestational age group may have been related to term milk providing inadequate nutrition for early preterm infants.[38] The sample size may again have been insufficient to detect growth differences.

Further evidence of preterm infant growth in response to human milk compared with formula came from an American study by Gross in 1983.[39] In this study, preterm infants (<1600 g; 27-33 weeks) were randomized to be fed early milk from mothers of preterm infants (n = 20), term donor milk (n = 20), or a whey-based formula (n = 20). All donor milk was pasteurized according to the Holder technique. For the group randomized to preterm donor milk, the milk was collected from mothers who gave birth before 35 weeks of gestation, and the postpartum week of gestation for the study infant corresponded to the postpartum week during which the milk was collected. The composition of the milks differed, and preterm milk changed over the 12 weeks of the study. Protein content of term milk was 1 g/dL; formula was 1.93 g/dL; and the protein content of preterm milk decreased from 2.26 g/dL in week 1 to 1.14 g/dL in week 12. Mineral content was higher in the formula compared with donor milk. Feedings began at a mean of day 3 of life and were initiated at 24 mL/kg/d. By day 8, all subjects were receiving 180 mL/kg/d. The number of days to regain birth weight was different between groups and was highest in infants receiving term milk (18.8 ± 1.7 days), compared with preterm milk (11.4 ± 0.8 days) and formula (10.3 ± 0.8 days) ($P < .001$). Rate of weight gain, linear growth, and head circumference were also higher in preterm milk-fed and formula-fed infants, compared with infants fed term milk. The author concluded that term milk alone is not a satisfactory source of nutrition for preterm infants.

In the same year, Tyson et al.[41] published the results of a second American study of VLBW (<1500 g) infants who were randomized to receive either pooled, raw unfortified donor milk (n = 34) or an enriched formula designed for preterm infants (n = 42), on postnatal days 10 to 30. Infants whose mother had an adequate supply of milk after day 10 were excluded from the study. Donor milk and formula were reported to have very different macronutrient profiles, with much higher concentrations of protein, fat, and carbohydrate in the formula (2.22, 4.02, 8.84 g/dL, respectively) compared with donor milk (1.09, 2.21, 7.72 g/dL, respectively). Mineral content was also higher in the formula. Infants were fed by bottle as much as their appetite would allow or by intermittent gavage if their suck was inadequate. Daily milk intake was higher in the donor milk group (197 mL/kg/d) compared with the formula group (165 mL/kg/d). The infants fed donor milk grew more slowly between days 10 and 30, in weight, length, and head circumference. The authors concluded that donor milk must be analyzed to be certain that it contains adequate concentrations of macronutrients for the preterm infant.

In another early 1980s study of growth and development, Swedish preterm infants were randomized to receive either a high-protein formula (3 g/100 kcal; n = 16), a lower-protein formula (2.3 g/100 kcal; n = 14) or human milk (donor, n = 6; mother's milk, n = 12). Svenningsen reported no statistically significant difference in growth parameters between the groups.[46] Differences may not have been detected as a result of the small sample size.

Lucas et al. conducted in the United Kingdom a series of elegant parallel, multicentered RCTs of varying feeding regimens for low birth weight (LBW) infants (<1850 g) in the 1980s.[47–50] The first trial was published in 1984, with early growth data from 194 preterm infants born at a mean of 31 weeks' gestation and a mean birth weight of 1364 g. Groups included exclusive feeding of a newly designed preterm formula (n = 33), exclusive donor milk (n = 29), mother's milk + preterm formula (n = 65), and mother's milk + donor milk (n = 67). The preterm formula contained 80 kcal/dL and 2 g/dL protein, and donor milk contained 46 kcal/dL and 1 g/dL protein. The median days to regain birth weight was greater in the exclusive donor milk group (16 days) compared with the preterm formula group (10 days). Linear growth, head circumference, and rate of weight gain was higher in the preterm formula group compared with the donor milk group. In the groups where mother's milk was supplemented, supplementation with preterm formula resulted in faster weight gain and linear growth rate compared with those in infants supplemented with donor milk.

By this point, in the mid-1980s, it had become abundantly clear that the growth of preterm infants was impeded by a diet of unfortified human milk—whether mother's milk or, most especially, pooled, pasteurized, term donor milk. The focus of much research at this point was on the commercial development of cow's milk formulas that provided improved growth.[34,41,48] This occurred concomitantly with the closure of the majority of milk banks throughout industrialized countries in the 1980s when it became apparent that HIV could be transmitted via human milk.[15] Research in human donor milk ceased for nearly 2 decades, and preterm infants who required supplementation to mother's milk were routinely fed preterm formulas.

As the study of the bioactive components of human milk evolved in the 1990s, and as evidence emerged regarding the benefits of human milk, including improved neurodevelopment and a reduction in the incidence of infection- and inflammation-related outcomes in preterm infants, such as NEC and sepsis,[51] a focus on human milk emerged in trials of infant feeding. Investigators sought to determine how infant growth could be optimized with the use of human milk, rather than by developing more nutrient-dense bovine-based formulas.[52] A more pragmatic approach to feeding evolved, with mother's milk provided whenever possible but fortified with a multinutrient bovine based fortifier. The first of these more recent trials using donor milk and multinutrient fortifiers, published by Schanler in 2005, represented the beginning of a shift in thinking in the clinical care of preterm and low-birth weight babies.[11] This study enrolled mothers who intended to breastfeed their preterm infants and randomly assigned the infants to receive either donor milk or preterm formula as a supplement, if the mother's milk supply was insufficient. The study compared three groups: (1) infants receiving exclusively their mother's milk (n = 70); (2) those receiving mother's milk + donor milk (n = 81); and (3) those receiving mother's milk + preterm formula (n = 92). Both mother's milk and donor milk were fortified with a bovine-based milk fortifier. The study duration was 90 days or until discharge from hospital, whichever was earlier. Early growth results in this study demonstrated that preterm infants fed fortified donor milk gained weight at a slower rate than those fed preterm formula; there was, however, no difference between groups in length or head circumference gains. Secondary to poor weight gain, 21% of the infants in the donor milk group crossed over to the preterm formula group. There were no crossovers from the preterm formula group. Weight gain over the study duration was highest in preterm formula-fed infants and lowest in donor milk-fed infants.

Sullivan et al.[37] hypothesized that health benefits (reduced duration of parenteral nutrition, sepsis, and NEC) might be observed if infants were fed an exclusively human milk-based diet, with fortification of mother's milk with a human milk-based fortifier, instead of the bovine milk-based fortifiers that had been investigated to date. To evaluate a human milk-based fortifier, infants (500-1250 g) whose mothers intended to breastfeed were recruited from 12 centers and randomized to receive human milk-based fortifier when their enteral intake was 40 mL/kg/d (n = 71), 100 mL/kg/d (n = 67), or bovine milk-based fortifier when enteral intake was 100 mL/kg/d (n = 69). The first two groups received donor milk if a supplement to mother's milk was required, whereas the final group received a preterm formula if a supplement was required. Feeding was initiated 1 to 4 days after birth, and once feeding at 10 to 20 mL/kg/d was tolerated for up to 5 days, milk volumes were increased by 10 to 20 mL/kg/d. No difference between groups in weight gain, length, or head circumference growth was observed. Because the majority of milk provided in this trial was mother's milk, Cristofalo et al. conducted a subsequent multicenter trial of similar design but with infants whose mother did not intend to provide their own milk.[35] The infants were randomized to be fed either a bovine milk-based preterm formula or pasteurized donor milk fortified with a human milk-based fortifier. Weight gain was not different over the study period between the two groups, but infants fed preterm formula had increased head and length growth compared with human milk-fed infants.

Recently, a human milk-derived cream has come on the market. Hair et al.[36] investigated the impact on the growth of feeding this supplement to preterm infants (750-1250 g; n = 78). Infants received mother's milk, supplemented with donor milk if required, and a human milk-based fortifier. Infants in the cream group also received human milk cream if the caloric content of the milk received was <67 kcal/dL based on a daily batched assessment. Weight and length gain was higher in the group receiving the cream supplement, and there were no differences in head circumference gains. The study did not include a preterm formula control group.

Finally, a large pragmatic, multicenter, double-blind, randomized trial of VLBW infants (<1500 g) was recently conducted in Canada.[10] This trial was entitled DoMINO (Donor Milk for Improved Neurodevelopmental Outcomes). Infants with a birth weight of <1500 g were enrolled in the first 96 hours of life. They were randomized to receive a supplement to mother's milk, as required, as either pasteurized donor milk with a bovine milk-based fortifier and modular protein supplement of 0.4 g/dL protein/dL (n = 181) or preterm formula (n = 182) for 90 days or until hospital discharge. No differences were observed between the groups in any anthropometric measures at the end of the feeding intervention even after controlling for the volume of mother's milk fed.

The 2014 Cochrane review of quasi-controlled trials and RCTs by Quigley and McGuire included studies of now-obsolete methods of feeding preterm infants, such as unfortified donor milk and term formula.[33] This systematic review and meta-analysis concluded that feeding donor milk resulted in slower gain in weight, head circumference, and length compared with formula feeding. The slower growth associated with the use of donor milk compared with formula in some early studies appears to have been attenuated or even ameliorated in recent clinical trials that employed various strategies for fortifying donor milk.

Late Growth

The large, multicenter randomized parallel trials led by Lucas and initiated in the early 1980s ultimately saw the enrollment of 926 preterm infants. In a series of reports, this group has subsequently examined the growth and health outcomes of these infants at 7.5 to 8 years of age and beyond. This larger cohort of now school-age children had been fed one of 4 feeding regimens during initial hospitalization when they were infants: (1) donor milk; (2) preterm formula; (3) mother's milk + donor milk; and (4) mother's milk + preterm formula.[53] Lucas et al. presented data from several time points: 9 months, 18 months, and 7.5 to 8 years.[47–50] Although significant differences in growth were observed in the neonatal period (as described previously), no significant differences in any measured parameters (weight, length, head circumference, skinfold thicknesses, body mass index) were identified at any of the follow-up points.

In the previously described Swedish trial by Svenningsen et al.,[48] infants were randomized to receive one of two formulas or human milk, and no differences were found in growth in the neonatal period; those authors also followed up their patients at ages 8 and 24 months.[46] There were similarly no differences in weight, length, or head circumference in any of the three feeding groups at the later time points, although the sample size was likely insufficient to detect differences that may have been present.

To date, no other studies of donor milk feeding in preterm infants have measured long-term effects on growth.

Metabolic Responses

Early studies of donor milk measured a variety of metabolic indices, including BUN, serum ammonia, serum albumin, blood glucose, and metabolic acidosis. In an early study by Raiha et al., infants with birth weights <2100 g (but few infants <1250 g) were randomized to either unfortified donor milk (0.96 g/dL protein) or one of four different formula preparations as previously described (1.5 versus 3.0 g/dL protein, whey/casein ratio of 60:40 or 18:82).[34] The feeding intervention lasted until the infants reached 2400 g. As expected, BUN values reflected the protein content of enteral feeds with infants in the unfortified donor milk group with the lowest values (mean values ≈3.6 nmol/L). Although the Raiha et al. study[34] found little evidence that the protein content of enteral feeds alone impacted growth, Arslanoglu et al. reported more recently that individually adjusting the protein content of enteral feeds to achieve a BUN concentration in the range of 3.6 to 7 mmol/L (versus <3.6 nmol/L) is best associated with optimal growth.[54] Raiha et al.[34] further found that BUN levels resulting from feeding the 1.5 g/dL protein whey-predominant (60:40) formula most closely mimicked the BUN of donor milk fed infants. Casein-predominant formulas (18:82; 1.5 and 3 g/dL) and the 3 g/dL whey-predominant formula (60:40; 3 g/dL) resulted in higher blood ammonia levels compared with donor milk feeding. Blood ammonia concentrations, urine osmolarity, and total serum protein were highest in the 3 g/dL protein formula groups and lowest in the donor milk group. Infants fed a high-casein 3 g/dL formula developed late acidosis for as long as 5 weeks, and feeding whey-predominant formulas resulted in nearly normal acid–base balance. In all measured metabolic parameters, feeding a whey-predominant, 1.5 g/dL protein formula most closely resembled donor milk feeding. In North America, standard preterm formulas for in-hospital use are whey predominant and contain 2.0 g/dL (67 kcal/dL) and 2.4 g/dL (80 kcal/dL) protein.

In 1980 Schultz et al. randomized 20 preterm infants to be fed either unfortified pooled donor milk (1.2 g/dL protein) or formula (2.6 g/dL protein).[40] Like the Raiha et al. study,[34] the BUN values among preterm infants fed formula were greater than those of infants fed unfortified donor milk. Infants in the formula group were also more likely to develop late acidosis in postnatal weeks 2 and 3. Plasma free amino acid concentrations were generally higher in formula-fed infants compared with donor milk-fed infants, particularly phenylalanine and lysine. This remained true throughout the 4-week study period.

To try to support growth at intrauterine rates but address the metabolic disturbances resulting from high-protein formula feeding, Tyson et al. fed a 2.2 g/dL protein (60:40 whey/casein ratio)–mineral–calorie–enriched formula and compared metabolic responses to unfortified donor milk feeding (1.1 g/dL protein) in 76 preterm infants (<1500 g).[41] No differences between the groups in serum albumin, protein, BUN, blood pH, or osmolarity were observed on postnatal days 20 and 30, although BUN did decrease from day 20 to day 30 in both groups. Few differences in plasma amino acids were noted (lower threonine on days 20 and 30, lower proline on day 20, and lower arginine and methionine on day 30 in the donor milk group). The authors attributed similarity in the metabolic response in the two groups to the use of whey-predominant formula and a more modest protein/calorie ratio compared with previous studies. In that same year, Gross reported similar findings after a feeding trial of unfortified term donor milk, unfortified early preterm donor milk, and a whey-predominant 1.9 g/dL protein infant formula (n = 20 per group).[39] No differences in BUN, blood pH, bicarbonate, serum calcium, serum total protein, or albumin were observed among the groups.

Necrotizing Enterocolitis and Late-Onset Sepsis

In the 1970s and 1980s, the predominant research focus for preterm infant nutrition was the development of an infant formula that would achieve better intrauterine growth rates while minimizing metabolic disturbances.[1] Feeding preterm formula became common practice in many North American NICUs. It was in these early studies that other ramifications of feeding preterm formula began to emerge, particularly in the rates of NEC and late-onset sepsis (LOS).

NEC affects preterm infants disproportionately, with the incidence highest in the earliest gestations (varying from 1.3%-12.9% in infants with <33 weeks' gestation within the Canadian Neonatal Network) and a peak occurrence at weeks 31 to 33 corrected gestational age.[55] NEC is marked by intestinal inflammation with or without infection and may lead to intestinal necrosis and perforation. It carries a mortality rate of 25% to 50% and is the leading cause for short bowel and multiorgan transplantation in childhood.[56] Staging of NEC is defined by the Bell criteria,[57] which have been modified as the understanding of NEC has evolved over the years.[58] Emerging research suggests that very preterm infants who develop NEC have an altered microbiome (dysbiosis) compared with very preterm infants who remain healthy.[59-63] The emergence of non–culture-based techniques for elucidating the intestinal microbiota have led to a clearer picture of the pathogenic events that precede NEC.[64] The mode of feeding preterm infants impacts the development of the microbiome along with other factors, such as mode of delivery and antibiotic exposure.[65-67]

By the 1980s, observational data became available, and these suggested that human milk may be protective against NEC.[68,69] No trial of feeding donor milk to preterm infants had yet investigated outcomes beyond growth. Tyson et al.[41] did mention in their discussion that two infants in the formula-fed group developed signs of NEC; they did not elaborate on the significance of this finding but suggested that future studies that "enroll sick infants shortly after birth" would be able to elaborate on the relationship between formula feeding and NEC.

Lucas et al.'s parallel multicenter clinical trials of the 1980s were the first to investigate the incidence of a number of sequelae to various feeding strategies for preterm infants beyond growth and biochemical indices.[47–50] Ultimately the trials included 926 infants, and clinical features of NEC developed in 51 subjects and was confirmed in 31 subjects. The differences observed among the groups were striking, with confirmed cases of NEC in 7.2% of formula-only group, 2.5% of formula + mother's milk group, and only 1.2% of the human milk only group (donor milk and mother's milk). Donor milk as a sole diet appeared to be as protective as mother's milk, but the sample size was limited for these analyses. Other risk factors identified for NEC included gestational age, respiratory disease, umbilical artery catheterization, and polycythemia, but significant differences in the incidence of NEC were observed between diet groups even after controlling for these variables.

Since 2005, there have been five published RCTs that examined the impact of either donor milk compared with preterm formula or an exclusive human diet on the incidence of NEC.[10,11,35,37,70] In the study by Schanler et al. (n = 243), the rate of NEC alone was not different between groups (6% in mother's milk + donor milk, 11% in mother's milk + preterm formula, 6% in mother's milk alone; P = .27 comparing donor milk group and preterm formula group).[11] When comparing the sum of death or any infection-related events, fewer events cases per 100 infants) occurred in the preterm infants fed exclusively mother's milk, but there was no difference between the donor milk supplemented group and the preterm formula supplemented group (77 ± 103 events in mother's milk plus donor milk, 85 ± 111 in mother's milk plus preterm formula, 47 ± 70 in mother's milk alone; P = .012 comparing mother's milk alone group and combined other groups).[11] In this trial, mother's milk and donor milk were enriched with nutrients with intact bovine-based fortifiers. The authors concluded that in a setting of high use of mother's milk, there was little advantage of donor milk over preterm formula when a supplement was required.

It was proposed that that the use of bovine milk-based fortifiers in donor milk may have impacted the findings in the Schanler et al. study[11] and that an exclusively human milk-based diet that includes not only mother's milk and donor milk as a supplement but also a fortifier derived from human milk may be of benefit. This hypothesis was tested in an RCT reported by Sullivan et al. in 2010.[37] As described previously, infants with a birth weight of 500 to 1250 g and whose mothers intended to breastfeed were randomized to one of three groups: (1) HM100 (infants fed mother's milk supplemented with donor milk and fortified with a human milk-based fortifier commencing at enteral tolerance of 100 mL/kg/d; n = 67); (2) HM40 (infants fed mother's milk supplemented with donor milk and fortified with a human milk-based fortifier commencing at enteral tolerance of 40 mL/kg/d; n = 71); and (3) BOV (infants fed mother's milk fortified with a bovine based fortifier at enteral tolerance of 100 mL/kg/d and supplemented with preterm formula as required; n = 69). When the rate of NEC was analyzed for only infants completing the study without any protocol violation, there were significant reductions in the human milk fortifier groups with rates of NEC of HM100 1.7%, HM40 3.2%, and BOV 15.3% (P = .006). What was unclear in the outcome of this trial is whether it was the lack of preterm formula, the lack of bovine fortifier, or both that led to the reduction in NEC in the exclusive human milk diet groups.[37]

The impact of an exclusive human milk diet was further studied in a trial of infants whose mother did not intend to breastfeed.[35] As described earlier, infants were randomized to receive either preterm formula (n = 24), or donor milk (n = 29) with a human-milk–derived fortifier. The incidence of NEC in infants fed preterm formula was significantly higher (21%) than in the group receiving donor milk (3%) (P = .04). In this study, the rate of NEC in the preterm formula group was much higher than the typical rates reported elsewhere and calls into question the difficulty of confirming cases of NEC in a blinded fashion. The previously described Hair et al. trial on human milk cream as a supplement had both study arms receiving an exclusively human milk-based diet (n = 78; birth weight 750-1250 g). There were no cases of NEC in either group.[36]

Two new trials comparing donor milk as a supplement with mother's milk were published in 2016, and these were the first trials to describe masking of the study feeds in amber-colored syringes.[10,70] In the trial by Corpeleijn et al.[70] from the Netherlands, 373 VLBW (<1500 g) infants were randomized to two supplement groups (183 to donor milk and 190 to preterm formula as a supplement) if mother's milk was not sufficiently available for the first 10 days after birth. There was a high mean intake of mother's milk during the intervention period (89.1% in the donor milk group and 84.5% in the preterm formula group). There was no difference in the combined incidence of NEC stage II or greater and/or serious infection to 60 days between groups (44.7% in the preterm formula group versus 42.1% in the donor milk group; mean difference 2.6%; 95% confidence interval [CI], −12.7% to 7.4%; adjusted hazard ratio [HR] 0.87; 95% CI 0.63-1.19; P = .37). The authors acknowledge that a longer duration of intervention should be studied.

5

The second donor milk trial published in 2016 was the Greater Toronto Area Donor Milk for Improved Neurodevelopmental Outcome (GTA DoMINO), a multicenter RCT by O'Connor et al.[10] Confirmed cases of NEC were adjudicated by a panel blinded to feeding assignments using the modified Bell criteria; stage 1 was defined as presence of consistent symptomatology, as defined by Bell, along with treatment for a minimum of 7 days (suspension of enteral feeds and antibiotics). Stage II or greater was defined by the presence of pneumatosis; portal venous air or bowel perforation on any of the radiographs or ultrasound scans or at the time of surgery; or bowel ischemia on histology. Preterm infants who received donor milk with bovine fortifier exhibited a lower rate of any stage NEC (7 of 181; 3.9%) compared with those receiving preterm formula (20 of 182; 11%) resulting in a risk difference of −7.1 (95% CI −12.5 to −1.8; $P = .01$). The rate of stage II or higher NEC was similarly lower in the donor milk group (3 of 181; 1.7%) compared with those receiving preterm formula (12 of 182; 6.6%), a risk difference of −4.9 (95% CI −9.0 to −0.9; $P = .02$).

Overwhelming evidence favors provision of human milk over provision of preterm formula for prevention of NEC. Numerous mechanisms have been proposed to explain why bovine milk causes higher rates of NEC, including increased intestinal permeability,[71] dysbiosis,[67] and direct cytotoxicity to the intestinal epithelial cells.[72]

Neurodevelopment

The trial by Svenningsen et al.[46] in 1982 with six donor milk-fed infants was the first to report long-term neurodevelopment in donor milk-fed infants. There was no difference noted at 2 years, although the specifics of the testing were not provided in the report and the number of infants studied was too small to detect meaningful clinical differences. Tyson et al.[41] in 1983 studied 76 VLBW infants fed either unfortified donor milk or preterm formula and measured neonatal behavior at 37 weeks corrected age according to the Brazelton Neonatal Behavioral Assessment Scale, a measure of 27 behavior-related indices, and 20 elicited responses.[73] The average score for the Brazelton orientation scales, which measure alertness and responsiveness to auditory and visual stimuli, was not different between the two groups (preterm formula 3.4 ± 1.4 versus donor milk 2.6 ± 1.0; $P < .10$). The groups did differ in their responses to inanimate objects, with a higher score observed in the formula group compared with the donor milk group (preterm formula 7.5 ± 3.0 versus donor milk 5.0 ± 2.1; $P < .02$).

One of the primary outcomes of the large multicenter feeding intervention trials of preterm infants conducted by Lucas et al. in the 1980s was neurodevelopment at 9 and 18 months.[49,50] At 9 and 18 months corrected age, 502 infants underwent follow-up examinations, including a developmental screening inventory by Knobloch et al.[74] This assessment tool tests five fields of behavior, for which the investigators adjusted the quotient for preterm birth: adaptive, gross motor, fine motor, language, and personal–social. Infants were also neurologically assessed and categorized as normal, equivocal, or impaired, according to the methods of Ameil-Tison and Grenier.[75]

At 9 months, there were no differences observed in neurologic status among the four feeding groups (donor milk alone [6% impaired] or as a supplement to mother's milk [5% impaired], preterm formula alone [14% impaired], or as a supplement to mother's milk [9% impaired]). There were no differences in overall development between the groups fed donor milk as the sole diet versus the group fed preterm formula as the sole diet. When groups were combined, however, to include infants fed donor milk as the sole diet and those fed donor milk as a supplement (n = 195), there were significant differences between the group fed preterm formula as a sole diet and that fed preterm formula as a supplement (n = 174) (donor milk developmental quotient mean 97.9 [SD 9.6] versus preterm formula 100.4 [SD 10.7], difference 95% CI 0.4-4.6; $P < .025$). This difference became more significant when subgroups were analyzed on the basis of infants receiving more than half of intake as a supplement or being small for gestational age (<10th percentile for birth weight). Among babies who received >50% of their intake as a supplement, there were 68 in the donor milk group and 56 in the preterm formula group (donor milk developmental quotient mean

96.5 [SD 9.9] versus preterm formula 101.4 [SD 10.5]; difference 95% CI 1.3-8.5; P < .01). Among babies who were born small for gestational age, there were 62 in the donor milk group and 68 in the preterm formula group (donor milk developmental quotient mean 94.3 [SD 8.7] versus preterm formula 99.6 [SD 10.7]; difference 95% CI 2.0-8.6; P < .01). Although the predictive validity of neurodevelopment results at 9 months corrected age is uncertain, these statistically significant differences do raise concerns about the impact of feeding unfortified donor milk on the neurodevelopment of preterm infants.

In their parallel trials that compared preterm formula to unfortified donor milk at 18 months, Lucas et al. followed up 422 infants by using the Bayley Scales of Infant Development (BSID).[49] The BSID is commonly used and is a validated tool to assess neurodevelopment in infancy and early childhood (from 1 to 42 months); version 1 yielded a composite score on the mental development index (MDI) and on the psychomotor development index (PDI).[76] No differences were observed in the MDI or the PDI at 18 months for infants fed preterm formula compared with those fed donor milk as the sole diet or as a supplement (95% follow-up rate in the donor milk group [n = 212] and 97% in the preterm formula group [n = 210]). For the donor milk group, the mean MDI ± standard error was 98.6 ± 1.3 and for the preterm formula group 100.1 ± 1.5, with a non-statistically significant mean difference of 1.5 (95% CI 2.4-5.4). For the donor milk group, the mean PDI ± standard error was 92.2 ± 1.2 and for the preterm formula group 90.9 ± 1.3, with a non-statistically mean difference of 1.25 (95% CI −4.8 to 2.3). A subgroup analysis of infants small for gestational age similarly showed no difference in the MDI or the PDI at 18 months corrected age. The authors had expected to see improved developmental outcomes for infants fed preterm formula compared with those fed donor milk on the basis of a higher nutrient content of the preterm formula. They speculated that the lack of difference between groups may be related to other biologic advantages of human milk and recommended that future research focus on the fortification of donor milk to further improve outcomes.

The long-term neurodevelopmental outcome after the use of fortified donor milk was the goal of the GTA DoMINO trial.[10] O'Connor et al. assessed neurodevelopment in preterm infants who had been randomized to receive either fortified donor milk or preterm formula as a supplement to mother's milk, whenever required.[10] The authors used the third edition of the Bayley Scales of Infant and Toddler Development (BSID III) to assess infants at 18 months of age.[77] This tool is designed to assess the cognitive, language, and motor development of infants up to 42 months of age. All of the assessors were blinded as to the intervention group and recertified to ensure >80% agreement on BSID III measures. Of the 363 infants randomized to receive either donor milk (n = 181) or preterm formula (n = 182), 37 died during initial hospitalization, and 299 were assessed at 18 months corrected age (92% follow-up rate of survivors). The mean (SD) birth weight was 995 (273) g in the donor milk group and 996 (272) g in the preterm formula group. Neurodevelopmental outcomes were analyzed by using logistic regression and then adjusted according to two different models. In the first model, the analyses were adjusted according to randomization strata, including the recruitment center and the birth weight group. In the second model, the analyses were adjusted according to the maternal education level and the percentage of total enteral feeds consumed by the infant as mother's milk during the intervention period. No significant difference was observed in mean (95% CI) cognitive composite scores with a score of 92.9 (range 89.8-95.9) in the donor milk group and 94.5 (range 91.4-97.5) in the preterm formula group. In the statistical model that adjusted for recruitment center and birth weight, the mean effect size was −1.6 (95% CI −5.5 to 2.2; P = .41). In the fully adjusted statistical model that included the maternal education level and the percentage of total enteral feeds as mother's milk, an effect size of −2.0 was observed (95% CI −5.8 to 1.8; P = .31). Children with a cognitive composite score of <85 were classified as having a neuroimpairment and those with <70 as having a disability. There were significantly more children with a neuroimpairment in the donor milk-fed group (27.2% versus 16.2%) with an adjusted risk difference of 10.6 (95% CI 1.5-19.6; P = .02). There was no difference between the two groups in those children classified as having a disability. No differences in the language composite (adjusted scores 87.3 in the donor milk group versus 90.3 in the formula group; fully adjusted mean difference -3.1 [95% CI −7.5 to 1.3]) or the motor composite (adjusted scores 91.8 in the donor milk group versus 94.0 in the formula group; fully adjusted mean difference −3.7 [95% CI −7.4 to 0.09]) were identified.

In summary, neither Lucas et al. nor O'Connor et al., the only two groups to describe neurodevelopmental outcomes in infants at 18 months corrected age, demonstrated a long-term benefit when donor milk is fed to VLBW infants, particularly in a setting that supports high use of mother's milk. This should therefore not be seen as a treatment goal in prescribing donor milk.

Retinopathy of Prematurity

Retinopathy of prematurity (ROP) remains a common morbidity in VLBW infants, with rates varying from 25% to 91% internationally, and about 25% of these infants require treatment with either laser or intravitreal antivascular endothelial growth factor.[78] A recent meta-analysis of observational studies reported a possible role for human milk in the prevention of ROP.[79] Results from RCTs comparing donor milk to formula do not support a benefit with donor milk in this outcome. O'Connor et al.,[10] Sullivan et al.,[37] and Cristofalo et al.[35] all did not see a difference in the occurrence of ROP between infants receiving donor milk as supplement versus those receiving preterm formula as supplement. Schanler et al. observed that stage 3 ROP occurred less frequently in infants fed mother's milk compared with those fed donor milk or preterm formula.[11] There were no differences between the groups with regard to requirement for surgery for the treatment of ROP.

Mortality

To date, none of the trials reporting mortality as an outcome has shown a difference between donor milk and formula; interpretation of these comparisons must, however, be done with caution because of the low event rate and sample size of available trials. Gross was the first to report on deaths in their trial in 1983, and they noted three deaths resulting from NEC, of which two occurred in infants who had been in the formula group and 1 in an infant in the mature donor milk group.[39] In the Lucas et al. study,[50] mortality was not a preplanned outcome measure, but these authors were the first to analyze the differences between groups. Of 502 infants randomized, those fed donor milk alone and those fed preterm formula alone had mortality rates of 8.4% and 11.8%, respectively. Infants fed donor milk and those fed preterm formula in addition to mother's milk had mortality rates of 7.1% and 8.7%, respectively. Neither difference was statistically significant.

Schanler et al.'s 2005 trial revealed no differences in mortality among feeding intervention groups receiving mother's milk (3%), donor milk (4%), or preterm formula (3%).[11] Mortality rates from Sullivan et al.'s trial comparing donor milk fortified at two different periods with preterm formula were not statistically analyzed for differences among groups, but the mortality rate was reported as 3 of 138 in the exclusive human milk-fed group and 5 of 69 in the bovine milk-fed group.[37] In the subsequent trial by Cristofalo et al., which only included infants whose mothers did not intend to breastfeed, differences in mortality were not significantly different (2 of 24 in the preterm formula-fed group and 0 of 29 in the human milk-fed group).[35]

In the Dutch trial by Corpelejin et al., comparing infants fed donor milk or preterm formula as a supplement to mother's milk (babies only fed mother's milk excluded) for the first 10 days, there was no difference between groups in mortality rate.[70] Mortality in the donor milk group was 13.7%, with a median day of death of 11.0 (interquartile range [IQR] 5.5-26.0) and for the preterm formula group 12.1%, with a median day of death of 9.0 (IQR 5.0-18.0). The adjusted HR was 1.15 (95% CI 0.64-2.05; $P = .63$).

Similarly, in the Canadian trial by O'Connor et al., which compared infants fed donor milk with those fed preterm formula as a supplement to mother's milk for 90 days or to hospital discharge found no significant difference among groups in mortality.[10] The mortality rate in the donor milk group was 17 of 181 (9.4%) and in the preterm formula group was 20 of 182 (11%), a risk difference of −1.0% (95% CI −9.7 to 7.6; $P = .82$). Further, there was no difference between groups in the mortality/morbidity index. The index was a dichotomous variable and was positive either for mortality or any one of a predetermined list of morbidities that included confirmed LOS (positive blood or cerebrospinal fluid culture), NEC (Bell stage ≥ II), chronic lung disease (oxygen support at 36 weeks) or retinopathy of prematurity (International stage 4/5, laser of intraocular antivascular injection). This index was positive for 43.1% of infants in the donor milk group and 40.1% in the preterm formula group, with a risk difference of 5% (95% CI −2.7 to 12.7; $P = .2$).

Nonrandomized Studies of Donor Milk

To date, four studies have been reported in the literature where donor milk and formula was provided to infants in a nonrandomized fashion. The results of these studies were not included in the primary review of clinical trials reported above; they do, however, provide further insight, and thus a brief discussion of each of these studies is provided here.

A controlled, prospective study conducted in New Delhi, India, by Narayanan et al. was also reported in 1982.[80] This is one of the few trials investigating the use of donor milk in a developing country, where milk banking had not been established at that time.[80] Low birth weight infants (birth weight 1000-2500 g) who were deemed prone to infection (n = 261) were enrolled in the study. Initially, allocation to one of four feeding groups was done randomly by block design; an analysis after one year, however, demonstrated that infants fed formula were developing significantly more infections (overall infection rate 48%). Thereafter ethics precluded further allocation of infants to this group, provided that human milk was available, and nonrandomized allocation was performed for the remainder of the study. The four feeding groups were (1) raw milk feeding during the day and pasteurized milk during the night; (2) raw milk during the day and formula at night; (3) colostrum three times per day with formula; and (4) formula alone. Human milk was a combination of mother's milk, if available, and donor milk. The rates of infection (diarrhea, pneumonia, septicemia, meningitis, conjunctivitis, pyoderma, thrush, and upper respiratory infection) were strikingly higher in the formula-alone group compared with all other groups. The group receiving human milk alone (n = 45) had only four cases of conjunctivitis and one of pyoderma and did not have any serious infections (overall infection rate 11%). The two groups that received a combination of human milk and formula milk both had higher rates of serious infections (overall infection rates: raw milk and formula 17%, colostrum and formula 21%).

Jarvenpaa et al., from the same Finnish hospital that published the first RCT of donor milk for preterm infants, reported in 1983 on a nonrandomized trial investigating the potential for improved metabolic outcomes resulting from feeding an infant formula fortified with taurine and cholesterol.[34,81] The group hypothesized that growth could be improved by increasing serum cholesterol; because the fat content of infant formula was derived from vegetable oils, the cholesterol content was substantially lower than that of mother's milk. Taurine, known to be involved in bile salt conjugation and therefore also relevant to cholesterol metabolism, was also low in formula milk at that time. Three isocaloric formulas were developed, each with 1.5 g/dL protein (60:40 whey/casein ratio), a control, one fortified with taurine, and one fortified with taurine and cholesterol. A control group of infants whose mothers wished to breastfeed was included; when mother's milk was insufficient, the infants in this group were fed donor milk. This group was therefore a self-selected and nonrandomized group. These infants were fed about 35% pasteurized mother's milk, 10% at the breast, and 65% donor milk. Forty-eight infants (nine in the group receiving mother's milk with donor milk) were followed up until 4 months of age. No differences in infection-related illnesses were noted among the groups, but episodes of conjunctivitis, thrush, constipation, colic, and eczema occurred only in the formula-fed groups. No consistent differences in growth measures were observed among the groups from birth weight to 2400 g. Infants fed formula tended to gain weight more quickly after a weight of 2400 g was achieved, whereas human milk-fed infants tended to gain weight more rapidly before achieving a weight of 2400 g. The authors concluded that neither taurine nor cholesterol content in formula was a limiting factor for growth.

Putet et al. reported, in 1984, on their study measuring growth and energy balance (by indirect calorimetry) of VLBW male infants fed either pooled pasteurized donor milk or preterm formula (2 g/dL protein).[82] The study included 12 infants, and the method of allocation to each group was not described in the paper and is therefore presumed to be nonrandom. As in all other studies of that time, weight and length gains were significantly higher in formula-fed infants compared with donor milk-fed infants; the weight gain, however, was already significantly higher in the preterm formula group at the time of study day 1, when the infants had reached a point of full oral tolerance. Energy balance studies demonstrated higher energy intake in the preterm formula group, with higher percentage of energy absorbed also in the formula group at 33 weeks' gestation (94% for formula and 84% for donor milk; $P < .001$) but similar energy absorbed at 36 weeks' gestation (95% both groups). Energy retention was about 50% in both groups, resulting in a fat accretion greater than the intrauterine rates. Nonprotein energy stored at 36 weeks' gestation was 48.0 ± 1.8 kcal/kg/d in the preterm formula group and 42.3 ± 8.7 in the donor milk group, and the difference was not significantly different. Protein accretion was similar to intrauterine rates for the preterm formula group and lower for the donor milk group (at 36 weeks' gestation 2.1 ± 0.2 versus 1.5 ± 0.2 g/kg/day; $P < .01$).

The South African group of Cooper et al. conducted a nonrandomized study, which was reported in 1984, where infants born before 36 weeks' gestation weighing between 1200 and 1500 g received either a bovine milk-based preterm formula containing 2.4 g/dL protein (60:40 whey/casein ratio; n = 19) or unfortified donor milk (n = 20).[83] At the time of the study, feeding donor milk exclusively was a standard practice. Rather than allocating infants randomly to feeding groups, infants were alternately assigned to the feeding groups. The authors reported that there was an outbreak of NEC in the hospital during the study period. In the formula group, two infants developed NEC, and thus at the request of physicians caring for the infants enrolled in the trial, allocation to the formula group was halted until the outbreak ceased, but infants were still enrolled into the donor milk group during that period. Formula feeding ultimately resumed in infants who would not normally be fed donor milk, and additional infants were also recruited from another hospital. Although this study was not an RCT, the results closely mirrored those of the previously described trials with more rapid weight gain (27.7 ± 4.6 g/d versus 17.2 ± 3.5 g/d; $P < .001$), head circumference growth (0.98 ± 0.23 cm/wk versus 0.81 ± 0.16 cm/wk; $P < .01$), and increased skinfold thicknesses from enrollment until a weight of 1800 g was reached (1.51 ± 1.00 mm versus -0.25 ± 1.13 mm; $P < .001$) in infants fed preterm formula compared with those fed donor milk.

Ongoing Trials

Numerous ongoing clinical trials are registered on national and international databases, including the U.S. National Institutes of Health (ClinicalTrials.gov)[84] and the WHO's International Clinical Trials Registry Platform[85] related to the study of donor milk. Many of these studies have been completed recently or will be completed by 2020. A great deal more information on the optimal feeding of preterm infants is thus anticipated to be reported in the scientific literature.

With a planned enrollment of 670 extremely preterm infants (<29 weeks gestational age) and a slated completion date of June 2019, The Milk Trial is an RCT that aims to determine the effect of donor milk compared with preterm formula on neurodevelopmental outcomes at age 22 to 26 months, as measured by the BSIDIII.[86] Secondary outcomes include growth, mortality, LOS, NEC, duration of parenteral nutrition, length of hospital stay, and bronchopulmonary dysplasia. This trial is funded by the Eunice Kennedy Shriver National Institute of Child Health and Human Development Neonatal Research Network.

The PREterM FOrmula Or Donor breast milk (PREMFOOD) for premature babies, commenced as a pilot study (n = 66) in the United Kingdom, recently completed its final data collection.[87] The trial included preterm infants born between 25 and 32 weeks' gestation. The pilot study had three study arms: mother's milk was fed when possible, and the shortfall in milk was made up by fortified donor milk, unfortified donor milk, or preterm formula. The study was designed to inform the practicality and feasibility of an intended very large (n = 4000) trial aimed at conclusively defining the optimal feeding strategy for preterm infants, with planned outcome measures of NEC, LOS, metabolic outcomes (e.g., obesity, type 2 diabetes), and neurodevelopment. This study has several unique aspects, including the evaluation of body composition using whole body magnetic resonance imaging, urine metabolomics, and blood microRNA profile.

A randomized, parallel group trial in India investigating the impact of fortification of donor milk on the rate of NEC in preterm infants in the first 28 days began enrollment in February 2016 (target n = 230).[88] All of the study subjects receive mother's milk, whenever available, and are randomized to receive either fortified, pooled, pasteurized donor milk or unfortified donor milk with nutritional supplements of vitamin D, calcium, iron, and vitamin E for 28 days or discharge, whichever is earlier. The primary outcome of the study is the development of NEC in the first 28 days of life. Secondary outcomes include severity of NEC, incidence of sepsis, mortality, duration of stay, number of days to full enteral feeds, and weight gain.

Besides the studies described here, there are multiple new research studies focusing on human donor milk. Of interest is the impact of donor milk on the developing microbiome as well as the immune-stimulating effects of donor milk. A group in Argentina commenced a clinical trial in 2012, of VLBW infants (<1500 g) to investigate the impact of donor milk as a supplement to mother's milk on the number of respiratory episodes occurring in preterm infants during the first year of life.[89] There are also open-label trials on the use of donor milk in children with Norovirus infection[90] and children under age 5 years undergoing bone marrow transplantation.[91] Additionally, an active area of research is the impact of processing on donor milk and potential new and innovative techniques. One group in Vienna, Austria, is exploring the impact of utilizing single-donor milk,[92] and another group from Baylor, Texas, is exploring the use of target fortification[93] with donor milk. Other novel uses where donor milk has been postulated to be of potential benefit are in feeding of infants of mothers with diabetes or infants with neonatal abstinence syndrome.[94]

Conclusions

The number of VLBW infants continues to increase, but their survival rate is improving. To ensure the best long-term health, development, and growth of these infants, meticulous care in the neonatal period is vital, and an understanding of optimal nutrition is key to this. There is ample evidence proving the health-protective effects of mother's milk in these fragile infants. Despite every effort, preterm infants continue to require a supplement to their mother's milk for a variety of reasons. Unfortunately, in North America, the majority of human milk banks closed in the mid-1980s, and research in this area also ceased. With the safety of donor milk ensured, milk banks are now opening at an unprecedented rate. Trials performed to date have indicated that donor milk is safe. In particular, more recent data suggest that multinutrient fortification of donor milk has helped address the slower rates of growth observed in babies fed donor milk compared with those fed preterm formula in early studies. There is consistent evidence that feeding donor milk to VLBW infants leads to a significant reduction in NEC. There is therefore scientific justification to feed donor milk to VLBW infants as a supplement to mother's milk during the risk period for NEC. To date, long-term outcomes after donor milk feeding have only been studied to 18 months corrected age, and no significant differences have been seen. Further research in longer-term outcomes will be important.

Acknowledgment

The authors wish to acknowledge the funding received from the Canadian Institutes of Health Research (MOP-102638 and FDN-143233) that supports their research in relation to the use of donor milk for VLBW infants.

REFERENCES

1. Greer FR. Feeding the premature infant in the 20th century. *J Nutr*. 2001;131(2):426S–430S.
2. Hess JH. Nutritional requirements and methods of feeding low birth weight infants. *Premature and Congenitally Diseased Infants*. Philadelphia, PA: Lea & Febiger; 1922:107–204.
3. Hansen JD, Smith CA. Effects of withholding fluid in the immediate postnatal period. *Pediatrics*. 1953;12(2):99–113.
4. Gordon HH, Levine SZ, Mc NH. Feeding of premature infants; a comparison of human and cow's milk. *Am J Dis Child*. 1947;73(4):442–452.
5. Lundeen E, Kunstadter RH. Body composition of premature infants: relation to nutrition. *Care of the Premature Infant*. Philadelphia, PA: J. B. Lippincott; 1958.
6. World Health Organization. *Donor Human Milk for Low-Birth-Weight Infants*. Geneva: Switzerland; 2016.
7. Eidelman AI. Breastfeeding and the use of human milk: an analysis of the American Academy of Pediatrics 2012 Breastfeeding Policy Statement. *Breastfeed Med*. 2012;7(5):323–324.
8. Committee on Nutrition, Section on Breastfeeding, Committee on Fetus and Newborn. Donor human milk for the high-risk infant: preparation, safety, and usage options in the United States. *Pediatrics*. 2017;139(1).
9. Kim J, Unger S. Human milk banking. *Paediatr Child Health*. 2016;15(9):595–602.
10. O'Connor DL, Gibbins S, Kiss A, et al. Effect of supplemental donor human milk compared with preterm formula on neurodevelopment of very low-birth-weight infants at 18 months: a randomized clinical trial. *JAMA*. 2016;316(18):1897–1905.
11. Schanler RJ, Lau C, Hurst NM, Smith EO. Randomized trial of donor human milk versus preterm formula as substitutes for mothers' own milk in the feeding of extremely premature infants. *Pediatrics*. 2005;116(2):400–406.
12. Husebye ES, Kleven IA, Kroken LK, Torsvik IK, Haaland OA, Markestad T. Targeted program for provision of mother's own milk to very low birth weight infants. *Pediatrics*. 2014;134(2):e489–e495.
13. Spatz DL, Froh EB, Schwarz J, et al. Pump early, pump often: a continuous quality improvement project. *J Perinat Educ*. 2015;24(3):160–170.
14. Fildes VA. *Wet Nursing: A History From Antiquity to The Present*. Oxford: Basil Blackwell; 1988.
15. Jones F, Human milk banking association of North America. History of North American donor milk banking: one hundred years of progress. *J Hum Lact*. 2003;19(3):313–318.
16. Barret C, Hiscox I. The collection and preservation of breast milk. *Canadian Nurse*. 1939;1:15–18.
17. Talbot F. An organization for supplying human milk. *N Engl J Med*. 1928;199:610–611.
18. Springer S. Human milk banking in Germany. *J Hum Lact*. 1997;13(1):65–68.
19. Hoobler R. Problems connected with the collection and production of human milk. *JAMA*. 1917;55:421–425.
20. Bednarek F. Supply side statistics of a human milk bank. In: Goldberg A, ed. *Human Milk Banking: Its Problems and Practices. AAP Symposium on Milk Banking*. New York, NY: AAP; 1982.
21. Sauve R, McIntosh D, Clyne A, Buchan K. *The Calgary Mothers Milk Bank*. Calgary, Alberta: Foothills Hospital; 1982.
22. PATH. *Strengthening Human Milk Banking: A Global Implementation Framework. Version 1.1*. Seattle, Washington, USA: Bill & Melinda Gates Foundation Grand Challenges initiative; 2013.
23. Braga LP, Palhares DB. Effect of evaporation and pasteurization in the biochemical and immunological composition of human milk. *J Pediatr (Rio J)*. 2007;83(1):59–63.
24. Ewaschuk JB, Unger S, Harvey S, O'Connor DL, Field CJ. Effect of pasteurization on immune components of milk: implications for feeding preterm infants. *Appl Physiol Nutr Metab*. 2011;36(2): 175–182.
25. Liebhaber M, Lewiston NJ, Asquith MT, Olds-Arroyo L, Sunshine P. Alterations of lymphocytes and of antibody content of human milk after processing. *J Pediatr*. 1977;91(6):897–900.
26. Ewaschuk JB, Unger S, O'Connor DL, et al. Effect of pasteurization on selected immune components of donated human breast milk. *J Perinatol*. 2011;31(9):593–598.
27. Silvestre D, Ruiz P, Martinez-Costa C, Plaza A, Lopez MC. Effect of pasteurization on the bactericidal capacity of human milk. *J Hum Lact*. 2008;24(4):371–376.
28. Groer M, Duffy A, Morse S, et al. Cytokines, chemokines, and growth factors in banked human donor milk for preterm infants. *J Hum Lact*. 2014;30(3):317–323.
29. Dutta S, Singh B, Chessell L, et al. Guidelines for feeding very low birth weight infants. *Nutrients*. 2015;7(1):423–442.
30. Rochow N, Landau-Crangle E, Fusch C. Challenges in breast milk fortification for preterm infants. *Curr Opin Clin Nutr Metab Care*. 2015;18(3):276–284.
31. Cooper AR, Barnett D, Gentles E, Cairns L, Simpson JH. Macronutrient content of donor human breast milk. *Arch Dis Child Fetal Neonatal Ed*. 2013;98(6):F539–F541.
32. Hamilton BE, Martin JA, Osterman MJ, Curtin SC, Matthews TJ. Births: final data for 2014. *Natl Vital Stat Rep*. 2015;64(12):1–64.
33. Quigley M, McGuire W. Formula versus donor breast milk for feeding preterm or low birth weight infants. *Cochrane Database Syst Rev*. 2014;(4):CD002971.

34. Raiha NC, Heinonen K, Rassin DK, Gaull GE. Milk protein quantity and quality in low-birthweight infants: I. Metabolic responses and effects on growth. *Pediatrics*. 1976;57(5):659–684.

35. Cristofalo EA, Schanler RJ, Blanco CL, et al. Randomized trial of exclusive human milk versus preterm formula diets in extremely premature infants. *J Pediatr*. 2013;163(6):1592–1595. e1591.

36. Hair AB, Blanco CL, Moreira AG, et al. Randomized trial of human milk cream as a supplement to standard fortification of an exclusive human milk-based diet in infants 750-1250 g birth weight. *J Pediatr*. 2014;165(5):915–920.

37. Sullivan S, Schanler RJ, Kim JH, et al. An exclusively human milk-based diet is associated with a lower rate of necrotizing enterocolitis than a diet of human milk and bovine milk-based products. *J Pediatr*. 2010;156(4):562–567. e561.

38. Davies DP. Adequacy of expressed breast milk for early growth of preterm infants. *Arch Dis Child*. 1977;52(4):296–301.

39. Gross SJ. Growth and biochemical response of preterm infants fed human milk or modified infant formula. *N Engl J Med*. 1983;308(5):237–241.

40. Schultz K, Soltesz G, Mestyan J. The metabolic consequences of human milk and formula feeding in premature infants. *Acta Paediatr Scand*. 1980;69(5):647–652.

41. Tyson JE, Lasky RE, Mize CE, et al. Growth, metabolic response, and development in very-low-birth-weight infants fed banked human milk or enriched formula. I. Neonatal findings. *J Pediatr*. 1983;103(1):95–104.

42. Hay WW, Thureen P. Protein for preterm infants: how much is needed? How much is enough? How much is too much? *Pediatr Neonatol*. 2010;51(4):198–207.

43. Ziegler EE. Meeting the nutritional needs of the low-birth-weight infant. *Ann Nutr Metab*. 2011; 58(suppl 1):8–18.

44. Franz AR, Pohlandt F, Bode H, et al. Intrauterine, early neonatal, and postdischarge growth and neurodevelopmental outcome at 5.4 years in extremely preterm infants after intensive neonatal nutritional support. *Pediatrics*. 2009;123(1):e101–e109.

45. Stephens BE, Walden RV, Gargus RA, et al. First-week protein and energy intakes are associated with 18-month developmental outcomes in extremely low birth weight infants. *Pediatrics*. 2009;123(5):1337–1343.

46. Svenningsen NW, Lindroth M, Lindquist B. Growth in relation to protein intake of low birth weight infants. *Early Hum Dev*. 1982;6(1):47–58.

47. Lucas A, Cole TJ. Breast milk and neonatal necrotising enterocolitis. *Lancet*. 1990;336(8730): 1519–1523.

48. Lucas A, Gore SM, Cole TJ, et al. Multicentre trial on feeding low birthweight infants: effects of diet on early growth. *Arch Dis Child*. 1984;59(8):722–730.

49. Lucas A, Morley R, Cole TJ, Gore SM. A randomised multicentre study of human milk versus formula and later development in preterm infants. *Arch Dis Child Fetal Neonatal Ed*. 1994;70(2):F141–F146.

50. Lucas A, Morley R, Cole TJ, et al. Early diet in preterm babies and developmental status in infancy. *Arch Dis Child*. 1989;64(11):1570–1578.

51. Schanler RJ, Shulman RJ, Lau C. Feeding strategies for premature infants: beneficial outcomes of feeding fortified human milk versus preterm formula. *Pediatrics*. 1999;103(6 Pt 1):1150–1157.

52. Reis BB, Hall RT, Schanler RJ, et al. Enhanced growth of preterm infants fed a new powdered human milk fortifier: a randomized, controlled trial. *Pediatrics*. 2000;106(3):581–588.

53. Morley R, Lucas A. Randomized diet in the neonatal period and growth performance until 7.5-8 y of age in preterm children. *Am J Clin Nutr*. 2000;71(3):822–828.

54. Arslanoglu S, Moro GE, Ziegler EE. Adjustable fortification of human milk fed to preterm infants: does it make a difference? *J Perinatol*. 2006;26(10):614–621.

55. Yee WH, Soraisham AS, Shah VS, et al. Incidence and timing of presentation of necrotizing enterocolitis in preterm infants. *Pediatrics*. 2012;129(2):e298–e304.

56. Shulhan J, Dicken B, Hartling L, Larsen BM. Current knowledge of necrotizing enterocolitis in preterm infants and the impact of different types of enteral nutrition products. *Adv Nutr*. 2017;8(1):80–91.

57. Bell MJ, Ternberg JL, Feigin RD, et al. Neonatal necrotizing enterocolitis. Therapeutic decisions based upon clinical staging. *Ann Surg*. 1978;187(1):1–7.

58. Lee JS, Polin RA. Treatment and prevention of necrotizing enterocolitis. *Semin Neonatol*. 2003;8(6):449–459.

59. Brower-Sinning R, Zhong D, Good M, et al. Mucosa-associated bacterial diversity in necrotizing enterocolitis. *PLoS One*. 2014;9(9):e105046.

60. Mai V, Young CM, Ukhanova M, et al. Fecal microbiota in premature infants prior to necrotizing enterocolitis. *PLoS One*. 2011;6(6):e20647.

61. McMurtry VE, Gupta RW, Tran L, et al. Bacterial diversity and Clostridia abundance decrease with increasing severity of necrotizing enterocolitis. *Microbiome*. 2015;3:11.

62. Raveh-Sadka T, Thomas BC, Singh A, et al. Gut bacteria are rarely shared by co-hospitalized premature infants, regardless of necrotizing enterocolitis development. *Elife*. 2015;4.

63. Torrazza RM, Ukhanova M, Wang X, et al. Intestinal microbial ecology and environmental factors affecting necrotizing enterocolitis. *PLoS One*. 2013;8(12):e83304.

64. Neu J, Pammi M. Pathogenesis of NEC: impact of an altered intestinal microbiome. *Semin Perinatol*. 2017;41(1):29–35.

65. Good M, Sodhi CP, Egan CE, et al. Breast milk protects against the development of necrotizing enterocolitis through inhibition of Toll-like receptor 4 in the intestinal epithelium via activation of the epidermal growth factor receptor. *Mucosal Immunol*. 2015;8(5):1166–1179.

5

66. Gregory KE, Samuel BS, Houghteling P, et al. Influence of maternal breast milk ingestion on acquisition of the intestinal microbiome in preterm infants. *Microbiome*. 2016;4(1):68.

67. Unger S, Stintzi A, Shah P, Mack D, O'Connor DL. Gut microbiota of the very-low-birth-weight infant. *Pediatr Res*. 2015;77(1–2):205–213.

68. De Curtis M, Paone C, Vetrano G, Romano G, Paludetto R, Ciccimarra F. A case control study of necrotizing enterocolitis occurring over 8 years in a neonatal intensive care unit. *Eur J Pediatr*. 1987;146(4):398–400.

69. Kliegman RM, Walsh MC. Neonatal necrotizing enterocolitis: pathogenesis, classification, and spectrum of illness. *Curr Probl Pediatr*. 1987;17(4):213–288.

70. Corpeleijn WE, de Waard M, Christmann V, et al. Effect of donor milk on severe infections and mortality in very low-birth-weight infants: the early nutrition study randomized clinical trial. *JAMA Pediatr*. 2016;170(7):654–661.

71. Taylor SN, Basile LA, Ebeling M, Wagner CL. Intestinal permeability in preterm infants by feeding type: mother's milk versus formula. *Breastfeed Med*. 2009;4(1):11–15.

72. Penn AH, Altshuler AE, Small JW, Taylor SF, Dobkins KR, Schmid-Schonbein GW. Digested formula but not digested fresh human milk causes death of intestinal cells in vitro: implications for necrotizing enterocolitis. *Pediatr Res*. 2012;72(6):560–567.

73. Als H, Tronick E, Lester BM, Brazelton TB. The Brazelton Neonatal Behavioral Assessment Scale (BNBAS). *J Abnorm Child Psychol*. 1977;5(3):215–231.

74. Knobloch H, Pasamanick B, Sherard Jr ES. A developmental screening inventory for infants. *Pediatrics*. 1966;38(6). [Suppl:1095–1108].

75. Ameil-Tison C, Grenier G. *Neurological Assessment During The First Year Of Life*. Oxford: Oxford University Press; 1986.

76. Bayley N. *Bayley Scales Of Infant Development*. New York, NY: The Psychological Corporation; 1969.

77. Bayley N. *Bayley Scales of Infant and Toddler Development*. 3rd ed. San Antonio, TX: Harcourt Assessment; 2006.

78. Darlow BA, Lui K, Kusuda S, et al. International variations and trends in the treatment for retinopathy of prematurity. *Br J Ophthalmol*. 2017;101(10):1399–1404.

79. Zhou J, Shukla VV, John D, Chen C. Human milk feeding as a protective factor for retinopathy of prematurity: a meta-analysis. *Pediatrics*. 2015;136(6):e1576–e1586.

80. Narayanan I, Prakash K, Prabhakar AK, Gujral VV. A planned prospective evaluation of the anti-infective property of varying quantities of expressed human milk. *Acta Paediatr Scand*. 1982;71(3):441–445.

81. Jarvenpaa AL, Raiha NC, Rassin DK, Gaull GE. Feeding the low-birth-weight infant: I. Taurine and cholesterol supplementation of formula does not affect growth and metabolism. *Pediatrics*. 1983;71(2):171–178.

82. Putet G, Senterre J, Rigo J, Salle B. Nutrient balance, energy utilization, and composition of weight gain in very-low-birth-weight infants fed pooled human milk or a preterm formula. *J Pediatr*. 1984;105(1):79–85.

83. Cooper PA, Rothberg AD, Pettifor JM, Bolton KD, Devenhuis S. Growth and biochemical response of premature infants fed pooled preterm milk or special formula. *J Pediatr Gastroenterol Nutr*. 1984;3(5):749–754.

84. ClinicalTrials.gov. Available at: https://clinicaltrials.gov/. Accessed March 28, 2017.

85. World Health Organization. *International clinical trials registry platform*. Available at: http://apps.who.int/trialsearch/Default.aspx. Accessed March 28, 2017.

86. ClinicalTrials.gov [Internet]. Bethesda (MD): National Library of Medicine (US). 2000. Identifier NCT01534481. *Donor milk vs. Formula in extremely low birth weight (ELBW) infants*. Available at: https://clinicaltrials.gov/ct2/show/NCT01534481?term=NCT01534481&rank=1. Accessed March 29, 2017.

87. ClinicalTrials.gov [Internet]. Bethesda (MD): National Library of Medicine (US). 2000. *Identifier* NCT01686477, *PREterM FOrmula or donor breast milk for premature babies*. Available at: https://clinicaltrials.gov/ct2/results?term=NCT01686477&Search=Search. Accessed March 29, 2017.

88. International Clinical Trials Registry Platform [Internet]. Geneva, Switzerland: Word Health Organization. Identifier CTRI/2016/04/006855. *Impact of human breast milk bank on the mortality and morbidity pattern in a NICU of a tertiary care hospital*. Available at: http://apps.who.int/trialsearch/Trial2.aspx?TrialID=CTRI/2016/04/006855. Accessed March 29, 2017.

89. ClinicalTrials.gov [Internet]. Bethesda (MD): National Library of Medicine (US). 2000. Identifier NCT01390753. *Role of human milk bank in the protection of severe respiratory disease in very low birth weight premature infants*. Available at: https://clinicaltrials.gov/ct2/show/NCT01390753?term=NCT01390753&rank=1. Accessed March 29, 2017.

90. ClinicalTrials.gov [Internet]. Bethesda (MD): National Library of Medicine (US). 2000. Identifier NCT02371538. *Human breastmilk in young children with norovirus infection of the gut*. Available at: https://clinicaltrials.gov/ct2/show/NCT02371538?term=NCT02371538&rank=1. Accessed March 29, 2017.

91. ClinicalTrials.gov [Internet]. Bethesda (MD): National Library of Medicine (US). 2000. Identifier NCT02025478. *Human breastmilk in children receiving a bone marrow transplant (MILK)*. Available at: https://clinicaltrials.gov/ct2/show/NCT02025478?term=NCT02025478&rank=1. Accessed March 29, 2017.

92. ClinicalTrials.gov [Internet]. Bethesda (MD): National Library of Medicine (US). 2000. Identifier NCT02216292. *Impact of preterm single donor milk in very low birth weight infants*. Available at: https://clinicaltrials.gov/ct2/show/NCT02216292?term=NCT02216292&rank=1. Accessed March 29, 2017.

93. ClinicalTrials.gov [Internet]. Bethesda (MD): National Library of Medicine (US). 2000. Identifier NCT02943746. *Targeted protein fortificiation in extrememely low birth weight preterm infants.* Available at: https://clinicaltrials.gov/ct2/show/NCT02943746?term=NCT02943746&rank=1. Accessed March 29, 2017.
94. ClinicalTrials.gov [Internet]. Bethesda (MD): National Library of Medicine (US). 2000. Identifier NCT02182973. *Donor human milk in neonatal abstinence syndrome (DHM&NAS).* Available at: https://clinicaltrials.gov/ct2/show/NCT02182973?term=NCT02182973&rank=1. Accessed March 29, 2017.

5

CHAPTER 6

Neonatal Necrotizing Enterocolitis

NEONATOLOGY QUESTIONS AND CONTROVERSIES

Lauren Astrug, MD, Erika Claud, MD

Introduction

Neonatal necrotizing enterocolitis (NEC) is a devastating disease that continues to remain poorly understood. NEC is an acquired gastrointestinal (GI) disease that mostly affects premature infants; the risk of development is the highest in infants born at <32 weeks' gestation and with birth weight of <1500 g. The diagnosis was first described in 1960, and it has remained challenging to understand, prevent, and manage despite dedication to research. The prevalence of the disorder is about 7% among infants born weighing 500 to 1500 g.[1] The rate of death resulting from complications of NEC is about 30%.[1] In this discussion, we will review the basics of NEC, the role of the infant microbiome, and controversial risk factors, including antibiotic exposure, medications, anemia and blood transfusions, feeding regimens, and the use of probiotics.

NEC—Back to Basics

NEC, which is a common risk for premature infants, increases mortality and morbidity, including, but not limited to, severe neurodevelopmental outcomes and prolonged hospital stays. The development of NEC is multifactorial. It typically occurs between 2 and 6 weeks of life, with the highest risk at 29 to 33 weeks corrected gestation age.[2] Classic signs and symptoms are nonspecific and include abdominal distension, poor tolerance of feeds, and hematochezia, along with subtle signs, such as activity change or increased occurrence of apnea. Early findings may be represented radiographically by notably dilated loops of bowel, paucity of bowel gas, fixed loops of bowel, and/or extraluminal air. However, an infant's condition can deteriorate rapidly to a septic shock–like appearance, including hemodynamic instability and acute respiratory failure.[2] The pathognomonic finding on abdominal radiography is pneumatosis intestinalis, or air tracking within the bowel wall. Management is only supportive, not specific, and includes bowel rest with intravenous (IV) nutrition, decompression of the abdomen, broad-spectrum antibiotics, and/or surgery. Surgery may involve placement of a peritoneal drain or laparotomy, with resection of the affected part of bowel.[3] Treatment options depend on the severity of the disease in each neonate. Bell et al. described a staging system in the 1970s, and that system has been modified over the years, with improvements in neonatal management and understanding of other neonatal morbidities that may have caused confusion in the stratification of NEC earlier.[2] The criteria are categorized into three stages and substages. Stage I is classified as suspected

Table 6.1   MODIFIED BELL'S CLINICAL STAGING CRITERIA FOR NEONATAL NECROTIZING ENTEROCOLITIS[4]

Bell's Stages	Clinical Findings	Radiographic Appearance	Gastrointestinal Symptoms
Stage I	Apnea/Bradycardia (A/B), temperature instability	Normal vs. mild ileus	Bloody stools, mild abdominal distension, poor toleration of feeds
Stage IIa	A/B, temperature instability	Ileus, dilated loops, focal pneumatosis	Grossly bloody stools, abdominal distension, no bowel sounds
Stage IIb	Thrombocytopenia, mild metabolic acidosis	Widespread pneumatosis, ascites, portal venous gas	Abdominal wall edema, palpable loops, tender examination
Stage IIIa	Mixed acidosis, oliguria, hypotension, coagulopathy	Prominent bowel loops, worsening ascites, no free air	Severe abdominal wall edema, erythema or abdominal color changes
Stage IIIb	Shock, sepsis, severe deterioration in vital signs and laboratory values	Pneumoperitoneum representing free air or perforation	Perforated bowel

NEC—manifesting as temperature instability, apnea, and slight changes in feeding tolerance. Stage II is classified as definite NEC and includes stage I symptoms plus significant changes in abdominal examination with radiographic findings of pneumatosis or portal venous air. Stage III is classified as advanced NEC—manifesting as significant septic shock–like appearance, severe abdominal extension, and ascites or free air as seen on the radiograph (Table 6.1).[4]

Despite much research and further advancements in the neonatal intensive care unit (NICU) setting, management has remained essentially unchanged because of limited knowledge about the pathophysiology of NEC. We do not know how to specifically prevent or treat this disease. There is only a general understanding of NEC, and merely overall systemic supportive measures are provided to the sick neonate. The development of NEC is thought to be multifactorial in nature, and these factors include prematurity, changes in the neonatal microbiome, enteral feeding, early antibiotic exposure, lack of bowel perfusion, and/or medication exposure.[4] A greater understanding of the pathogenesis of this disease is needed to tie together the seemingly disparate risk factors, to reliably predict patients at highest risk, and to provide specific therapies to prevent and treat this disease. A possible link is the microbiome of the newborn intestine. In this chapter, we will discuss a few of the most common theories about the triggers or influences that may increase the risk for NEC and their connection to the microbiome (Fig. 6.1).

Microbiome

It was once thought that NEC could be caused by a direct insult to the intestine, whether from altered intestinal perfusion, infection, or other etiology. Research has revealed more areas of consideration and understanding of the dynamic community of the GI tract. The intestinal microbiome comprises all of the bacteria within the intestine, ideally with a balance among organisms, living symbiotically in a healthy environment.

Although bacteria appear to play a role, NEC is not an infection in the classic sense and cannot be isolated to one infecting agent or pathogen. In fact, in most cases, blood culture results are negative for infectious agents. A large cohort study in the 1980s reviewed all blood culture samples drawn from infants with NEC and noted that only about 30% of these culture samples showed bacterial growth.[5] A more recent study in 2012 further demonstrated that <15% of blood cultures from infants with NEC were positive for bacteria.[6]

The concept of one pathogen causing the insult has given way to questioning whether a community of organisms cause NEC. With advancements in technology during the 1990s, the microbiome began to be studied in depth. Molecular profiling of the microbiota, through sequencing of the highly conserved 16S small subunit bacterial ribosomal RNA genes, now allows identification of previously undetectable

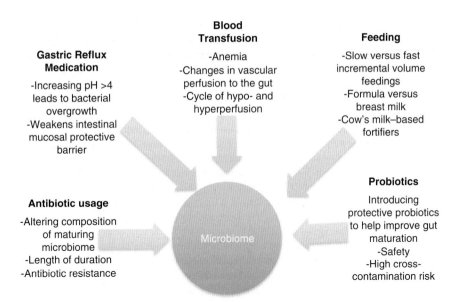

Gastric Reflux Medication

-Increasing pH >4 leads to bacterial overgrowth
-Weakens intestinal mucosal protective barrier

Blood Transfusion

-Anemia
-Changes in vascular perfusion to the gut
-Cycle of hypo- and hyperperfusion

Feeding

-Slow versus fast incremental volume feedings
-Formula versus breast milk
-Cow's milk–based fortifiers

Antibiotic usage

-Altering composition of maturing microbiome
-Length of duration
-Antibiotic resistance

Microbiome

Probiotics

Introducing protective probiotics to help improve gut maturation
-Safety
-High cross-contamination risk

Fig. 6.1 Neonatal necrotizing enterocolitis—clinical controversies and factors impacting the developing microbiome.

microbes.[7] The composition of these microbes within the GI tract is dynamic, influenced by the environment, and undergoes changes in infancy. It was once thought that infants were born from a sterile environment because investigators were unable to grow bacteria from the amniotic fluid or from the surface culture samples from newborn infants directly after delivery.[8] It was believed that bacteria begin to populate in the infant only after delivery. With further development of technologies, as previously discussed, the presence of bacterial species from the phyla Firmicutes, Tenericutes, Proteobacteria, Bacteriodes, and Fusobacteria have been found on the basal plate of the placenta (shared maternal–fetal interface).[8] In multiple studies, bacteria have also been identified in low amounts within the umbilical cord and meconium of infants before initiation of feedings.[9,10] It is, therefore, likely that the gut begins to colonize with bacteria in utero. Over time, the community becomes more complex so that by adulthood, the human intestinal microbiome consists of 10 to 100 trillion different microbial species.[8]

A healthy microbiome is characterized by a high diversity of bacteria in balance, providing redundancy in function and protection against disease. Bacteria that are out of balance, a state termed *dysbiosis*, lose the ability to function at full capacity and to provide protection against disease. It is not surprising to find that the microbiomes of preterm and term infants differ.[11] Several factors, including oxygen exposure altering the viability of anaerobic bacteria, the mode of delivery (vaginal delivery results in exposure to maternal vaginal flora versus cesarean section results in exposure to maternal skin flora), type of feedings, and exposure to medications, affect the development of the microbiome.[11-13] For example, the microbiome of infants delivered via cesarean section does not harbor strict anaerobes and a large amount of facultative anaerobes, such as *Clostridium* species.[14,15] The developing microbiome of all infants is influenced by all of these factors; in premature infants, however, development is being completed in the context of this microbiome. They are additionally exposed to unnatural settings, such as sterile hospital environments, medical instrumentation (nasogastric tubes, endotracheal tubes, intravenous lines, etc.), and feedings initiated at an earlier developmental stage than in term infants.[8] All of these exposures lead to atypical development of the microbiome, which may place premature infants at a higher risk for developing NEC. Claud et al. compared the intestinal microbiome of healthy premature infants without NEC to that of healthy, vaginally delivered, breastfed, full-term infants.[16] Stool samples were collected weekly over the first 8 weeks of life and sequenced by using the 16S rRNA process to document the evolving bacterial microbiome. Samples from full-term infants were found to be clustered with similar bacteria at all time points.[16] In contrast, healthy premature infants revealed clustering at particular intervals including <2 weeks of age, 3 to 5 weeks of age, and >6 weeks of age.[16] This suggests that the time course of the development of the microbiome may be important in premature infants.

Microbiota in healthy term infants is established in a stepwise process, starting with facultative anaerobes.[17] Within a few weeks of life, *Bifidobacterium* species become highly prevalent. Diversity of the infant's gut increases with time and undergoes a major shift during weaning.[17] In contrast, preterm infants are exposed to prenatal and postnatal environmental insults while the microbiome is still undergoing development. The initial microbiome has low diversity.[18] The microbiome is then influenced by the NICU environment, and community shifts may have an influence on the risk of NEC. In particular, a further decrease in species diversity and a bloom of gamma-proteobacteria has been demonstrated weeks before the actual clinical development of the disease.[19]

In 2016 a case study published by Hourigan et al.[20] highlighted the importance of the microbiome in twins, with only one of them developing NEC. Diamniotic and dichorionic twins (boy and girl) exhibited similar early NICU courses undergoing a course of antibiotics, total parental nutrition, and the initiation of feeds. Twin A had an uncomplicated case and was discharged from the NICU around the time of the expected due date; twin B had a complicated course, including medical closure of her patent ductus arteriosus and feeding intolerance, and ultimately developed NEC in the ileum with multiple perforations.[20] Stools for each infant had been collected before twin B developed NEC, and each stool specimen was sequenced by using 16S rRNA sequencing technologies. Twin B had a much more diverse microbiome in earlier stages of life, but this diversity was abruptly lost weeks before the development of clinical NEC.[20] Twin A had a prominence of *Firmicutes* in all samples (>95%), whereas twin B had both *Proteobacteria* and *Firmicutes*, with an increasing amount of *Proteobacteria* weeks before developing NEC.[20] This case report highlighted the potential disparity between twins in microbiome development and clinical course despite their similar intrauterine and early environmental exposures.[20] The ever-changing composition of specific bacteria may create an unbalanced microbiome with both increase in pathogens and decrease in protective species, leading to susceptibility to NEC. Can monitoring of the development of the microbiome in premature infants help identify those at higher risk of developing NEC? Could this be the strategy used in the near future to map those at a higher risk of developing NEC based on changes in the microbiome?

Furthermore, the microbiome plays a major role in immune system development and in protection against disease. The microbiota promotes epithelial cell regeneration, modulating epithelial permeability, as well as promoting angiogenesis, remodeling the intestinal vascular system.[17] Preterm infant dysbiosis may contribute to gut dysmotility, immature barrier function, and poorly controlled immune responses, thus increasing the risk of NEC development.[17,21]

As an example, growth is a parameter that can be clinically monitored in premature infants as a sign of health.[22] In 2015 a study used a humanized gnotobiotic mouse model to investigate the functioning of the microbial community in preterm infants. Microbiota samples extracted from stools from a premature infant with appropriate growth and an infant with poor growth, both with the same gestational age and at <2 weeks of life, were gavaged to gnotobiotic pregnant dams.[22] Both microbiomes were quite similar at the phylum level.[22] The delivered pups acquired the designated microbiota from each infant naturally through birth and nursing from the newly colonized dams. The pup with the microbiota from the infant with poor growth was found to have significant upregulation of genes related to inflammatory response and the innate immunity.[22] There was an increase in the baseline serum inflammatory cytokine levels even without an actual inflammatory insult. The pup with the microbiota from the properly growing infant showed downregulation of these genes. This finding suggests that a particular microbiome does modulate inflammatory responses, potentially protecting the premature infant and supporting healthier development.[22]

Furthermore, the pups from dams receiving the stools from the normally growing preterm infant had statistically significant longer small intestines, along with greater villus height and crypt depths.[22] There were also more proliferating cells and decreased apoptosis along all sections of the intestinal tract in comparison with those pups from dams with microbiota from poorly growing preterm infants. The differentiation of cells differed significantly, including higher concentrations of goblet cells and Paneth cells within the microbiota of appropriately growing preterm infants.[20] All these improved variables indicated an overall process of protection within the intestinal tract and better-developed mucosal defense and function.[17] A healthy microbiome enhances intestinal development, protects against disease, and is influenced by the environment. What routine aspects of neonatal care influence the microbiome and NEC risk?

Antibiotics

Medications may disrupt microbiome balance. Antibiotics are the most common medications used in the NICU. Antibiotics have been investigated as a preventative measure against NEC. In the 1990s, double-blind randomized control trials, such as that by Siu et al., studied the use of oral vancomycin versus placebo in the prevention of NEC. Of the 71 premature infants included in the study by Siu et al., 13% developed NEC in the vancomycin group compared with 28% of those who received the placebo.[23] Despite these significant results, prophylactic antibiotics for NEC have not been widely studied because of concerns about development of resistant bacteria.[24] Furthermore, despite their possible effectiveness, antibiotics can have a significant impact on the microbiome. Most premature infants receive broad-spectrum antibiotics covering the most common neonatal pathogenic bacteria to prevent infection. However, studies have demonstrated alterations in microbiome balance in premature infants exposed to antibiotics. La Rosa et al. analyzed fecal samples from 58 infants over the course of their stay in the NICU and identified overall a common initial presence of *Bacillus* species transforming to higher amounts of *Clostridia* species weeks later.[25] During this time, abrupt changes in bacterial species were noted in the microbiome. It is noteworthy that antibiotics were given to these neonates around the time of these identified abrupt changes.[25]

Prolonged use of therapeutic agents influence initial intestinal colonization, and thus the length of antibiotic therapy may increase morbidity. A study by Cotten et al. reviewed 5693 extremely low–birth weight infants admitted to 19 different centers; 96% of infants were treated with a combination of two antibiotics with a median of 3 to 9.5 days of therapy, with more than 50% receiving more than 5 days of treatment.[26] Longer durations of initial empirical antibiotic treatment were more likely to be associated with NEC and/or death compared with shorter durations.[26] There was a 4% increase in the risk of NEC or death with each additional day of empirical antibiotic coverage.[26] The increase in the risk of NEC alone almost doubled to a 7% increase for each additional day of coverage. The risk of NEC and/or death and the risk of death were increased with initial empirical antibiotic treatment lasting >5 days.[26] Research on the specific effects of antibiotic use on microbiome development in preterm infants is ongoing, and more focus is needed before making changes to practice. However, available data indicate the need for caution regarding the potential adverse effects of certain empirical treatments.

Antireflux Medications

Another highly controversial topic is the use of antireflux medications, including proton pump inhibitors (PPIs) and histamine-2 (H2) blockers in the NICU. Although it is recommended that these medications be reserved for neonates who have evidence of pathologic exposure to acid reflux episodes, these medications tend to be overused.[27] Two thirds of neonatologists use antireflux medications to treat apnea despite limited data demonstrating any association between reflux and cardiorespiratory events.[28] Furthermore, these medications have potential adverse effects. Gastric acid inhibitors may increase the risk of NEC by altering the gastric pH, thus manipulating the protective properties of stomach acid and causing alteration in bacterial colonization.[29] Physiologically, gastric pH is around 1.4 in adults.[29] Any pH <4 has bactericidal effects on ingested acid-sensitive bacteria.[29] Studies in rats and humans have shown a change in lower intestinal bacteria after exposure to a PPI increasing gastric pH to >4.[29] Facultative and obligate anaerobic bacteria belonging to seven genera—*Prevotella*, *Atopobium* group, *Clostridium coccoides* group, *Veillonella*, *Lactobacillus* group, *Enterobacteriaceae*, and *Bacteroides fragilis*—were found in much higher levels in rats that received H2 blocker treatment compared with rats not exposed to a gastric acid inhibitor.[29] The study also compared the use of a PPI versus an H2 blocker and found that use of a PPI had a statistically significant dose-dependent effect, increasing the populations of both *Lactobacillus* and *Veillonella* species.[30] Interestingly, these two bacterial species originate in the oropharyngeal region, suggesting that failure of the gastric acid barrier possibly increased the load of bacteria entering the intestines.[29,30]

These medications also delay gastric emptying and thin the viscosity of mucus, allowing easy bacterial overgrowth. Without a strong acidic environment, the immature humoral immune system cannot function at full capacity.[31] The process of chemotactic response and leukocyte reactions to antigens is limited by the lack of the necessary acidic environment.[31] There is decreased adhesion of leukocytes to endothelial cells in environments with a higher pH. There is reduction in bactericidal killing of microbes, and phagosomes no longer function, and this allows bacterial overgrowth.[31] Wandall investigated the effects of omeprazole on polymorphonuclear neutrophil chemotaxis, superoxide generation, and degranulation and translocation of cytochrome b, which are important immunologic defenses.[32] This study demonstrated that a higher concentration of omeperazole leading to a more alkalotic environment inhibited this process.[32] With changes to pH, there is a change in bacterial species found within the microbiome, as well as inhibition of natural immune defenses, possibly leaving the intestinal mucosa vulnerable to pathogenic changes.

In August 2012, More et al. evaluated the association between exposure to H2 inhibitors and the incidence of NEC and infections in preterm infants.[33] Guillet et al.[33a] evaluated 10,903 infants, of whom 72.2% were on H2 blockers. In the study by Terrin, of the 274 preterm infants included, 33.2% were on H2 blockers.[33a] The overall incidence of NEC was 7.1% and the risk of NEC was 6.6-fold higher in infants on H2 blockers.[33] Overall, H2 blockers affect the protective barrier of the gastric lining and allow for bacterial overgrowth, altering the microbiome and increasing inflammation within the mucosal lining. These alterations may increase the risk of NEC.

Blood Transfusions

About 40% of preterm infants with birth weight of 1000 to 1500 g and 90% of infants weighing <1000 g receive blood transfusion at least once.[34] Transfusions are used to enhance oxygen delivery; however, no target hematocrit or hemoglobin for transfusion has been specifically identified. Guidelines have been based on the hemoglobin and/or hematocrit levels combined with the clinical condition of the infant (respiratory status, requiring respiratory support, age of the infant, hemodynamic stability, etc.).[35] Premature infants commonly receive transfusions because of decreased production of red blood cells (RBCs), frequent laboratory blood draws, and overall grave clinical status. However, there is concern that blood transfusions are associated with the development of NEC.

It is difficult to determine whether NEC is truly caused by anemia or if there is an association because the average age at which NEC develops is typically around the same time premature infants become anemic and require blood transfusions. Are these events associated, or do they occur independently around the same corrected gestational age? A meta-analysis of randomized control trials did identify an increase in NEC with RBC transfusions in infants with lower hemoglobin levels; however, no temporal relationship between transfusion and the time of onset of NEC has been identified.[36]

It is possible that chronic anemia, coupled with intermittent blood transfusions, may lead to a hypoperfusion–hyperperfusion cycle at the GI vascular level.[36] Alternatively, active mediators, such as free hemoglobin, cytokines, or broken red cell fragments, in the blood transfused may trigger an immunologic reaction in the gut mucosa, leading to mucosal injury and inflammation and thus increasing the risk of NEC.[37,38] It is also possible that the initial anemia results in lack of perfusion to the gut via the mesenteric vessels, thus increasing hypoxic events and mucosal injury.[39] Each of these factors could alter microbial colonization. Agwu and Narchi compared 111 preterm infants who developed NEC stage >2a with 222 matched controls, and 28 clinical variables, including hematocrit and number of blood transfusions, were recorded.[39] After controlling for confounding variables, a lower hematocrit level was associated with increased risk of NEC, and blood transfusions had a temporal relationship with the onset of NEC at 24, 48, and 96 hours.[40]

It has been hypothesized that vasoactive responses associated with blood transfusions cause intestinal mucosal injury, potentially increasing susceptibility to NEC.[40] Intestinal mucosal injury before and after blood transfusions has been measured by utilizing urinary levels of intestinal fatty acid binding protein, a sensitive and specific marker for mucosal injury.[40] This retrospective study included 62 infants with gestational ages ranging from 24 to 28 weeks and found that infants who received blood transfusions and went on to develop NEC had elevated urinary levels of intestinal fatty acid binding protein both before and after transfusion.[40] The transfusions were therefore likely not the cause of alteration in the intestinal environment; rather, the mucosal injury had occurred before the transfusion.[41] A recent analysis of studies examining the effects of small volume (10-20 mL/kg) RBC transfusion identified no significant differences between restrictive and liberal transfusions.[42] Another study reported in 2017 attempted to identify the effects and complications from RBC transfusions. That study enrolled 641 very low–birth weight infants, 37.6% of whom were of extremely low–birth weight, with mean gestational age of 29.4 weeks.[34] Overall, 42% had received a transfusion at least once within the first 28 days of life.[34] The mean pretransfusion hemoglobin was 9.6 ± 1.1 g/dL.[34] Of the total number of infants who had received transfusions (194 infants), only 3% developed NEC, whereas 2% of those who had not received transfusions (47 infants) developed NEC; in all cases, NEC had developed at least 48 hours after RBC transfusion. This study did not show an association between transfusions and NEC development.[34]

Consistent data to provide confirmation of a causal relationship between RBC transfusions and NEC or to provide exact guidelines for RBC transfusions are lacking. Links among anemia, altered intestinal perfusion and microbial colonization or translocation are still being investigated.

Feedings

Enteral feeds have been associated with the development of NEC. The majority of infants with NEC are started on enteral feeds, and most reach full feeds before the disease develops. Feeding practices have been extensively studied as a potential intervention to decrease NEC risk. Most NICUs have feeding protocols targeting nonaggressive feeds for premature infants who weigh less than 1500 g, starting with small volumes and increasing in small amounts daily as tolerated. These trophic feeds are important because a delay in feeding and prolonged use of total parental nutrition can increase intestinal atrophy and inflammatory responses, which can potentially lead to increased severity of NEC.[43] A meta-analysis of nine randomized control trials comprising a total of 949 infants reviewed feeding schedules and volume increments of feeds in and showed no statistically significant difference in NEC incidence between infants fed at slower rates (15-24 mL/kg/day) versus faster rates (30-40 mL/kg/day).[44] In fact, infants who were fed at slower rates reached full feeding volumes later compared with those fed at faster incremental rates, and this was associated with shorter duration of total parental nutrition and a higher risk of late-onset invasive infection.[44] The infants also reached their birth weight much later compared with those fed at faster incremental rates.[44]

Type of feeding must also be considered. Since the 1970s, the focus of constituting formulas for preterm infants has been nutrition content. Initial formulations had high protein concentrations, with casein protein being dominant.[45] These formulations caused protein intolerance in many infants, azotemia, metabolic acidosis and growth failure.[45] Formulas for preterm infants have undergone several modifications and currently contain more whey (60%) than casein (40%). Whey is easier to digest, does not slow gastric emptying, and has faster amino acid absorption, reducing the risk of metabolic acidosis.[46] High osmolar formulas were also once thought to put a strain on the GI tract of the immature preterm infant and increase mucosal injury. This may not be true because recent research suggests that the increased osmolality of high osmolar formulas within the upper portion of the GI tract becomes diluted and balanced when reaching the intestinal tract by the natural process of osmosis and diffusion through GI transit.[47]

The impact of feeding extends beyond nutrition. Many studies have demonstrated that infants receiving mother's milk have not only a decreased risk of NEC but also improved feeding tolerance and motility. Protective elements in breast milk encourage improvement of gut immunity. Human breast milk contains immunoglobulins (specifically IgA), growth factors, lysozyme, lactoferrin, polyunsaturated fatty acids, oligosaccharides, cytokines, and other protective agents.[48,49] Healthy flora, specifically *Lactobacillus* and *Bifidobacterium*, which are commonly found in high concentrations in a healthy balanced microbiome, are supported by prebiotics.[50] Prebiotics are mainly oligosaccharides found in human milk as lactoferrin and lactalbumin milk proteins and are nondigestible.[50,51] These factors are lacking in formula and pasteurized donor milk. A meta-analysis of two recent trials included 260 infants with birth weight <1500 g receiving diets ranging from 100% human milk to 100% cow milk.[52] The percentage of cow milk in the diet was a predictor of both overall NEC and surgical NEC. For each 10% increase in the intake of diet based on milk other than human milk, the risk of NEC increased by 11.8% (95% confidence interval [CI] 0.2%-24.8%) and the risk of surgical NEC increased by 21% (95% CI 4.2%-39.6%).[52] In 2012 Penn et al.[53] evaluated gut mucosal injury associated with breast milk versus formula feeds in rats. Different formulas were digested either with pancreatic lipase, proteases, lipase, and protease together or with rat small intestinal luminal fluid. The resulting products were tested on intestinal epithelial cells, endothelial cells, and neutrophils.[53] It was found that the products of digestion of formula, not human milk–based products, caused significant death of neutrophils (47%-99% with formula, up to 6% with human milk), epithelial and endothelial cells.[53] These insults can lead to a cascade of events increasing the risk for NEC.[54]

The increased availability of donor milk has led to additional studies. Because of ethical reasons, there are no recent prospective studies; however, trends have been reviewed retrospectively. A meta-analysis found that donor human milk feeding was associated with significantly reduced relative risk of NEC. Infants receiving donor milk were three times less likely to develop NEC compared with those receiving formula milk.[55] A randomized trial evaluating extremely premature infants who were fed either pasteurized donor milk or preterm formula as supplements to their own mothers' milk, found that in infants who received a higher percentages of mothers' own milk, the incidence of NEC was 50% lower.[56] Cow's milk–based products, including bovine milk–based milk fortifiers and cow's milk formula, lead to mucosal injury and inflammation.[57] Studies on the long-term effects of donor milk beyond NEC risks are ongoing. Emphasizing the importance of feeding infants their own mothers' milk, encouraging mothers to breastfeed or pump, and providing extra resources to help mothers in these efforts are of primary importance in preventing NEC.

Probiotics

The most recent controversial topic related to NEC is the use of probiotics. Antibiotics, reflux medications, transfusions, and feeding are clinical practices that aim to optimize benefits and prevent harm, and the use of probiotics are currently of interest as an active therapeutic or preventive measure against NEC. Probiotics are bacteria that have a beneficial effect beyond their nutritive value. Probiotics encompass many species, including *Lactobacillus*, *Bifidobacterium*, *Streptococcus*, *Escherichia*, *Enterococcus*, *Bacillus*, and *Saccharomyces*.[58] *Lactobacillus* and *Bifidobacteria* are the most common. *Lactobacillus acidophilus* is commonly found in food and supplements, it can withstand a wide range of pH and temperature, and it has been shown to decrease the severity of NEC in rat models of NEC.[59] This probiotic has antibacterial properties against a wide range of bacteria and secretes anti-inflammatory factors that inhibit induction of an inflammatory process.[60] *Bifidobacteria* will colonize in the presence of human milk and uses human milk as its energy source. It, too, has anti-inflammatory properties that have been shown to decrease the incidence of NEC.[61] *Bifidobacteria* has been shown to activate B cells of innate immunity to mature into secretory IgA plasma cells. This results in protection against pathogens penetrating the mucosal barrier by coating the gut mucosa with IgA.[62]

In an initial study by Hoyos, probiotics (*Lactobacillus* and *Bifidobacterium*) were administered daily during the entire hospital stay to every baby in the NICU in Bogota, in Colombia, for 1 year. The incidence of NEC was significantly decreased in comparison with previous years.[63] A recent meta-analysis by Goncalves et al. examined over 35 randomized controlled trials comprising a total of 5559 premature infants receiving probiotics and 5513 infants receiving either a placebo or blinded nontreatment.[59] Using stage ≥2 NEC as the primary outcome of interest, probiotics were found to reduce the incidence of NEC to 3.3% in infants receiving probiotics compared with 6.1% in control infants.[58] A meta-analysis in 2016 by Sawh et al. aimed to review the efficacy and safety of preterm exposure to probiotics.[64] A total of 37 randomized control trials, comprising 10,520 infants, with the primary outcome of NEC were identified. The incidence of the disease was notably decreased in infants receiving probiotics in comparison with those receiving the placebo.[64,65] All infants were of gestational age <37 weeks and weighed <2500 g. However, when extremely low–birth weight infants (<1000 g) were highlighted, similar results were found compared with all infants.[64] Other factors, such as culture-positive sepsis, did not differ between the two groups; specifically, sepsis was not found to be caused by a particular probiotic species in any positive culture.[64] Furthermore, it was notable that infants receiving probiotics had shorter hospital stays, increased weight gain, and shorter duration in reaching goal feeds.[64] The incidence of NEC was not affected by the time of starting probiotics, whether within 48 hours of birth or within the initiation of feeds.[64]

However, despite positive outcomes, there are true risks for preterm infants receiving probiotics in the NICU setting. When administered to premature infants with a developing intestinal mucosa and mucosal barrier, probiotics can increase the risk of intestinal microbial translocation leading to sepsis.[65] There have been a few reports of *Saccharomyces boulardii* sepsis after infants received probiotics.[65] Currently, there is also no U.S. Food and Drug Administration approval for a pharmaceutical-grade probiotic because probiotics are considered nutritional supplements and not a medication.[66] Probiotic supplement products have been found to contain varying concentrations of particular probiotic species, as well as other species that are not considered probiotics. Probiotics have also been found to have a risk of cross-contamination in the NICU, affecting infants not receiving these supplements.[66] If the goal of probiotics is to optimize the microbiome to prevent NEC, other means, such as breast feeding and limiting antibiotics, as discussed above, are currently considered safer means to accomplishing this goal.

Conclusion

NEC, which has been an important area of study in Neonatology for several years, continues to cause high morbidity and mortality in NICUs, specifically in very low–birth weight premature infants. The diagnosis remains the same; the understanding of the pathophysiology of the development of NEC, however, has evolved with research. Ultimately, we do not fully understand the pathology of NEC, we do not know which direct insults leave premature infants at a higher risk for developing this disease, and we do not know how to prevent it. We believe many answers lie within the microbiome. A healthy microbiome facilitates the continued maturation process of the preterm gut. Antibiotics can alter this microbiome, certainly with longer periods of exposure. Changes in environmental variables as a result of medications can also lead to bacterial overgrowth, upsetting the balance of the microbiome. Enteral feeding is important for gut development, and multiple factors in mother's milk contribute to an optimized microbiome and decreased incidence of NEC. Probiotics may be beneficial, but at present, there are no regulated products that have been investigated not only for the short-term outcomes of NEC and sepsis but also for the potential long-term effects of microbiome manipulation in these vulnerable patients. An increased understanding of the importance of the microbiome in health and disease will help provide better clinical recommendations. Protecting the developing microbiome through human milk feeding, limiting the use of antibiotics, and considering the impact of clinical interventions on the microbiome may collectively be an effective measure to decrease NEC incidence.

REFERENCES

1. Neu J, Walker WA. Necrotizing Enterocolitis. *NEJM*. 2011;364:255–264.
2. Caplan MS, Fanaroff A. Necrotizing: a historical perspective. *Semin Perinatol*. 2016:1–3.
3. Moss RL, et al. Laparotomy versus peritoneal drainage for necrotizing enterocolitis and perforation. *NEJM*. 2006;354:2225–2234.
4. Gordon P, Christensen R, Weitkamp JH, Maheshwari A. Mapping the new world of necrotizing enterocolitis (NEC): review and opinion. *J Neonatol Res*. 2012;2:4.
5. Stoll BJ, Kanto Jr WP, Glass RI, Nahmias AJ, Brann Jr AW. Epidemiology of necrotizing enterocolitis: a case control study. *J Pediatr*. 1980;96:447–451.
6. Clark RH, Gordon P, Walker WM, Laughon M, Smith PB, Spitzer AR. Characteristics of patients who die of necrotizing enterocolitis. *J Perinatol*. 2012;32:278–285.
7. Turnbaugh PJ, Ley RE, Gordon JI. The human microbiome project: exploring the microbial part of ourselves in a changing world. *Nature*. 2007;449(7164):804–810.
8. Elgin TG, Kern SL, McElroy SJ. Development of the neonatal intestinal microbiome and its association with necrotizing enterocolitis. *Clin Ther*. 2016;38:706–715.
9. Jimenez E, Marin ML, Martin R, et al. Is meconium from healthy newborns actually sterile? *Res Microbiol*. 2008;159:187–193.
10. Jimenez E, Fernandez L, Marin ML, et al. Isolation of commensal bacteria from umbilical cord blood of healthy neonates born by cesarean section. *Curr Microbiol*. 2005;51:270–274.
11. Palmer C, Bik EM, DiGiulio DB, Relman DA, Brown PO. Development of the human infant intestinal microbiota. *PLoS Biol*. 2007. https://doi.org/10.1371/journal.pbio.0050177.
12. Stark PL, Lee A. The microbial ecology of the large bowel of breastfed and formula-fed infants during the first year of life. *J Med Microbiol*. 1982;15:189–203.
13. Biasucci G, Benenati B, Morelli L, Bessi E, Boehm G. Cesarean delivery may affect the early biodiversity of intestinal bacteria. *J Nutr*. 2008;138:17965–18005.
14. Dominguez-Bello MG, Costello EK, Contreras M, et al. Delivery mode shapes the acquisition and structure of the initial microbiota across multiple body habitats in newborns. *Proc Natl Acad Sci USA*. 2010;107(26):11971–11975.
15. Gronlund MM, Lehtonen OP, Eerola E, Kero P. Fecal microflora in healthy infants born by different methods of delivery: permanent changes in intestinal flora after cesarean delivery. *J Pediatr Gastroenterol Nutr*. 1999;28(1):19–25.
16. Claud EC, Keegan KP, Brulc JM, et al. Bacterial community structure and functional contributions to emergence of health or necrotizing enterocolitis in preterm infants. *Microbiome*. 2013;1(1):20.
17. Yu Y, Lu L, Sun J, Petrof EO, Claud EC. Preterm infant gut microbiota affects intestinal epithelial development in a humanized microbiome gnotobiotic mouse model. *Am J Physiol Gastrointest Liver Physiol*. 2016;311(3):G521–G532.
18. Wang Y, Hoenig JD, Malin KJ, et al. 16S rRNA gene-based analysis of fetal microbiota from preterm infants with and without necrotizing enterocolitis. *ISME J*. 2009;3(8):944–954.
19. Mai V, Young CM, Ukhanova M, et al. Fecal microbiota in premature infants prior to necrotizing enterocolitis. *PLoS One*. 2011;6(6):e20647.
20. Hourigan SK, Ta A, Wong WS, et al. The microbiome in necrotizing enterocolitis: a case report in twins and minireview. *Clin Ther*. 2016;4:747–753.
21. Hunter CJ, Upperman JS, Ford HR, Camerini V. Understanding the susceptibility of the premature infant to necrotizing enterocolitis (NEC). *Pediatr Res*. 2008;63(2):117–123.
22. Lu L, Yu Y, Guo Y, Wang Y, Chang EB, Claud EC. Transcriptional modulation of intestinal innate defense/inflammation genes by preterm infant microbiota in a humanized gnotobiotic mouse model. *PLoS One*. 2015;10(4):e0124504.
23. Siu YK, Ng PC, Fung SC, et al. Double blind, randomized, placebo controlled study of oral vancomycin in prevention of necrotizing enterocolitis in preterm, very low birth-weight infants. *Arch Dis Child Fetal Neonatal Ed*. 1998;79:F105–F109.

24. Bury RG, Tudehope D. Enteral antibiotics for preventing necrotizing enterocolitis in low birth weight or preterm infants. *Cochrane Database Syst Rev.* 2001;1:CD000405.

25. La Rosa PS, Warner BB, Zhou Y, et al. Patterned progression of bacterial populations in the premature infant gut. *Natl Acad Sci.* 2014;111:12522–12527.

26. Cotten CM, Taylor S, Stoll B, et al. Prolonged duration of initial empiric antibiotic treatment is associated with increased rates of necrotizing enterocolitis and death for extremely low birth weight infants. *Pediatrics.* 2009;123(1).

27. Vandenplas Y, Rudolph C, DiLorenzo C, et al. Pediatric gastroesophageal reflux clinical practice guidelines: joint recommendations of the North American Society for Pediatric Gastroenterology, Hepatology, and Nutrition (NASPGHAN) and the European Society for Pediatric Gastroenterology, Hepatology and Nutrition (ESPHGHAN). *J Pediatr Gastroenterol Nutr.* 2009;49:498–547.

28. Fiore JD, Arko M, Herynk, Martin R, Hibbs AM. Characterization of cardiorespiratory events following gastroesophageal reflux in preterm infants. *J Perinatol.* 2010;30:683–687.

29. Safe M, Chan WH, Krishan U. Widespread use of gastric acid inhibitors in infants: are they needed? Are they safe? *World J Gastrointest Pharmacol Ther.* 2016;7:531–539.

30. Kanno T, Matsuki T, Oka M, et al. Gastric acid reduction leads to an alteration in lower intestinal microflora. *Biochem Biophys Res Commun.* 2009;381:666–670.

31. Canani B, Roberto, Terrin, Gianluca. Gastric acidity inhibitors and the risk of intestinal infections. *Gastroenterology.* 2010;26:31–35.

31a. Terrin G, Passariello A, De Curtis M, et al. Ranitidine is associated with infections, necrotizing enterocolitis, and fatal outcome in newborns. *Pediatrics.* 2012;129:e40–e45.

32. Wandall JH. Effects of omeprazole on neutrophil chemotaxis, super oxide production, degranulation, and translocation of cytochrome b-245. *Gut.* 1992;33:617–621.

33. More K, Athalye-Jape G, Rao S, Patole S. Association of inhibitors of gastric acid secretion and higher incidence of necrotizing enterocolitis in preterm very low-birth-weight infants. *Am J Perinatol.* 2013;30(10):849–856.

33a. Guillet R, Stoll BJ, Cotten CM, et al. National Institute of Child Health and Human Development Neonatal Research Network. Association of H2-blocker therapy and higher incidence of necrotizing enterocolitis in very low birth weight infants. *Pediatrics.* 2006;117:e137–e142.

34. Ghirardello S, Dusi E, Cortinovis I, et al. Effects of red blood cell transfusions on the risk of developing complications or death: an observation study of a cohort of very low birth weight infants. *Am J Perinatol.* 2017;34(01):88–95.

35. Kirplani H, Whyte R, Andersen C, et al. The premature infants in need of transfusion (pint) study: a randomized, controlled trial of a restrictive (LOW) versus liberal (HIGH) transfusion threshold for extremely low birth weight infants. *J Pediatr.* 2006:301–307.

36. Kirpalani H, Zupancic JA. Do transfusions cause necrotizing enterocolitis? The complementary role of randomized trials and observational studies. *Semin Perinatol.* 2012;36(4):269–276.

37. Mohamed A, Shah PS. Transfusion associated necrotizing enterocolitis: a meta-analysis of observational data. *Pediatrics.* 2012;129(3):2011–2872.

38. Blau J, Calo JM, Dozor D, Sutton M, Alpan G, La Gamma EF. Transfusion-related acute gut injury: necrotizing enterocolitis in very low birth weight neonates after pack red blood cell transfusion. *J Pediatrics.* 2011;158(3):403–409.

39. Agwu J, Narchi H. In a preterm infant, does blood transfusion increase the risk of necrotizing enterocolitis? *Arch Dis Child.* 2005;90:102–103.

40. Singh R, Visintainer PF, Frantz III D, et al. Association of necrotizing enterocolitis with anemia and packed red blood cell transfusions in preterm infants. *J Perinatol.* 2011;31:176–182.

41. Hyung N, Campwala I, Boskovic D, et al. The relationship of red blood cell transfusion to intestinal mucosal injury to premature infants. *J Pediatr Surg.* 2016;10:49.

42. Keir A, Pal S, Trivella M, et al. Adverse effects of red cell transfusions in neonates: a systematic review and meta-analysis. *Transfusion.* 2016:13785.

43. Moss RL, Kalish LA, Duggan C, et al. Clinical parameters do not adequately predict outcome in necrotizing enterocolitis: a multi-institutional study. *J Perinatol.* 2008;28:665–674.

44. Morgan J, Young L, McGuire W. Slow advancement of enteral feed volumes to prevent necrotizing enterocolitis in very low birth weight infants. *Cochrane Database Syst Rev.* 2015;10:1–32.

45. Snyderman S, Holt LE, Norton PM, Roitman E, Phansalkar SV. The plasma aminogram. I. Influence of the level of protein intake and a comparison of whole protein and amino acid diets. *Pediatr Res.* 1968;2:131–144.

46. Hay WW, Hendrickson KC. Preterm formula use in the preterm very low birth weight infant. *Semin Fetal Neonatal Med.* 2016;10:1–16.

47. Radmacher PG, Adamkin MD, Lewis ST, Adamkin DH. Milk as a vehicle for oral medications: hidden osmoles. *J Perinatol.* 2012;32:227–229.

48. Frost BL, Jilling T, Lapin B, Maheshwari A, Caplan MS. Maternal breast milk transforming growth factor-beta and feeding intolerance in preterm infants. *Pediatr Res.* 2014;76:386–393.

49. Caplan MS, Amer M, Jilling T. The role of human milk in necrotizing enterocolitis. *Adv Exp Med Biol.* 2002;503:83–90.

50. Grady NG, Petrof EO, Claud EC. Microbial therapeutic interventions. *Semin Fetal Neonatal Med.* 2016;21(6):418–423.

51. Coppa GV, Zampini L, Galeazzi T, Gabrielli O. Prebiotics in human milk: a review. *Dig Liver Dis.* 2006;38:291–294.

52. Abrams SA, Schanler RJ, Lee M, Rechtman D. *Breastfeed Med.* 2014;9(6):281–285.

53. Penn AH, Altshuler AE, Small JW, Taylor SF, Dobkins KR, Schmid-Schonbein GW. Digested formula but not digested fresh human milk causes death of intestinal cells in vitro: implications for necrotizing enterocolitis. *Pediatr Res*. 2012;72:560–567.

54. Cristofalo EA, Schanler RJ, Blanco CL, et al. Randomized trial of exclusive human milk versus preterm formula diets in extremely premature infants. *J Pediatr*. 2013;163:1592–1596.

55. McGuire W, Anthony MY. Donor human milk versus formula for preventing necrotizing enterocolitis in preterm infants: systematic review. *Arch Dis Child Fetal Neonatal Ed*. 2003;88:11–14.

56. Schanler RJ, Lau C, Hurst NM, Smith EO. Randomized trial of donor human milk versus preterm formula as substitutes for mothers' own milk in the feeding of extremely premature infants. *Pediatrics*. 2005;116:400–406.

57. Sullivan S, Schanler RJ, Kim JH, et al. An exclusively human milk-based diet is associated with a lower rate of necrotizing enterocolitis than a diet of human milk and bovine milk-based products. *J Pediatr*. 2010;156:562–567.

58. Underwood M. Impact of probiotics on necrotizing enterocolitis. *Semin Perinatology*. 2016: S0146–S0005(16).

59. Goncalves FL, Soares LM, Figueira RL, Simoes AL, Gallindo RM, Sbragia L. Evaluation of the expression of I-FABP and L-FABP in a necrotizing enterocolitis model after the use of Lactobacillus acidophilus. *J Pediatr Surg*. 2015;50(4):543–549.

60. Borthakur A, Bhattacharyya S, Kumar A, Anbazhagan AN, Tobacman JK, Dudeja PK. Lactobacillus acidophilus alleviates platelet-activating factor-induced inflammatory responses in human intestinal epithelial cells. *PLoS One*. 2013;8(10):e75664.

61. Wickramasinghe S, Pacheco AR, Lemay DG, Mills DA. Bifidobacteria grown on human milk oligosaccharides downregulate the expression of inflammation-related genes in Caco-2 cells. *BMC Microbiol*. 2015;15:172.

62. Bertelsen RJ, Jensen ET, Ringel-Kulka T. Use of probiotics and prebiotics in infant feeding. *Best Practice Res Clin Gastroenterol*. 2016;30(1):39–48.

63. Hoyos AB. Reduced incidence of necrotizing enterocolitis associated with enteral administration of Lactobacillus acidophilus and Bifidobacterium infantis to neonates in an intensive care unit. *Int J Infect Dis*. 1999;3(4):197–202.

64. Sawh SC, Deshpande S, Jansen S, Reynaert CJ, Jones PM. Prevention of necrotizing enterocolitis with probiotics: a systematic review and meta-analysis. *PeerJ*. 2016;4:e2429.

65. Chioukh FZ, Ben Hmida H, Ben Ameur K, Toumi A, Monastiri K. Saccharomyces cerevisiae fungemia in a premature neonate treated receiving antibiotics. *Med Mal Infect*. 2013;43(8):359–360.

66. Dani C, Biadaioli R, Bertini G, Martelli R, Rubaltelli FF. Probiotics feeding in prevention of urinary tract infection, bacterial sepsis and necrotizing enterocolitis in preterm infants: a prospective double-blind study. *Biol Neonate*. 2002;82:103–108.

CHAPTER 7

Nutrition for the Surgical Neonate

Holly J. Engelstad, MD, Brad W. Warner, MD

Introduction

Surgical procedures are not infrequent among patients admitted to regional neonatal intensive care units. It is estimated that 24.1% of referrals are for surgical evaluation and management and that 32% of admitted neonates undergo minor or major operations.[1] Adequate nutrition in the newborn period, especially during times of critical illness and "stress," is necessary to decrease the morbidity and mortality associated with malnutrition. Additionally, many surgical patients are at risk for long-term growth failure and nutritional deficiencies. This chapter aims to address critical elements in understanding the metabolic stress response and the nutritional management of surgical neonates.

Growth in Surgical Neonates

Somatic growth is an important marker of appropriate nutritional support and the general health of infants and children. Growth has classically been monitored as weight gain over time; however, as more attention has been given to weight gain and nutrition, there has been a shift toward a focus on linear growth and body composition.[2] Linear growth and fat free mass represent protein accretion, lean body mass, and organ development. Inflammation and prolonged illnesses have been proposed to disrupt normal linear growth velocity and therefore are associated with stunting.[2] Surgical neonates represent a special population at risk for growth failure, given the heightened inflammatory response to surgical stress, risk for malabsorption, and other comorbidities, which place them at risk for infection, such as with central venous access. Infants with gastroschisis, congenital diaphragmatic hernia (CDH), and short gut syndrome (SGS) (including infants with gastroschisis, intestinal atresia, and necrotizing enterocolitis [NEC] as primary diagnoses) have all been associated with poor weight gain, linear growth, and head circumference during the first year of life.[3-6] This is in contrast to the usual presentation of malnutrition, which disproportionately affects weight and typically spares height and head circumference. Linear growth stunting has been identified as an independent predictor of neurodevelopmental delay in premature infants,[7] but few studies have examined the long-term effects of failure to thrive in the surgical cohort of patients.

Surgical Stress Response to Operative Trauma and Critical Illness

After injury or trauma the body undergoes a series of hormonal and metabolic alterations known as the *metabolic stress response*. This effect has been most extensively studied in adults and has been shown to increase pituitary hormone secretion, sympathetic nervous system stimulation, and activate a proinflammatory cascade. Pituitary hormones, such as adenocorticotropic hormone and arginine vasopressin, are released to initiate catabolism and maintain cardiovascular homeostasis.[8] Neonates are also able to mount a metabolic response after surgical stress that results in increased catecholamines, cytokines, and counterregulatory hormones, such as glucagon and cortisol, which further stimulate catabolism.[9] However, this response is often more severe and of shorter duration compared with that in older children and adults.[10,11] The increased metabolic response directly opposes the anabolic actions of insulin, growth hormone, and insulin-like growth factor 1.[12] During catabolism, protein from muscle is degraded to release free amino acids for the synthesis of proteins needed for the inflammatory response (cytokines, acute phase reactants) and tissue repair.[13] The remaining carbon skeletons are then converted to glucose through gluconeogenesis in the liver. Factors affecting the surgical stress response include age, fasting status before surgery, degree of operative stress, anesthesia, and the surgical approach.[11,14]

Energy Requirements During Stress

Energy homeostasis is the balance of energy influx and outflow. Providing the appropriate amount of energy to meet the needs of energy homeostasis is important in the nutritional management of the surgical neonate. Underestimation of energy needs can result in malnutrition, loss of muscle mass, and poor wound healing,[15] whereas overestimation can result in increased risk of infection, liver damage, and hyperglycemia.[16] This may be particularly challenging in the surgical neonate because energy expenditure is variable, making the use of standard predictive equations generally inaccurate.

Total energy expenditure comprises three main components: resting energy expenditure (REE), energy required for physical activity, and diet-induced thermogenesis.[17] Surgical infants are generally considered to be at rest for 80% to 90% of the time; therefore energy needs are primarily dependent on REE.[18]

The gold standard for the measurement of REE is direct calorimetry whereby patients are placed in a thermally isolated chamber that measures dissipated heat for a certain period. It is impractical to use direct calorimetry in hospitalized patients. However, through the use of breath measurements, indirect calorimetry offers a portable and equivalent alternative.[19] Indirect calorimetry measures the amount of oxygen consumed (VO_2) and the amount of carbon dioxide produced (VCO_2) and then uses a correction factor based on urinary nitrogen excretion, which calculates the overall rate of energy production. Indirect calorimetry also provides the measurement of the respiratory quotient (RQ), which is determined by the ratio of VCO_2 to VO_2 and is a marker of substrate use.[20] The RQ generally ranges from 0.85 to −1.0, with values >1.0 indicating the presence of lipogenesis, typically as a result of overfeeding.[21] It is important to note that indirect calorimetry is not accurate in the setting of air leaks around the endotracheal tube, ventilator circuit, or chest tube, or in those with a fraction of inspired oxygen >0.6.[22]

Indirect calorimetry can be technically challenging to perform; therefore its use should be reserved for special populations of infants. The use of predictive energy expenditure equations, such as the Schofield, Harris-Benedict, or World Health Organization equations, have been proposed but have largely been found to be inaccurate because of individual variation in energy expenditure.[23] As a practical guide, estimated energy requirements for comparable "nonstressed" neonates are used as a starting point to determine energy provisions for the stressed neonate. Generally, newborns require 40 to 70 kcal/kg/day for maintenance metabolism, 50 to 70 kcal/kg/day for growth, and 20 kcal/kg/day for fecal and urinary losses.[17] The total energy requirement of an enterally fed term newborn infant is therefore in the range of 100 to 120 kcal/kg/day. Preterm infants may require even more energy than term infants. Parenterally fed newborns do not have losses of energy or diet-induced thermogenesis and therefore their energy requirement is about 80 to 100 kcal/kg/day.[17] It is recognized that this may be quite inaccurate, and careful monitoring of head circumference, weight, length, and weight for length is therefore necessary.

The REE in surgical neonates is only moderately elevated postoperatively, and this increase is short-lived. Conflicting reports about REE after surgical procedures in neonates have been published[24-27]; however, this likely the result of different timings of the studies in relation to surgery and small sample sizes. REE has been shown to increase 15% to 25% by 4 hours after major abdominal surgery in infants and return to normal by 12 to 24 hours postoperatively.[25] Therefore studies occurring >24 hours postoperatively would not show an elevation in REE. However, there is paucity of data regarding REE in neonates who remain critically ill and are dependent on parenteral nutrition for a prolonged time. In adults, REE can be increased by 20% to 80% and remain elevated for >30 days after major trauma to compensate for the energy required for tissue repair.[28] It is thought that the minimal change in energy expenditure seen in infants is a result of diversion of protein and energy normally spent on growth to tissue repair and healing, placing surgical infants at risk for growth retardation during metabolic stress. Careful monitoring of head circumference, weight, length, and weight for length is necessary over time. Surgical neonates may benefit from more exact measurement of their REE by indirect calorimetry to provide the appropriate energy prescription.

Macronutrient Metabolism and Requirements During Stress

Amino acids, carbohydrates, and lipids are the three macronutrients needed for growth and metabolism. The processing of macronutrients changes to support the body's new metabolic needs after surgery or periods of "stress."

Nearly 98% of amino acids are found in proteins with the remainder available as free amino acids. Through protein turnover, amino acids are released from protein breakdown and are available for protein synthesis to meet physiologic needs. This dynamic process makes amino acids the most important building blocks used for tissue growth and recovery. Neonates have high protein turnover rates (6-12 g/kg/day) and need to remain in a positive nitrogen balance to achieve appropriate growth and development.[29] This is in contrast to adults, who are not in a period of active growth. Their protein turnover is less (4 g/kg/day),[30] and they remain in a neutral nitrogen balance.

An 80% increase in protein turnover is noted in critically ill neonates and persists throughout the duration of illness.[31] Similarly, infants with cardiopulmonary failure who are supported on extracorporeal life support (ECLS) exhibit nearly double the amount of protein turnover compared with stable patients.[32] The accelerated protein turnover during stress facilitates the redistribution of amino acids from skeletal muscle to injured tissues. The enhanced catabolism of skeletal muscle is the fastest way to provide amino acids and glucose for ill neonates. However, protein stores in neonates are considerably less than in adults, and when protein turnover predominates over synthesis, it places critically ill neonates in a state of negative nitrogen balance.[33] This is clinically evident as skeletal muscle wasting, impaired growth, delayed immune response, and poor wound healing.

Amino acid supplementation improves nitrogen balance in surgical patients by supporting protein synthesis.[34] The minimum amino acid requirement of term surgical patients to prevent protein catabolism is 1 to 1.5 g/kg/day of amino acids; however, infants who received 2.5 g/kg/day had improved nitrogen balance without evidence of protein intolerance.[34] Even higher protein administration may be tolerated in this subgroup of patients, as it is known to be beneficial and safe to provide intravenous (IV) amino acid solutions of 3.5 to 4 g/kg/day to very low–birth weight preterm neonates,[35,36] but amino acid infusions at this rate have not been studied in the neonatal surgical population. Some neonates who have extensive protein losses through ostomies or who are already severely malnourished may require additional protein supplementation.

Protein provides 4 cal/g of amino acid and therefore is limited in the amount of energy that can be prescribed by protein administration. Carbohydrates in parenteral nutrition also provide 4 cal/g of carbohydrate but can be infused at a higher rate than amino acids. Lipids provide a more concentrated amount of calories at 9 cal/g of lipid. Therefore the oxidation of both carbohydrates and lipids provides the primary sources of energy as adenosine triphosphate, whereas protein is utilized for protein synthesis and growth.

The most important carbohydrate is glucose. Glucose is the primary substrate used in nearly all organs but is of particular importance in the brain, renal medulla, and red blood cells, where it is used as an obligate energy source.[17] Adults are easily able to mobilize glucose from glycogen during times of increased energy requirement. However, glycogen stores are limited in the term neonate and even more so in the preterm population. The limited availability of glycogen necessitates an exogenous supply of glucose, which is commonly administered as D-dextrose, a monohydrate form for IV use.[37] However, during times of stress, endogenous glucose production continues despite administration of IV glucose.[38] Endogenous glucose is produced through glycogenolysis, gluconeogenesis from protein catabolism, and peripheral insulin resistance, which can result in hyperglycemia.[39] Indeed, hyperglycemia has been identified postoperatively in patients with NEC and is associated with increased morbidity and mortality.[40] Currently there are no recommendation regarding the routine administration of exogenous insulin to treat stress-induced hyperglycemia.[41] Insulin administration may be considered when hyperglycemia persists despite reduction in glucose infusion rate (GIR) and correction of other underlying causes of hyperglycemia, such as sepsis. No changes in morbidity and mortality have been seen in postoperative cardiac cases with tight glycemic control.[42] Careful monitoring of blood glucose during provision of insulin therapy is necessary to prevent hypoglycemia. Because of extreme sensitivity to insulin, however, its use in neonates is rare.

Glucose provided in excess of energy needs or in excess of the rate of glucose oxidation (RGO) will be converted to fat through the process of lipogenesis, which may increase the baseline energy expenditure.[17] This process can result in metabolic acidosis, increase in VCO_2 and can induce hepatic steatosis through the inability to export very-low-density lipoproteins at the same rate it is produced.[17] In term surgical neonates and infants on long-term parenteral nutrition, the RGO has been found to be 18 g/kg/day,[43] which corresponds to a GIR of 12 mg/kg/min. Therefore it is not recommended to exceed this amount in supplementation through parenteral nutrition in the surgical neonate.

Energy provided exclusively through carbohydrates has been associated with increased VCO_2, VO_2, and energy expenditure.[25] The untoward effects of excess glucose administration can be minimized by diversifying the nonprotein energy source through providing a lipid emulsion.[43-46] It is recommended to provide 25% to 40% of nonprotein calories as lipids, which generally can be translated to 2 to 4 g/kg/day of IV lipid emulsion.[47] Lipids are calorically dense and isosmotic, and this makes them appropriate to be delivered peripherally if no central access can be obtained. Soy-based lipids provide the essential fatty acids (EFAs) linoleic (an omega-6 fatty acid [FA]) and alpha-linolenic (an omega-3 FA), which are necessary to prevent EFA deficiency, which can occur rapidly in preterm neonates because of limited stores of lipids.[48]

During times of critical illness and stress, lipids are used preferentially in oxidation.[33] Increased lipid metabolism can result in lipid peroxidation and free radical formation, which may be an important mediator in oxygen-induced tissue damage.[49,50] However, it has been shown that exogenous lipid administration is tolerated during times of stress[51] and does not need to be stopped during times of stress or sepsis. Many have concern regarding the development of hypertriglyceridemia with IV infusion of lipid emulsions and the potential adverse effects of elevated serum triglyceride levels, such as impaired oxygenation from lipid microemboli,[52] altered pulmonary vascular tone,[53] displacement of bilirubin from albumin causing hyperbilirubinemia,[54] and immunosuppression.[55] Monitoring of triglyceride levels could be considered during times of critical illness and adjustments made if lipid accumulation is identified.[47] Many practitioners would consider lipid intolerance at >150 to 250 mg/dL in the preterm neonate. However, there are no data regarding the maximum triglyceride concentrations that would be considered unsafe in a surgical neonate.

One significant side effect of long-term administration of parenteral nutrition is cholestasis, defined as a conjugated bilirubin ≥2 mg/dL.[17] Cholestasis can start as steatosis, progress to bile duct proliferation and fibrosis, and ultimately result in cirrhosis and liver failure. The incidence of cholestasis is >50% in infants maintained on parenteral nutrition for >2 months[56-58]; this risk is higher in the surgical subpopulation with SGS, including those with gastroschisis, intestinal atresia, and NEC.[58,59]

IV lipids have been implicated as a causative agent in the development of parenteral nutrition–associated cholestasis (PNAC). Until recently, the only available lipid emulsion in the United States was derived from soybean oil (Intralipid). Plant-based lipid emulsions contain phytosterols and a greater amount of proinflammatory omega-6 FAs compared with the anti-inflammatory omega-3 FAs. Both the phytosterols and omega-6 FAs have been implicated in the pathogenesis of PNAC.[60,61] Current strategies in reversing cholestasis include lipid reduction (1 g/kg lipid 1-3 times per week) and advancement of enteral nutrition, if tolerated. However, if lipid reduction is undertaken, it is important to not compensate for decreased caloric intake by increasing the GIR over the RGO (18 g/kg/day) as previously mentioned. This will only increase the RQ to >1.0 and result in lipogenesis. In these cases it may be preferential to allow lower caloric intake. Other strategies that have evolved in recent years include alternative lipid emulsions, including fish oil (Omegaven)[62] and combination oils (SMOF, Clinolipid).[63] Fish oil contains a greater amount of omega-3 FAs compared with omega-6 FAs and do not contain phytosterols. Additionally, fish oil contains a greater amount of alpha-tocopherol, a vitamin E isoform that acts as a potent anti-inflammatory molecule that inhibits lipid peroxidation and oxidative stress.[64] Fish oil has been shown to reverse the effects of cholestasis,[65] but there is insufficient evidence in the prevention of cholestasis. Currently the fish oil emulsion, Omegaven, is only available in the United States through the Food and Drug Administration (FDA) under a compassionate use protocol; therefore it is not widely available. In 2016 the FDA approved the use of SMOFlipid in adults. SMOFlipid is a combination oil composed of 30% soy oil, 30% medium-chain triglycerides, 25% olive oil, and 15% fish oil. It contains intermediary amounts of EFAs, omega-6 FAs, omega-3 FAs, alpha-tocopherol, and phytosterols compared with pure soy and fish oils, but has shown to have some benefit in reversing cholestasis compared with soy oil in small studies.[63,66] The surgical neonatal subpopulation may benefit from the use of alternative lipid emulsions; however, larger randomized trials are needed to further study safety and efficacy in the neonatal and pediatric populations.

Micronutrient Metabolism and Requirements

Micronutrients are composed of vitamins and trace elements that are essential for many of the metabolic processes in the body. In surgical neonates, the metabolism of these micronutrients may be altered during times of stress, or these infants may experience excessive loss through diarrhea or ostomy output.[67] Essential trace elements include zinc, iron, copper, selenium, manganese, iodide, molybdenum, and chromium. Vitamins can be divided into water soluble (ascorbic acid, thiamine, ribo-flavin, pyridoxine, niacin, folate, vitamin B_{12}) and fat soluble (vitamins A, E, D, K). These vitamins and minerals are routinely administered through parenteral nutrition while advancing enteral nutrition. Other trace minerals, such as iodine and iron, are not typically provided in parenteral nutrition. In the surgical neonate iron is obtained through periodic blood transfusions[67] or additional supplementation, whereas iodine is absorbed through application of skin disinfectants, such as betadine.[67]

During times of critical illness and hypermetabolism, certain micronutrients, such as vitamins C and E and the trace element selenium, become important as antioxidants neutralizing the effects of reactive oxygen species produced through increased oxidative metabolism. Surgical neonates suffering from diarrhea or excessive ostomy losses may require increased supplementation of micronutrients, specifically zinc and selenium.[68] Selenium deficiency has been associated with an increased risk of infections in neonates.[69] Zinc deficiency has also been associated with predisposition to infection in addition to failure to thrive, poor wound healing, and impaired immune function, making zinc one of the most important micronutrients to the surgical neonate.[67,68,70]

Copper and manganese are both excreted through the biliary system and may accumulate in the liver of surgical neonates with hepatic failure from parenteral nutrition–associated cholestasis.[67] This may contribute to toxic levels of copper and manganese, and therefore supplementation with these minerals should be reduced or discontinued when the direct bilirubin reaches >2 mg/dL.

Periodic monitoring of trace vitamins and minerals is recommended in surgical neonates at risk for micronutrient deficiencies or toxicities. Either supplementation or reduction in micronutrients may be required in the surgical neonate.

Fluid and Electrolyte Requirements

Drastic fluid shifts and electrolyte imbalances can be seen in the immediate post-operative period in neonates undergoing surgical interventions. These changes are most evident in neonates who are critically ill and undergoing operations, such as those with NEC. They often experience third spacing of fluid and electrolytes as a result of capillary leak and may develop tachycardia and hypotension requiring fluid bolus administration. These infants require careful monitoring of serum electrolytes (Na^+, K^+, Ca^{2+}, Cl^-, HCO_3^-, Mg^{2+}, P^-) and fluid balance with adjustment in IV fluid components, as needed.

In the surgical neonate, metabolic acidosis can be caused by a variety of mechanisms. Metabolic acidosis can be the result of poor tissue perfusion after surgical procedure, or it can be caused by gastrointestinal (GI) losses of bicarbonate as seen in infants with ostomies.[71] It is important to recognize the cause of the metabolic acidosis because they are treated differently. Surgical intervention in a critically ill neonate may result in hypotension and poor tissue perfusion. This is oftentimes managed by replacing chloride with acetate in IV fluids because hyperchloremia can exacerbate metabolic acidosis. However, in this setting, providing a base will not correct the underlying cause of acidosis and may cause hypercarbia.[72] In this case, providing volume resuscitation and vasoactive medications to improve tissue perfusion may be required. Additionally, acute metabolic acidosis as seen in critically ill neonates causes hyperkalemia through the shifting of intracellular potassium to the extracellular space to buffer hydrogen ions into the cell. Correcting the underlying acidosis will correct the hyperkalemia in most situations, but careful monitoring of potassium is required. Potassium may need to be removed from IV fluids if urine output ceases.

GI losses of electrolytes through ostomy output generally represent more chronic loss rather than critical illness after surgical intervention. These patients require electrolyte replacements and are primarily at risk for sodium and bicarbonate losses.[73] GI fluid and electrolyte losses can be exacerbated by the osmotic load of enteral nutrition known as "dumping" syndrome which may prevent the advancement of enteral nutrition. An average of 3.3 mEq/kg/day of sodium may be lost through normal ostomy output.[74] In cases of extreme sodium losses, aldosterone stimulates absorption of sodium in the proximal renal tubules. This leaves little sodium to participate in the sodium–hydrogen ion exchange in the distal renal tubule, thereby limiting the kidney's ability to correct the metabolic acidosis caused by GI bicarbonate loss.[75] An equation to assist in calculating sodium supplementation is "Na intake" = 1.2 mEq + (0.13 × ostomy output in mL/kg/day). Another common consequence of sodium deficits and metabolic acidosis is failure to thrive that improves after adequate sodium supplementation with or without bicarbonate supplementation.[75] Patients with ostomies should be monitored closely with measurement of ostomy output, urine sodium, and serum sodium, bicarbonate, and chloride on a regular basis until stable.[74,75] A urine sodium >10 mEq/L indicates adequate serum sodium reaching the distal renal tubules. Sodium chloride supplementation should be considered if urine sodium <10 mEq/L.

Routes of Nutrient Provision

Enteral nutrition is the preferred route of nutrient delivery in the surgical patient with intact GI function. Enteral nutrition stimulates the intestine to release regulatory polypeptides and GI hormones that stimulate gut motility, enzyme release, mucosal growth, and blood flow.[76,77] These factors are required to coordinate the systemic digestive processes that occur with ingestion of nutrients.

Enteral nutrition is integral in maintaining normal villus structure and epithelial cell barrier function.[78] The villi and microvilli increase the absorptive surface area of the intestine and are absorbed into blood vessels that are able to transfer nutrients systemically. Lack of enteral nutrition causes villus atrophy and disruption in barrier function.[78] Infants unable to tolerate enteral nutrition have an increased risk of infection and immunologic complications.[79] However, villus atrophy improves when even a small amount of enteral nutrition is provided.[78] Additionally, enteral nutrition plays an important role in the process of intestinal adaptation in patients who have had a massive intestinal resection.[80,81]

For neonates, the preferred enteral nutrition is maternal breast milk. However, if maternal breast milk is unavailable, then donor breast milk could be considered, especially in low–birth weight premature infants with a history of NEC. Breast milk carries important immunologic and anti-infective properties. However, when breast milk is not available, the ideal enteral formula would be one that is easily digestible and provide appropriate nutrients.[17,81] Many surgical neonates have issues with malabsorption, specifically fat malabsorption,[17,82] and may require an elemental formula that provides amino acids, glucose, and medium-chain triglycerides. It is not recommended to immediately fortify formula or breast milk because this increases the osmolality and may worsen malabsorption. Fortification may be considered once volume tolerance has been established to provide adequate vitamins, minerals, and calories to promote growth.

Enteral nutrition should be initiated as small volume continuous feeds and advanced as tolerated.[81,83] In patients with motility, reflux or malabsorption issues, continuous feeds are better tolerated and allow for continuous saturation of carrier proteins.[83] Careful monitoring of stool output is required in patients with ostomies. Stool output approaching 30 to 40 mL/kg/day should be advanced cautiously, and it is generally a contraindication to advance feeds if stool output reaches >40 mL/kg/day. If there is concern about aspiration, then post-pyloric feeds can be initiated via nasojejunal or surgical insertion of a gastrojejunal or jejunal tube.[81] Post-pyloric feedings should always be delivered continuously, whereas gastric feeds can be transitioned to bolus feedings if full continuous feeds are tolerated. Bolus feedings are the most physiologic and allow for normal functioning of the extrahepatic biliary tree and stimulation of GI hormones. In patients on continuous feeds, the gallbladder becomes enlarged and noncontractile,[84] but upon initiation of bolus feedings, the gallbladder begins normal feeding-associated contraction.[85]

Parenteral nutrition is initiated when enteral nutrition cannot support the energy demands of the neonate. Patients with short bowel syndrome and other surgical patients with obstructive or motility issues, such as gastroschisis, atresia, or long-segment Hirschsprung disease represent a specific cohort of patients who are at risk for negative effects associated with long-term parenteral nutrition.[59] Parenteral nutrition is associated with increased risk of sepsis and venous thrombosis, given the need for central IV access.[86] The components of parenteral nutrition may have detrimental effects as previously discussed, the most significant being cholestasis associated with the use of soybean oil as an IV lipid emulsion. In addition to various lipid strategies outlined above, the most effective treatment for parenteral nutrition–associated cholestasis or intestinal failure–associated liver disease is advancement of enteral nutrition and cessation of parenteral nutrition.

Medications and Supplements

The surgical neonate often has long-term issues with feeding intolerance because of malabsorption or dysmotility; in many instances, alteration in feeding strategies is not sufficient to overcome a limited intestinal absorptive surface area. Therefore additional agents that assist in motility, absorption, and adaptation could be useful. However, there is limited evidence to support the use of medications, such as pancreatic enzymes, probiotics, bile acids, growth factors, antimotility agents, and antisecretory agents, to assist in the nutritional support of the surgical neonate.[87] Additionally, medication pharmacokinetics may be abnormal because of the varying degrees of absorption and bowel integrity.

In cases of cholestasis associated with parenteral nutrition in the surgical neonate, ursodiol, a bile acid that enhances hepatic bile flow, may be useful in correcting the biochemical alterations, but its long-term efficacy has not been studied.[87] A trial of ursodiol may be considered in patients with intestinal failure–associated liver disease. The only caveat is that patients must be able to tolerate some enteral nutrition because ursodiol is an oral medication.

Oral fish oil is a promising supplement in patients with SGS or in those who otherwise require prolonged parenteral nutrition and are at risk for cholestasis.[64] Enteral fat is isosmotic and therefore does not contribute to GI fluid losses as do hyperosmotic fluids, such as fortified formulas. It is also calorically dense and has been shown to decrease the need for intravenously supplemented fat.[80] Enteral fish oil provided as a combination of omega 6 and omega 3 FAs has been shown to improve weight and height velocity, decrease conjugated bilirubin, and result in fewer episodes of sepsis compared with standard parenteral nutrition without oral fat supplementation.[88] However, further studies are needed to confirm safety and efficacy before oral fish oil can be recommended.

Special Disease Considerations

Necrotizing Enterocolitis

NEC remains one of the most devastating complications of prematurity. The incidence of NEC overtime has remained relatively stable, ranging from 7% to 15% of premature infants <1500 g.[89] Approximately 27% of infants with NEC undergo a surgical procedure because of NEC, which may result in loss of bowel length and altered intestinal motility.[90] Whether the bowel is placed in continuity or discontinuity as well as the location and amount of resected bowel is important.[91] These factors affect the nutritional support patients with NEC require postoperatively. The duodenum and the jejunum are the primary digestive and absorptive sites of macro- and micronutrients, whereas the ileum is the primary site of absorption of fat-soluble vitamins (A, E, D, and K), vitamin B_{12}, and zinc.[92] Nutrient deficiencies should be anticipated on the basis of the site of resection but may change over time because of the process of adaptation. In general, the ileum is better able to undergo adaptation compared with the duodenum and the jejunum, in both the structure and function of the intestine.[92] For infants with substantial bowel loss, feeds ideally composed of breast milk should be initiated as small-volume continuous feeds.[81,83] Strictures and adhesions are common in these patients, and therefore if feeds are not tolerated, then a contrast study or exploratory laparotomy should be performed to evaluate for persistent obstruction.

Abdominal Wall Defects

Neonates with gastroschisis and omphaloceles represent a cohort of patients with anterior abdominal wall defects. Those patients with small omphaloceles reach full enteral feedings faster than those with giant omphaloceles (4 days versus 8 days, respectively).[93] The sac covering the intestine in these patients is protective of the bowel. The intestine in patients with omphalocele (other than being abnormally rotated) is functionally normal. As such, feeding advancement is infrequently delayed except in the immediate perioperative period of abdominal wall closure. In contrast, the intestine of patients with gastroschisis is frequently damaged because of amniotic fluid exposure as well as ischemia induced by the small opening in the abdominal wall, resulting in constriction of the blood supply. The degree of intestinal injury ranges from mild swelling to frank necrosis. Patients with gastroschisis are typically slow to reach full enteral feeding volumes because of intestinal dysmotility or the presence of intestinal atresia or short gut.[94] The median time to reach full enteral feedings in gastroschisis patients is 30 days (5-160 days).[95,96]

Intestinal Atresia

Infants with intestinal atresia overall have low mortality but may have variable morbidity during the time it takes for transition from parenteral to enteral nutrition based on location of atresia.[97] Data suggest a median of 10 days (7-20 days) for infants with duodenal atresia, 17 days (9-40 days) for jejunal or ileal atresia, and 4 days (0-20 days) for colonic atresia.[97]

Short Gut Syndrome

SGS is a malabsorptive state occurring after bowel resection or as a result of congenital bowel anomalies. The etiologies of SGS include NEC (35%), complicated meconium ileus (20%), abdominal wall defects (12.5%), intestinal atresia (10%), and volvulus (10%).[98] SGS can be divided into three anatomical subtypes: (1) small bowel resection (SBR) with intestinal–colonic anastomosis; (2) SBR and partial colon resection with enterocolonic anastomosis; and (3) SBR with high-output jejunostomy.[98] Patients with type 1 subtypes have the best potential for adaptation and ability to wean from parenteral nutrition, whereas those with type 3 are the most nutritionally challenging due to high rates of dumping syndrome and risk of dehydration and malnutrition.[98] Patients with SGS are at risk for macro- and micronutrient deficiencies, depending on the site of resection. These patients should be monitored closely for signs of malnutrition and dehydration. Many patients with SGS are dependent on partial or total parenteral nutrition to prevent malnutrition and dehydration. These patients are at risk for developing intestinal failure associated liver disease or PNAC, defined as an elevated conjugated bilirubin >2 mg/dL. Cholestasis may result in hepatic steatosis, fibrosis, or failure that may necessitate liver transplantation or may result in death. Lipids have been implicated as a potential cause of cholestasis, as previously described. These patients should be monitored closely for signs of cholestasis and adjustments in parenteral nutrition should be made as tolerated. Another special consideration in patients with SGS is small bowel bacterial overgrowth (SBBO), which may cause feeding intolerance, abdominal distension, diarrhea, or high ostomy output.[99] This may disrupt enteral feedings and contribute to prolonged need for parenteral nutrition. In patients with SBBO, it is recommended that antibiotics be cycled or enteral nutrition decreased to prevent overgrowth symptoms.[99]

Congenital Diaphragmatic Hernia

Infants with CDH are at risk for failure to thrive in the short term and the long term.[3,4,100] Immediately after birth, these patients are placed under fluid restriction and are therefore unable to receive adequate calories through parenteral nutrition. Exact timing of initiation of enteral feedings in patients with CDH is variable, and no consensus statement exists. This, in part, results from variable clinical courses and timing of surgical repair. In the long term, patients with CDH often have feeding intolerance because of gastroesophageal reflux and oral aversion.[100,101] These patients may require fundoplication and gastrostomy tube placement to receive adequate calories.

Extracorporeal Life Support

Optimal feeding practices for infants on ECLS have not been well established. The primary populations of infants requiring ECLS in the newborn period are those with CDH, respiratory failure most commonly from pulmonary hypertension, or congenital heart disease.[102] Early nutrition in this population is important because the infants experience greater protein catabolism and may require up to 3 g/kg/day of protein supplementation given parenterally.[32] However, their overall energy requirement is similar to that of healthy newborns,[24] and therefore they should receive similar goal calories. With regard to enteral nutrition, there is a theoretical concern about splanchnic hypoperfusion disrupting the intestinal integrity of patients who require ECLS.[103] There have been a few small studies evaluating the safety of enteral nutrition in neonatal and pediatric patients on ECLS, and no significant differences in outcomes were found when compared with the outcomes of those receiving full parenteral nutrition.[104,105] One of the main limitations in providing adequate nutrition in a patient supported on ECLS is volume restriction, which is typically 100 mL/kg/day, with up to 20 mL/kg/day of the total volume dedicated to continuous infusion of medications.[105] A potential solution could be excluding initial enteral feeds from total fluid calculations until they exceed 30 to 40 mL/kg/day; however, the safety and efficacy of this has not been studied. Current practice is to start nutritional support promptly with parenteral nutrition and to introduce enteral nutrition when the infants exhibit normal GI function and are no longer hemodynamically labile.[103]

Summary

Surgical neonates represent a special population at risk of nutrient deficiencies and growth failure, given the stress response to surgery and critical illness, as well as short-term and long-term feeding challenges. Adequate nutrition in the newborn period is crucial to prevent these deficiencies and to promote appropriate growth during early life. Although many advancements have been made over time to help support these patients during the perioperative period and beyond, further studies are needed to guide the care of these neonates. Many of the studies performed to identify protein, carbohydrate, and fat requirements in surgical neonates included only small numbers of patients several years ago and therefore should be repeated to accurately reflect current clinical management strategies and nutritional support. No studies have been recently performed to identify the appropriate composition of amino acid solutions; and although it has been proven that 2.5 g/kg/day of amino acid supplementation is safe in the surgical neonate, many of these patients may require even higher amount of supplementation to support adequate somatic growth. Additionally there are many new lipid emulsions, such as SMOF and Omegaven, that offer promising results in the treatment and prevention of cholestasis associated with conventional soy-based lipid emulsions, but further studies are needed to establish safety and efficacy in the surgical neonate before the widespread use of these products can be endorsed.

Overall, nutritional support remains challenging in this population, and attention to both short-term and long-term growth, including weight and length, in these infants is important. Recently more attention has been paid to the effects of linear growth failure and the potential association between impaired neurodevelopmental outcomes and linear stunting. Long-term outcomes, such as linear growth, body composition, and neurodevelopment, need to be evaluated in the surgical subpopulation to help guide the nutritional management of these infants.

REFERENCES

1. Murthy K, et al. The children's hospitals neonatal database: an overview of patient complexity, outcomes and variation in care. *J Perinatol*. 2014;34(8):582–586.
2. Dougherty KA, Stallings VA. *Growth and body composition in children with chronic disease*. 2013:3–11.
3. Haliburton B, et al. Long-term nutritional morbidity for congenital diaphragmatic hernia survivors: failure to thrive extends well into childhood and adolescence. *J Pediatr Surg*. 2015;50(5):734–738.

4. Leeuwen L, et al. Growth in children with congenital diaphragmatic hernia during the first year of life. *J Pediatr Surg*. 2014;49(9):1363–1366.
5. Minutillo C, et al. Growth and developmental outcomes of infants with gastroschisis at one year of age: a retrospective study. *J Pediatr Surg*. 2013;48(8):1688–1696.
6. De Cunto A, et al. Impact of surgery for neonatal gastrointestinal diseases on weight and fat mass. *J Pediatr*. 2015;167(3):568–571.
7. Pfister KM, Ramel SE. Linear growth and neurodevelopmental outcomes. *Clin Perinatol*. 2014;41(2):309–321.
8. Desborough J. The stress response to trauma and surgery. *Br J Anaesth*. 2000;85:109–117.
9. Anand K, et al. Can the human neonate mount an endocrine and metabolic response to surgery? *J Pediatr Surg*. 1985;20(1):41–48.
10. Ward Platt M, Tarbit M, Aynsley-Green A. The effects of anesthesia and surgery on metabolic homeostasis in infancy and childhood. *J Pediatr Surg*. 1990;25(5):472–478.
11. McHoney M, Eaton S, Pierro A. Metabolic response to surgery in infants and children. *Eur J Pediatr Surg*. 2009;19(5):275–285.
12. Letton R, et al. Early postoperative alterations in infant energy use increase the risk of overfeeding. *J Pediatr Surg*. 1995;30(7):988–993.
13. Owens JL, Hanson SJ, McArthur J. Nutritional considerations for infants and children during critical illness and surgery. In: Watson R, Grimble G, Preedy V, et al., eds. *Nutrition in Infancy*. Totowa, NJ: Humana Press; 2013:213–230.
14. Anand K, Sippell W, Aynsley-Green A. Randomised trial of fentanyl anaesthesia in preterm babies undergoing surgery: effects on the stress response. *Lancet*. 1987;1:62–66.
15. Zhong JX, Kang K, Shu XL. Effect of nutritional support on clinical outcomes in perioperative malnourished patients: a meta-analysis. *Asia Pac J Clin Nutr*. 2015;24(3):367–378.
16. Mehta NM. Energy expenditure: how much does it matter in infant and pediatric chronic disorders? *Pediatr Res*. 2015;77(1-2):168–172.
17. Pierro A, Eaton S. Metabolism and nutrition in the surgical neonate. *Semin Pediatr Surg*. 2008;17(4):276–284.
18. Pierro A, et al. Partition of energy metabolism in the surgical newborn. *J Pediatr Surg*. 1991;26(5):581–586.
19. Bell EF, Johnson KJ, Dove EL. Effect of body position on energy expenditure of preterm infants as determined by simultaneous direct and indirect calorimetry. *Am J Perinatol*. 2016.
20. McClave S, et al. Clinical use of the respiratory quotient obtained from indirect calorimetry. *J Parenter Enteral Nutr*. 2003;27(1):21–26.
21. McClave S, Snider H. Use of indirect calorimetry in clinical nutrition. *Nutr Clin Pract*. 1992;7(5):207–221.
22. Lev S, Cohen J, Singer P. Indirect calorimetry measurements in the ventilated critically ill patient: facts and controversies – the heat is on. *Crit Care Clin*. 2010;26(4):e1–e9.
23. Mehta NM, et al. Cumulative energy imbalance in the pediatric intensive care unit: role of targeted indirect calorimetry. *J Parenter Enteral Nutr*. 2009;33(3):336–344.
24. Jaksic T, et al. Do critically ill surgical neonates have increased energy expenditure? *J Pediatr Surg*. 2001;36(1):63–67.
25. Jones MO, et al. The metabolic response to operative stress in infants. *J Pediatr Surg*. 1993;28(10):1258–1263.
26. Shanbhogue R, Jackson M, Lloyd DA. Operation does not increase resting energy expenditure in the neonate. *J Pediatr Surg*. 1991;26(5):578–580.
27. Powis M, et al. Effect of major abdominal operations on energy and protein metabolism in infants and children. *J Pediatr Surg*. 1998;33:49–53.
28. Grodner M, Roth S, Walkingshaw B. Nutrition and metabolic stress. In: Grodner M, Escott-Stump S, Dorner S, eds. *Nutritional Foundations and Clinical Applications*. St. Louis, MO: Elsevier; 2011:341–356.
29. Beaufrère B. Protein turnover in low birth weight (LBW) infants. *Acta Paediatr Suppl*. 1994; 405:86–92.
30. Millward DJ. Protein: synthesis and turnover. In: Allen LH, Prentice A, Caballero B, eds. *Encyclopedia of Human Nutrition*. San Diego, CA: Elsevier Science; 2013:139–146.
31. Cogo PE, et al. Protein turnover, lipolysis, and endogenous hormonal secretion in critically ill children. *Crit Care Med*. 2002;30(1):65–70.
32. Keshen TH, et al. Stable isotopic quantitation of protein metabolism and energy expenditure in neonates on- and post-extracorporeal life support. *J Pediatr Surg*. 1997;32(7):958–963.
33. Coss-Bu J, et al. Energy metabolism, nitrogen balance, and substrate utilization in critically ill children. *Am J Clin Nutr*. 2001;74:664–669.
34. Reynolds RM, Bass KD, Thureen PJ. Achieving positive protein balance in the immediate postoperative period in neonates undergoing abdominal surgery. *J Pediatr*. 2008;152(1):63–67.
35. Thureen PJ. Effect of low versus high intravenous amino acid intake on very low birth weight infants in the early neonatal period. *Pediat Res*. 2003;53(1):24–32.
36. Ibrahim HM, et al. Aggressive early total parental nutrition in low-birth-weight infants. *J Perinatol*. 2004;24(8):482–486.
37. Carbohydrates. *J Pediatr Gastroenterol Nutr*. 2005;41:S28–S32.
38. Long C, Kinney J, Geiger J. Nonsuppressability of gluconeogenesis by glucose in septic patients. *Metabolism*. 1976;25(2):193–201.
39. Dungan K, Braithwaite S, Preiser J. Stress hyperglycemia. *Lancet*. 2009;373:1798–1807.

7

40. Hall NJ, et al. Hyperglycemia is associated with increased morbidity and mortality rates in neonates with necrotizing enterocolitis. *J Pediatr Surg*. 2004;39(6):898–901.
41. Arsenault D, et al. A.S.P.E.N. clinical guidelines: hyperglycemia and hypoglycemia in the neonate receiving parenteral nutrition. *J Parenter Enteral Nutr*. 2012;36(1):81–95.
42. Agus MS, et al. Tight glycemic control versus standard care after pediatric cardiac surgery. *N Engl J Med*. 2012;367(13):1208–1219.
43. Jones MO, et al. Glucose utilization in the surgical newborn infant receiving total parenteral nutrition. *J Pediatr Surg*. 1993;28(9):1121–1125.
44. Van Aerde J, et al. Effect of replacing glucose with lipid on the energy metabolism of newborn infants. *Clinical Sci*. 1989;76:581–588.
45. Pierro A, et al. Metabolism of intravenous fat emulsion in the surgical newborn. *J Pediatr Surg*. 1989;24(1):95–102.
46. Bresson JL, et al. Energy substrate utilization in infants receiving total parenteral nutrition with different glucose to fat ratios. *Pediatr Res*. 1989;25(6):645–648.
47. Lipids. *J Pediatr Gastroenterol Nutr*. 2005;41(2):s19–s27.
48. Friedman Z, et al. Rapid onset of essential fatty acid deficiency in the newborn. *Pediatrics*. 1976;58(5):640–649.
49. Basu R, et al. Free radical formation in infants: the effect of critical illness, parenteral nutrition, and enteral feeding. *J Pediatr Surg*. 1999;34(7):1091–1095.
50. Pitkanen O, Hallman M, Andersson S. Generation of free radicals in lipid emulsion used in parenteral nutrition. *Pediatr Res*. 1991;29(1):56–59.
51. Caresta E, et al. Oxidation of intravenous lipid in infants and children with systemic inflammatory response syndrome and sepsis. *Pediatr Res*. 2007;61(2):228–232.
52. Levene M, Wigglesworth J, Desai R. Pulmonary fat accumulation after intralipid infusion in the preterm infant. *Lancet*. 1980;316(8199):815–819.
53. Prasertsom W, et al. Pulmonary vascular resistance during lipid infusion in neonates. *Arch Dis Child Fetal Neonatal Ed*. 1996;74(2):F95–F98.
54. Amin SB, et al. Intravenous lipid and bilirubin-albumin binding variables in premature infants. *Pediatrics*. 2009;124(1):211–217.
55. Sweeney B, Puri P, Reen DJ. Modulation of immune cell function by polyunsaturated fatty acids. *Pediatr Surg Int*. 2005;21(5):335–340.
56. Kelly D. Liver complications of pediatric parenteral nutrition-epidemiology. *Nutrition*. 1998;14(1):153–157.
57. Nghiem-Rao TH. Potential hepatotoxicities of intravenous fat emulsions in infants and children. *Nutr Clin Pract*. 2016;31(5):619–628.
58. Lauriti G, et al. Incidence, prevention, and treatment of parenteral nutrition-associated cholestasis and intestinal failure-associated liver disease in infants and children: a systematic review. *JPEN J Parenter Enteral Nutr*. 2014;38(1):70–85.
59. Christensen RD, et al. Identifying patients, on the first day of life, at high-risk of developing parenteral nutrition-associated liver disease. *J Perinatol*. 2007;27(5):284–290.
60. Nandivada P, et al. Mechanisms for the effects of fish oil lipid emulsions in the management of parenteral nutrition-associated liver disease. *Prostaglandins Leukot Essent Fatty Acids*. 2013;89(4):153–158.
61. Llop JM, et al. Phytosterolemia in parenteral nutrition patients: implications for liver disease development. *Nutrition*. 2008;24(11-12):1145–1152.
62. Le HD, et al. Parenteral fish-oil-based lipid emulsion improves fatty acid profiles and lipids in parenteral nutrition-dependent children. *Am J Clin Nutr*. 2011;94(3):749–758.
63. Rayyan M. Short-term use of parenteral nutrition with a lipid emulsion containing a mixture of soybean oil, medium chain triglycerides, and fish oil: a randomized double-blind study in preterm infants. *JPEN*. 2012;36(1):81S–94S.
64. Warner BB, Warner BW. A fish tale worth telling: enteral fat for management of short gut syndrome. *J Pediatr*. 2014;165(2):226–227.
65. Rollins M, et al. Elimination of soybean lipid emulsion in parenteral nutrition and supplementation with enteral fish oil improve cholestasis in infants with short bowel syndrome. *Nutr Clin Pract*. 2010;25(2):199–204.
66. Muhammed R, et al. Resolution of parenteral nutrition-associated jaundice on changing from a soybean oil emulsion to a complex mixed-lipid emulsion. *J Pediatr Gastroenterol Nutr*. 2012;54(6):797–802.
67. Burjonrappa SC, Miller M. Role of trace elements in parenteral nutrition support of the surgical neonate. *J Pediatr Surg*. 2012;47(4):760–771.
68. Suita S, et al. Zinc and copper requirements during parenteral nutrition in the newborn. *J Pediatr Surg*. 1984;19(2):126–130.
69. Darlow BA, Austin NC. Selenium supplementation to prevent short-term morbidity in preterm neonates. *Cochrane Database Syst Rev*. 2003;(4):CD003312.
70. Diaz-Gomez N, et al. The effect of zinc supplementation on linear growth, body composition, and growth factors in preterm infants. *Pediatrics*. 2003;111(5):1002–1009.
71. Weise WJ, et al. Acute electrolyte and acid-base disorders in patients with ileostomies: a case series. *Am J Kidney Dis*. 2008;52(3):494–500.
72. Aschner JL, Poland RL. Sodium bicarbonate: basically useless therapy. *Pediatrics*. 2008;122(4):831–835.

73. Nightingale J, et al. Guidelines for management of patients with a short bowel. *Gut.* 2006;55(suppl 4):iv1–iv12.
74. Schwarz K, et al. Sodium needs of infants and children with ileostomy. *J Pediatr.* 1983;102(4):209–513.
75. Bower T, Pringle K, Spoper R. Sodium deficit causing decreased weight gain and metabolic acidosis in infants with ileostomy. *J Pediatr Surg.* 1988;23(6):567–572.
76. Murphy KG, Bloom SR. Gut hormones and the regulation of energy homeostasis. *Nature.* 2006;444(7121):854–859.
77. Sharman-Koendjbiharie M, et al. Gut hormones in preterm infants with necrotizing enterocolitis during starvation and reintroduction of enteral nutrition. *J Pediatr Gastroenterol Nutr.* 2002;35:675–679.
78. Yang H, et al. Enteral versus parenteral nutrition: effect on intestinal barrier function. *Ann N Y Acad Sci.* 2009;1165:338–346.
79. Moore F, et al. TEN versus TPN following major trauma–reduced septic morbidity. *J Trauma.* 1989;29(7):916–923.
80. Goulet O. Short bowel syndrome in pediatric patients. *Nutrition.* 1998;14(10):784–787.
81. Olieman JF, Jsselstijn HI, de Koning BA, et al. Short bowel syndrome: management and treatment. In: Watson R, Grimble G, Preedy V, et al., eds. *Nutrition in Infancy.* Totowa, NJ: Humana Press; 2013:43–55.
82. Jeejeebhoy KN. Management of short bowel syndrome: avoidance of total parenteral nutrition. *Gastroenterology.* 2006;130(2 suppl 1):S60–S66.
83. Joly F, et al. Tube feeding improves intestinal absorption in short bowel syndrome patients. *Gastroenterology.* 2009;136(3):824–831.
84. Jawaheer G, et al. Gall bladder contractility in neonates: effects of parenteral and enteral feeding. *Arch Dis Child Fetal Neonatal Ed.* 1995;72(3):F200–F202.
85. Jawaheer G, Shaw NJ, Pierro A. Continuous enteral feeding impairs gallbladder emptying in infants. *J Pediatr.* 2001;138(6):822–825.
86. Goutail-Flaud M, et al. Central venous catheter-related complications in newborns and infants: a 587-case survey. *J Pediatr Surg.* 1991;26(6):645–650.
87. Miller M, Burjonrappa S. A review of enteral strategies in infant short bowel syndrome: evidence-based or NICU culture? *J Pediatr Surg.* 2013;48(5):1099–1112.
88. Yang Q, et al. Randomized controlled trial of early enteral fat supplement and fish oil to promote intestinal adaptation in premature infants with an enterostomy. *J Pediatr.* 2014;165(2):274–279.e1.
89. Robinson JR, et al. Surgical necrotizing enterocolitis. *Semin Perinatol.* 2016.
90. Holman R, et al. Necrotising enterocolitis hospitalisations among neonates in the United States. *Paediatr Perinat Epidemiol.* 2006;20:498–506.
91. Andorsky DJ, et al. Nutritional and other postoperative management of neonates with short bowel syndrome correlates with clinical outcomes. *J Pediatr.* 2001;139(1):27–33.
92. Tappenden KA. Pathophysiology of short bowel syndrome: considerations of resected and residual anatomy. *JPEN J Parenter Enteral Nutr.* 2014;38(1 suppl):14S–22S.
93. Haug S, et al. The impact of breast milk, respiratory insufficiency and GERD on enteral feeding in infants with omphalocele. *J Pediatr Gastroenterol Nutr.* 2016.
94. Abdullah F, et al. Gastroschisis in the United States 1988-2003: analysis and risk categorization of 4344 patients. *J Perinatol.* 2007;27(1):50–55.
95. Driver CP, et al. The contemporary outcome of gastroschisis. *J Pediatr Surg.* 2000;35(12):1719–1723.
96. Huh NG, Hirose S, Goldstein RB. Prenatal intraabdominal bowel dilation is associated with postnatal gastrointestinal complications in fetuses with gastroschisis. *Am J Obstet Gynecol.* 2010;202(4):396 e1–e6.
97. Piper HG, et al. Intestinal atresias: factors affecting clinical outcomes. *J Pediatr Surg.* 2008;43(7):1244–1248.
98. Wales PW, Christison-Lagay ER. Short bowel syndrome: epidemiology and etiology. *Semin Pediatr Surg.* 2010;19(1):3–9.
99. Vanderhoof J, et al. Treatment strategies for small bowel bacterial overgrowth in short bowel syndrome. *J Pediatr Gastroenterol Nutr.* 1998;27(2):155–160.
100. Pierog A, et al. Predictors of low weight and tube feedings in children with congenital diaphragmatic hernia at 1 year of age. *J Pediatr Gastroenterol Nutr.* 2014;59(4):527–530.
101. Muratore CS, et al. Nutritional morbidity in survivors of congenital diaphragmatic hernia. *J Pediatr Surg.* 2001;36(8):1171–1176.
102. Desmarais TJ, et al. Enteral nutrition in neonatal and pediatric extracorporeal life support: a survey of current practice. *J Pediatr Surg.* 2015;50(1):60–63.
103. Jaksic T, et al. A.S.P.E.N. clinical guidelines: nutrition support of neonates supported on extracorporeal membrane oxygenation. *JPEN.* 2010;34(3):247–253.
104. Wertheim HF, et al. The incidence of septic complications in newborns on extracorporeal membrane oxygenation is not affected by feeding route. *J Pediatr Surg.* 2001;36(10):1485–1489.
105. Hanekamp MN, et al. Routine enteral nutrition in neonates on extracorporeal membrane oxygenation. *Pediatr Crit Care Med.* 2005;6(3):275–279.

7

CHAPTER 8

Controversies in Short Bowel Syndrome

Jacqueline J. Wessel, Med, RDN, CNSC, CSP, CLE, LD

Short bowel syndrome (SBS) is defined as reduced small bowel length that leads to intestinal failure. *Intestinal failure* (IF) is defined as a condition caused by inadequate intestinal absorption of nutrients, water, or electrolytes, resulting in the inability to maintain hydration and provide sufficient nutrition to support health, growth, and development, needing at least partial parenteral nutrition (PN) for a minimum of 90 days.[1] IF includes motility problems as well. SBS usually is the consequence of intestinal resection or atresia; however, there are limited reports of congenital short bowel. Because patients with IF may not always have reduced bowel length, the two terms are not synonymous. The approaches to care, however, are very similar and are termed *intestinal rehabilitation*. Patients with SBS generally require specialized nutritional support: first PN, followed by PN plus enteral nutrition (EN), then EN, and ultimately transition to all feedings by mouth, as possible.

This chapter attempts to deal with some of the leading controversies of the present decade affecting the management of this challenging population of patients by neonatologists, pediatric surgeons, pediatric gastroenterologists, nurses, dietitians, therapists, and others.

Controversy 1: Lipid Minimization versus Lipid Modification

Before the development of parenteral lipid formulations 50 years ago, patients had essential fatty acid deficiency, hepatic steatosis, and hyperglycemia.[2] This formulation was composed of soybean oil emulsified in an egg yolk-derived phospholipid layer to simulate enteral fat absorption.

Toxic Effects of Lipids

Although numerous factors play a role in the development of IF-associated liver disease (IFALD), attention has been focused on the contribution of parenteral lipid emulsions to the pathogenesis of IF. The use of parenteral lipids has been associated with development of severe and often life-threatening liver disease. A higher incidence of cholestasis and liver fibrosis has been reported in patients receiving high doses of parenteral lipids (>2 g/kg/day).[3] Lipid overload syndrome has been reported in infants receiving parenteral lipids at doses of >4 g/kg/day, manifesting as coagulopathy, elevated liver enzymes, hepatosplenomegaly, and thrombocytopenia.[4,5]

The etiology of the potential toxic effect of parenteral lipids remains unclear. Evidence points toward phytosterols, which are plant-derived sterols similar in structure to cholesterol. Phytosterols cause a reduction of bile flow in animal models. Furthermore, phytosterol levels appear to be elevated in children with cholestasis, although it is not clear whether this elevation is the cause or the result of liver disease.[6] Other studies implicate a role of the ω-6 fatty acids, the major components of plant-derived lipid preparations, such as the soybean-based product, Intralipid. The ω-6 fatty acids are generally proinflammatory, and experts speculate that these fatty acids promote hepatic inflammation and injury. A key mechanism of injury has been established in animal models, in which stigmasterol, one of the major sterols in soybean oil emulsion, inhibits farnesoid X receptor *(FXR)* target genes.[7] FXR is the hepatocyte nuclear receptor for bile acids and mediates cytoprotection by suppression of bile acid uptake, reduction of bile acid synthesis, and enhancement of bile acid efflux through the bile salt excretory protein.[6]

Clinical Approaches to Minimizing Lipid Toxicity

Two evolving lipid management strategies appear to play a role in minimization of IFALD. Lipid minimization is one such approach that may result in prevention of liver disease. Although IFALD has been reported without use of intravenous (IV) lipid, IFALD is more likely to be associated with clinical and histologic complications in individuals receiving IV fat emulsions at doses >1 g/kg/day.[7] Cober and Teitelbaum[8] examined the effects of a lipid minimization strategy in a neonatal intensive care unit population. In their preliminary report, neonates with cholestasis receiving 3 g/kg or more of IV lipid were enrolled in a lipid minimization protocol to receive 1 g/kg of IV lipid twice weekly. A significant negative trend in bilirubin was observed in the lipid reduction group compared with a similar recent historical cohort. One fourth (8 of 31) of these neonates developed biochemical evidence of mild essential fatty acid deficiency (triene-to-tetraene ratio of 0.2-0.5), but all the infants responded to increased lipid administration while maintaining lipid minimization strategies.[8] In a small retrospective study, Colomb et al. also reported normalization of serum bilirubin with the temporary reduction or elimination of IV fat emulsion.[9] Rollins et al.,[10] in a prospective trial of surgical infants given 1 g/kg parenteral lipid versus 3 g/kg, also found a slower rate of rise of direct bilirubin. No infant in this study became deficient in essential fatty acids.[10] Whether this beneficial effect of lipid reduction results from reduction of phytosterols (or another component of parenteral lipid preparations) remains unclear. With this strategy of lipid reduction, a higher glucose infusion rate is required for adequate calorie provision in neonates.

A control cohort study by Sanchez et al. compared surgical neonates with use of lipid restricted to 1 g/kg/day and an earlier cohort of infants with use of lipid 3 g/kg/day, and they found a significant reduction of cholestasis 22% versus 43% ($P = 0.002$).[11] Calkins et al., however, found no difference when 1 g/kg/day lipid restriction was used.[12]

Most clinicians that adopt lipid restriction use 1 g/kg/day of lipid; the author of this chapter has not seen essential fatty acid deficiency at this dose. There has been concern that there could be some neurodevelopmental sequelae even at this level of lipid restriction. A 2-year study by Ong et al.[13] on neurodevelopment and growth compared infants on 1 g/kg lipid versus the traditional 3 g/kg dose. There was no difference in neurodevelopment and growth outcomes except for a higher 12-month cognitive scaled score in the 1 g/kg group.[13] For background information, in a study on neurodevelopmental and cognitive outcomes in children, 80% of infants and children with IF scored within normal limits, with risk factors for problems being prematurity and repeat operations.[14] However, in the National Institute of Child Health and Human Development retrospective cohort analysis, major surgery in very low–birth weight infants was associated with a 50% increased risk of death or neurodevelopmental impairment.[15]

Another strategy involves use of fish oil lipid emulsions in the management of IFALD. Fish oil or ω-3 fatty acid–based parenteral lipid infusions, such as Omegaven, may have beneficial effects on IFALD. Proponents of Omegaven cite the potential detrimental effects of conventional plant-derived IV lipid emulsions mentioned previously. Gura et al. first reported improvement in two infants with cholestasis after they were given Omegaven.[16] Improvement was subsequently seen in 18 infants with SBS when they were switched to Omegaven after they developed cholestasis compared with 21 historical cohorts receiving soybean oil.[17] Use of fish oil in the latter study was not associated with clinical evidence of essential fatty acid deficiency, hypertriglyceridemia, coagulopathy, infections, or growth delay.[17]

Interpretation of this study is complicated by the fact that the infants received the IV ω-3 fatty acid emulsion at doses lower than those of conventional plant-based lipid preparations. Improvement in this fish oil cohort with liver disease may therefore be the result of lipid reduction as well. Many studies have now demonstrated improvement in infants with cholestasis with use of Omegaven, a 10% lipid solution administered over 12 hours at 1 g/kg/day.[18,19] In some infants, cholestasis is not resolved despite administration of Omegaven therapy.[20] The effects of Omegaven on liver histology are also unclear. Two reports described infants with persistent portal fibrosis on liver biopsy despite resolution in cholestasis after treatment with ω-3 fatty acid lipid.[21,22]

Nevertheless, use of Omegaven in doses of 1 g/kg/day appears to improve biochemical disease in most cases. It is still not approved by the U.S. Food and Drug Administration (FDA) and can only be obtained after approval of applications to the FDA, a veterinary application to the U.S. Department of Agriculture, the Institutional Review Board, and an order to the company in Hamburg, Germany. The medication costs $50 to $100 per day per child, and unless special permission is granted for use as an experimental drug, the cost of the drug cannot be billed to the patient, and the institution has to bear the cost.[23]

The strategies of lipid minimization and use of ω-3 fish oil preparations do suggest some role of conventional parenteral lipid preparation in IFALD. Nevertheless, several other nutrients have been implicated over the years in PN-associated liver injury, including amino acids, iron, choline deficiency, and endotoxin. IFALD is likely to have a multifactorial etiology, and IFALD and cholestasis were noted historically before the introduction of parenteral lipids. SMOF, a new lipid combining soy, medium-chain triglyceride (MCT) oil, olive, and fish, has recently been approved for use in adults. It has been shown to be safe and well tolerated in preterm infants[24] and currently is being studied in the United States to obtain FDA approval for pediatrics. It has been hoped that with this formulation, higher doses of IV lipid could be given without the side effect of cholestasis. Recent results of the NEON (Nutritional Evaluation and Optimisation in Neonates) trial, however, have indicated that use of SMOF, at a dose of 3 g/kg, in neonates did not reduce intrahepatic lipid accumulation.[25] Further studies investigating the role of ω-3 fatty acids and lipid reduction are necessary to clarify the optimal lipid strategy.

Controversy 2: Is Septicemia in Short Bowel Syndrome Caused by Bacterial Translocation or by Suboptimal Central Line Care?

Parenteral Nutrition and Epithelial Integrity

The long-term use of central indwelling catheters for the administration of PN places infants at an increased risk for bacteremia and sepsis. Translocation of enteric bacteria through the bowel wall and into the bloodstream, generally referred to as *bacterial translocation* (BT), may also play a role in septicemia. Clinically, it is not always possible to determine the source of infection (direct catheter contamination versus BT) because the isolation of enteric organisms from central indwelling catheters is not proof of BT.[26,27] In addition, PN fluids are conducive to microbial growth because of their nutritional components.[28] Nevertheless, there is no *direct* evidence in humans that PN promotes bacterial overgrowth, impairs neutrophil function, or causes villus atrophy.[29] However, in studies in piglets, a large-animal model that is more similar to humans than rodent models, the switch from enteral nutrition to PN produces atrophy of the villi and a decrease in crypt cell proliferation rate, along with increased crypt and villus cell apoptosis.[30]

The beneficial trophic effect of feeding has been carefully studied in piglets exposed to an isocaloric diet containing 0%, 10%, 20%, 40% 60%, 80%, or 100% of total nutrient intake enterally, with the rest given parenterally.[31] In this model, Burrin et al. demonstrated that intestinal mucosal mass increased when a minimum of 40% of calories were given enterally.[31] Between 60% to 80% of calories were required by the enteral route before normal villus height, brush border enzyme (e.g., disaccharidase) activity, mucosal blood flow, and trophic hormone levels were noted.

Microbial Ingress: Mechanisms and Clinical Evidence

The role of the intestinal tract as a central organ in systemic infections and multiorgan failure was proposed more than 20 years ago.[32,33] Major mechanisms promoting bacterial translocation include intestinal bacterial overgrowth, deficiencies in host immune defenses, increased intestinal permeability, and damage to the intestinal mucosal barrier. BT has been identified in several diseases in humans (demonstrated by positive mesenteric lymph node cultures). These include burns, intestinal transplantation, hemorrhagic pancreatitis, malignancy, cardiopulmonary bypass, and obstructive jaundice.[34]

Septic complications are linked to the carriage of abnormal microorganisms.[35,36] Bacterial growth in the bowel is controlled by several mechanisms, including gastric acidity, pancreatic enzyme activity, enterocyte turnover, normal peristaltic activity in the small intestine, and the presence of an ileocecal valve.[26] These factors can be altered in individuals with SBS. Bowel dilation and reduced peristalsis may develop as adaptive mechanisms to improve enteral absorption, but these factors may also promote bacterial overgrowth by reducing the bowel's ability to expel microorganisms. Moreover, the intestinal endotoxin pool may increase in infants without an ileocecal valve. Increased endotoxin level has been shown to impair liver function affecting the body's bactericidal activity.[37] Endotoxins, such as lipopolysaccharide, also stimulate Kupffer cells (liver macrophages) to produce increased amounts of inflammatory mediators.[37]

The mucosal barrier (tight junctions) of the intestinal epithelium in patients with SBS is overall intact, even though BT to mesenteric lymph nodes is markedly increased in patients with SBS.[38] The immune response to intestinal bacteria also appears to be altered in SBS. The reasons for this are unclear, but atrophy of gut-associated lymphoid tissue may play some role. Alterations in lymphocyte function may also play a role in susceptibility to translocation. In a mouse model, elimination of enteral feeding resulted in changes in intraepithelial lymphocyte (IEL) profile, with reduced numbers of circulating CD4$^+$, CD8$^-$ helper cells, CD4$^+$, CD8$^+$ cytotoxic T cells, CD8αβ$^+$ thymus-dependent, and CD8$^+$, CD44$^+$ mature

IELs. There were also major changes in gut cytokine profile.[39] Therefore bacterial overgrowth and impaired mucosal immunity are factors that place patients with SBS at risk for BT.

Bacterial Profiling

A link between bacterial overgrowth (of aerobic gram-negative bacilli) and septicemia in infants has been shown in some studies.[40,41] In these studies, the authors found that the episodes of septicemia occurred after the acquisition of specific bacteria. Thus the carriage of abnormal flora increased the risk for septicemia and sepsis, whereas the incidence of septicemia in the infants with normal flora was significantly lower. Potentially pathogenic microorganisms (PPMs) included *Klebsiella, Proteus, Morganella, Enterobacter, Citrobacter, Serratia, Acinetobacter* species, *Pseudomonas aeruginosa,* and *Candida albicans.* The types of bacteria that translocate are mainly aerobic (gram-positive and gram-negative) bacteria. A recent retrospective study reported that infants <1 year of age with IF had an incidence of sepsis of 68%, with most episodes caused by gram-positive organisms, especially *Staphylococcus* (60%) and *Enterococcus* (18%). The most common gram-negative isolates were *Klebsiella* (13%), *Enterobacter* (11%), *Escherichia coli* (10%), and *Pseudomonas* (5%).[42]

Many clinicians believe that septicemia is not caused by abnormal carriage of microbiota but, instead, by factors related to central venous line care. There could be either a scenario in which PPM colonization of the gut is followed by entry through the skin or one in which PPM colonization of the gut is followed by translocation.

Central line–associated bloodstream infections (CLABSIs) are a frequent and challenging complication occurring in infants with IF.[43] CLABSIs, along with necrotizing enterocolitis (NEC), have been seen to negatively affect somatic growth in infants as both are inflammatory conditions.[44] Preventive measures in pediatrics now include ethanol lock prophylaxis, which has been shown to be well tolerated and to decrease CLABSIs.[45] From the practical standpoint, for neonatology versus pediatrics, most infants will not be able to tolerate a window if the infant is on lipid restriction or is receiving Omegaven because the glucose infusion rate (GIR) becomes too high to provide sufficient calories unless the infants are able to absorb significant enteral feedings. The GIR becomes even higher with time off PN for ethanol instillation. The infants at greatest risk for CLABSIs are often the ones who cannot be enterally fed. Many institutions are using ethanol locks, but not yet for infants under 6 months of age.

What else can we do to address this problem? One commonly accepted approach is to initiate enteral feedings in infants with SBS. Enteral feeding appears to be the single most important factor in restoring gut-related immunity,[46] reducing the incidence of infection,[47] improving intestinal permeability,[48] and enhancing macrophage function.[49,50]

Controversy 3: What Is Wrong with the Intestinal Microbiota in Short Bowel Syndrome?

Abnormal Microbial Colonization

16S ribosomal RNA (rRNA) gene sequencing enables analysis of the entire microbial community within a sample. This technique has enabled researchers to describe the abnormal colonization of patients with SBS compared with healthy controls.

Lilja et al.[51] analyzed stool from 11 children with SBS, age 1.5 to 7 years. All but one had been premature. The comparison group comprised seven healthy siblings, 2 to 13 years of age. Five were still on PN, all did not have an ileocecal valve, and four were being treated for small bowel bacterial overgrowth (SBBO). The children still on total parenteral nutrition (TPN) were consuming a lactose-free hydrolyzed protein formula and age-appropriate solid foods, with the only modification being a reduction in disaccharide content. The Shannon Diversity Index (SDI) was used to illustrate the variability in diversity. Of the patients with SBS, those still on TPN had the lowest SDI score. *Enterobacteriaceae* was the predominant taxonomic family in four of five PN-dependent children, and one had a relative abundance of *Lactobacillaceae*, with *Enterobacteriaceae* being the second most predominant. These families totally dominated the microbiota of the PN-dependent infants. Overall, *Enterobacteriaceae* was evident in relatively high amounts in 6 of 11 patients with SBS. Only one of the patients with SBS reached the same SDI score as that of the controls. In the other children with SBS, all off PN, there was more diverse microbiota with more uniform distribution of taxonomic families.

Severe gut dysbiosis has been associated with poor growth in children with IF. A unique gut microbiota signature deficient in *Firmicutes* (anti-inflammatory *Clostridia* and *Lactobacillus* spp.) was observed in children with SBS with poor growth compared with those with good growth by Piper et al.[52] The functional output of bacteria, such as short-chain fatty acids (SCFAs), are now recognized not only as a preferred gut fuel for the colon but also an important source of calories, a stimulant of vascular flow and motility, and a means to increase sodium absorption.[53]

Davidovics et al.[54] showed a clear difference between infants and children with SBS (ages 4 months to 4 years) and healthy controls. They observed relative abundance of species from the phyla Proteobacteria and the class Gammoproteobacteria as well as the class Bacilla, with *Escherichia Shigella* and *Streptococcus* being the most notable. Patients with SBS were subcategorized into those experiencing diarrhea and those not experiencing diarrhea. *Lactobacillus* was in greater abundance in those with diarrhea. All of the SBS group had been treated for SBBO within the previous 6 months, and seven out of nine had been treated with metronidazole.[54]

In some studies, a relative abundance of Gammaproteobacteria was observed in the stools of premature infants who developed necrotizing enterocolitis.[55-57] A thorough discussion of the pathogenesis of NEC and the relationship to microbiota has been provided by Neu and Pammi.[58]

Lactobacillus has been observed in abundance in adults with SBS as well.[59] The microbiota of these patients with SBS was found to be dominated by lactobacilli, with a subdominant presence and poor diversity of *Clostridium* species (primarily *Clostridium leptum* and *Clostridium coccoides*) and poor diversity of Bacteroidetes. One species, *Lactobacillus mucosae,* was detected in the mucosa and feces of patients with SBS but was not found in the stool of any of eight normal volunteers.[59]

Studies primarily in adults showed a marked reduction in fecal concentration of SCFAs, the primary anions of normal stool. The highly acidic stools had lactate concentrations that were found to run as high as 60 mmol/L, in contrast to levels <1 mmol/L in normal volunteers' stools.[60] In addition, an enormous osmotic gap (the difference between Na^+ plus K^+ minus Cl^- in stool) was found to be produced by severe malabsorption of osmotically active particles, especially carbohydrates.

Stool cultures indicated a major shift from anaerobes (with virtually undetectable levels of *Bacteroides* and *Clostridium*) to high levels of aerotolerant enterobacteria. At the lower pH levels seen in children with SBS (5.0-5.5), *Bacteroides* species were uncultivatable from stools of patients with a short gut, whereas lactobacilli predominated.[61] In one study of patients with SBS, the total population of bifidobacteria plus lactobacilli added up to 91% of the total microbial population, whereas the populations of *Bacteroides* species, Enterobacteriaceae, and *Clostridium* species were 100-fold to 1000-fold less abundant.[62]

Metabolic Impact of the Altered Microbiota in Short Bowel Syndrome

The importance of the microbiota in patients with SBS is related not only to the tendency of some (Enterobacteriaceae) to invade systemically but also to the powerful metabolic capacity of the microbial community that is able to supply up to 1000 kcal/day. Lactobacilli are of major importance for two reasons. One is that they have a unique tendency to produce lactic acid (both L-lactate and D-lactate, the latter of which is not produced by human tissues). The second reason is the relationship with vitamin B_{12}.

A serious complication of adults and children with SBS is the development of D-lactic acidosis, a condition associated with confusion, speech disturbances, a severe metabolic acidosis (with increased anion gap), and sometimes shock.[63] The underlying pathophysiology has been described by Halperin and Kamel.[64] Both D-lactic acid and L-lactic acid are the products of this rapid bacterial metabolism in the colon, which is contingent on the predominant bacterial population. If there is insufficient exposure time, the bacteria have insufficient time to metabolize D- or L-lactic acid to final products, such as acetic acid. Thus acetic acid predominates in normal individuals, whereas lactic acid is a major anion in individuals with SBS. Lactic acid, when fully oxidized, per mole of adenosine triphosphate, yields 70% more hydrogen ions compared with acetic acid.[64] This may help explain the propensity of children with SBS to develop severe perianal dermatitis as well as acidosis.

One other metabolic consequence of the *Lactobacillus*-dominated flora is vitamin B_{12} deficiency. Certain lactobacilli require vitamin B_{12} for growth and therefore compete with the human host for its uptake. A 14-year-old with SBS with an intact ileum and an intact ileocecal sphincter developed severe macrocytic anemia and generalized fatigue.[65] He was found to have overwhelming overgrowth with bifidobacteria and lactobacilli and vitamin B_{12} deficiency.

It is very rare for patients with SBS to develop bacteremia caused by lactobacilli or bifidobacteria despite their predominance in the gut lumen. Although reports of *Lactobacillus* species in central blood cultures have been published, reports of bifidobacteremia are not available. "Lactobacillemia"[66,67] has been reported to occur, but is not common, and in most cases was associated with probiotic administration. In some large series, the three most important infectious agents associated with septicemia in patients with SBS (in order of frequency) were gram-positive cocci, especially coagulase-negative staphylococci, gram-negative rods, and fungi, especially *C. albicans*.[68,69] However, clinicians in Houston, Texas, have noted that infections with enteric organisms greatly outnumber infections with skin organisms (e.g., staphylococci, *Candida*).[70] During a 1-year period, at the University of Texas, Houston, babies who had SBS and were receiving PN developed 23 central line infections with enteric organisms compared with 14 infections with skin organisms (62% versus 38%). Of note, 17 of 23 episodes were associated with blood cultures positive for gram-negative rods. Similarly, Weber found that 81% of episodes of SBS-associated sepsis were associated with gram-negative rods in enterally fed children.[71]

Controversy 4: Should Small Bowel Bacterial Overgrowth Prophylaxis Be Given?

The ileocecal sphincter provides a mechanical barrier to bacterial migration into the small intestine but also assists in regulating the exit of fluid and nutrients into the colon. Loss of the ileocecal sphincter can lead to small bowel bacterial overgrowth, a condition associated with diarrhea and fat and vitamin (B_{12}) malabsorption, both resulting from bile salt deconjugation, along with fluid loss, abdominal cramps, and liver injury.[72,73] Furthermore, bacterial overgrowth of the small intestine in human babies with SBS is associated with proximal intestinal inflammation.[74] Whether it is the cause or the effect, children with SBS have nonspecific immune system activation. In one study, there were elevated concentrations of soluble tumor necrosis factor (TNF) receptor-II and interleukin (IL)-6 in urine and serum in patients with SBS and increased TNF-αcompared with healthy controls.[43] Infants with SBBO are at higher risk for bloodstream infections and have higher levels of fecal calprotectin. Cole et al. saw an inverse relationship between percentage of enteral nutrition calories and levels of proinflammatory cytokines, TNF-α, IL-6, IL-8, and IL-ß.[43]

The use of antimotility agents, such as loperamide, is not always recommended in children with SBS because slower transit may exacerbate SBBO.[75]

After bacterial overgrowth has been confirmed by intestinal microbiota analysis (duodenal) or hydrogen breath testing, SBBO treatment could be considered. Goulet and Ruemmele recommended the use of intermittent antimicrobial therapy based on oral metronidazole, either alone or in association with trimethoprim-sulfamethoxazole.[76] However, anaerobic organisms are depleted in children with SBS, and aerobic gram-negative rod coverage with medications, such as amoxicillin-clavulanate or ciprofloxacin, may be preferred. The response can be determined by assessing clinical improvement and feeding tolerance. Broad-spectrum antibiotics should be used cautiously, given the risk for emergence of multiresistant strains of bacteria and the effects on colonic bacterial flora. There are no prospective trials comparing the outcome in infants with SBS treated with prophylactic antibiotics versus placebo. The optimal duration and schedule of cyclic antibiotic prophylaxis for preventing SBBO is not standardized across intestinal rehabilitation centers.

The counterpoint to consider when treating SBBO is that reports in the literature have suggested that SBBO treatment may not help and could even make things worse. In the study by Piper et al., five children with SBS treated for SBBO had poorer growth and a lower quantity of a subset of bacteria producing SCFAs, the A_{1C} that stimulates the gut to make anti-inflammatory cytokines, such as IL-10 and colonic regulatory T cells.[52] These cells can dampen intestinal inflammation. Deficiencies in SCFA-producing bacteria can lead to more inflammation, worse absorption and, with that, poorer growth.

Galloway et al. evaluated anti-flagellin (FLiC) and anti-lipopolysaccharide (LPS) immunoglobulins in infants and children with SBS, about half of them receiving cycled antibiotics for SBBO treatment.[77] Antibodies against LPS and (FLiC) were statistically elevated at baseline in those who received a prophylactic regimen compared with those not on a regimen. In theory, during prophylactic treatment against the gram-positive anaerobes that deconjugate bile acids and are responsible for malabsorption, the genera of bacteria in SBBO are suppressed. There is then the likelihood that the remaining gram-negative aerobes proliferate and consequently translocate across the mucosal barrier into the portal circulation. This increased rate of translocation could lead to more activation of inflammatory pathways and a greater number of bloodstream infections.

Probiotics are microorganisms, which, when given orally in adequate quantities, have health-promoting properties. One might wonder whether prophylaxis against SBBO with probiotics to "out-compete" the enteric flora that tend to produce SBBO would be beneficial. However, because of the reports, albeit rare, of probiotic organisms in the circulating blood of patients with SBS and central lines, currently the recommended treatment of patients with SBS is with probiotics. With further research, we may find out specific strains deficient in infants and children with SBS and gather more information about very specific targeted and effective therapy.[52,78]

Controversy 5: What Is the Optimal Way to Feed?

Enteral nutrition is the key factor for initiating and maintaining the adaptation of the intestine.[79-82] Intestinal adaptation, a process by which the remaining intestine increases its ability to absorb nutrients, is highly individualized, encompassing structural and functional changes.[83] Food in the intestinal lumen works directly by providing energy and protein for the developing mucosa and indirectly by stimulating gastrointestinal (GI) hormones that regulate pancreatic, gastric, and intestinal functions.[84-86]

There is very little literature regarding how infants with SBS should be fed. There are two published studies, one in infants[87] and one in adults,[88] illustrating the benefit of continuous feeding in individuals with short or damaged gut. Parker et al. found benefit in absorption with continuous feedings compared with bolus intermittent feeds in infants.[88] There was noted difference in weight gain (168 g ± 16 g/72 h versus −171 ± 26 g/72 h), and absorption of fat (22 ± 2.0 g/ to 13 ±

0.8 g/24 h), nitrogen (1.7 ± 0.2 to −0.63 ± 0.2 g/24 h), calcium (145 ± 4 to −63 ± 20 mg/24 h), zinc (1.3 ± 0.2 to −0.57 ± 0.2 mg/24 h), and copper (0.21 ± 0.02 to −0.09 ± 0.03 mg/24 h).[81] In adults, Joly et al. found improved absorption using continuous tube feedings (compared with oral feeds) was seen in protein (72% ± 13% versus 57% ± 15%), lipids (69% ± 25% versus 41% ± 27%), and energy (82% ± 12% versus 65% ± 16%).[89] This method can achieve the greatest delivery of nutrients by constant saturation of carrier proteins.[90] On the basis of this information, continuous feedings is recommended as part of the enteral regimen to enhance absorption.

Others feel that bolus feedings are preferable to mimic the gastric filling and emptying in normal feeding.[76] Although bolus feeds are more physiologic, they can present intermittent high, osmotic loads to the intestines, leading to osmotic diarrhea.[82] Bolus feeding has one beneficial physiologic feature: improved gallbladder emptying.[91] Gallstones are a known complication of SBS.[92] For premature infants without gut issues, there are reports supporting a metabolic advantage to continuous feedings.[93] Others have described no difference in growth and macronutrient retention.[94]

Because of the need for normal oral motor development, it would seem important to adopt a combination of both methods,[95] with continuous feeding for enhanced absorption and small-volume bolus feeding to develop normal feeding development. Infants with SBS often develop an oral aversion. Interventions such as as "sham" feedings may allow for earlier oral feeding and may be crucial for the development of normal feeding skills. The skills of nurses, occupational therapists, and speech pathologists are essential to maximize oral motor therapy for these infants.

The addition of solid spoon-fed food at a developmentally appropriate age, usually 4 to 6 months corrected age, is recommended.[95] The Cincinnati Children's Hospital Intestinal Rehabilitation group has developed recommendations for introduction of solid foods and a daily food guide;[96] the ASPEN's Pediatric Intestinal Failure group also has developed handouts on fluids and electrolytes and foods for clinicians and for families of infants with SBS.[97]

The composition of the diet can affect how the intestine adapts to feeding. The ideal formula to promote intestinal adaption and to wean the infant from parental nutrition has not been determined. The options that exist for infants are maternal or donor breast milk, premature infant formula with intact proteins, whole-protein formulas, partial hydrolysates (hydrolyzed until the taste changes), completely hydrolyzed formula, and amino acid formulas.

Breast milk is the recommended feeding for all infants, with fortification used if the infant is premature.[98] The use of breast milk in SBS appears to be advantageous, with a retrospective review of infants with SBS showing the benefit of breast milk feedings over an amino acid formula.[99] This benefit may be related to an increase in secretory immunoglobulin A and other immune factors in the breast milk; glutamine/glutamate; and/or growth factors (e.g., epidermal growth factor and transforming growth factor-α). All these factors are important for adaptation and are highly abundant in human milk.[100-102]

If breast milk is unavailable, donor milk can be used. There are differences between mother's milk and donor milk, not only because of the lack of specific immune protection from the mother's exposure that can be conveyed to her infant and differences in the stage of lactation and the age of the baby but also because of the effects of Holder pasteurization.[103]

Based on experience and the findings of small studies, when human milk is not available, use of amino acid–based (elemental) formulas has demonstrated feeding tolerance, which helps increase the chances of weaning the infant off PN.[104] The paper by the Pediatric Intestinal Failure Consortium reported that human milk was given to 19% of infants, and that 20 different formulas were used as the initial diet and 40 different formulas used overall.[105] Clearly, in the period 2000 to 2004, a lot of variation was observed.[106] A recent paper duplicated the same survey, and there is now greater consensus, with more emphasis on the use of human milk.[107]

Although studies have been performed on the choice of formula components, their findings are slightly misleading because those studies were performed in older infants or children. A key factor may be the age at which the products were tried. The intestine changes over time, not only in the premature and term infants but during the time after any insult to the intestine or any resection performed. An algorithm for the best enteral feedings depending on these components may be the best approach to determine what to feed, when, and under which circumstances.

Whole-protein formulas or hydrolyzed formulas provide either full proteins or dipeptides/tripeptides and are thought to confer benefit in terms of enhanced adaptation with optimal paracrine stimulation.[8] The more complex diets may enhance the levels of luminal growth factors, which can influence mucosal growth.[108,109] Animal studies have shown that a more complex diet is associated with increased signs of adaptation (functional and morphologic) compared with an elemental diet. Hydrolyzed protein formulas have not been shown to be superior to whole-protein formulas when tested at age 4 months.[110]

Although studies indicate benefit of luminal feeding, the optimal diet has yet to be determined. Some studies have demonstrated that early dietary advancement, complex formulas, and the addition of solids (in older patients with SBS) has no adverse effect on adaptation.[111,112] In some cases of SBS, there is an increased risk for developing colitis, presumably related to increased intestinal permeability, allowing for the development of allergic sensitization.[113] In such cases, an amino acid formula may be beneficial to avoid "SBS colitis." The author's center encourages mothers to pump milk, with mother's milk being the first choice and donor milk the second choice.

The composition of fat in the diet can also affect growth and adaptation. MCTs are often employed to help improve fat absorption and are particularly useful in patients with bile acid or pancreatic insufficiency.[86,114] The addition of dietary long-chain triglycerides (LCTs; microlipids) was shown to slow gut motility, reduce ostomy output, and perhaps contribute to feeding advancement and weight gain.[115] Formulas with LCTs promote enterocyte proliferation and mucosal adaptation better than those with a high MCT content.[116] However, in patients with significant ileal resection, there may be decreased bile acid formation and therefore impairment of the ability to absorb LCTs.[117] In summary, there is no general consensus, but the author would prefer the use of mother's milk, with donor human milk as a backup, followed by use of an amino acid formula and then transition over time to a more complex formula and diet as the infant's clinical condition permits, always keeping in mind the ultimate goal of weaning from PN. Some clinicians do not see any advantage in the use of amino acid or casein hydrolysate formulas and prefer the use of premature infant formulas, even though it slows down enteral advancement. A key concept is that even term enteral formulas have more minerals available compared with those that can be put into PN because of precipitation concerns. Whether the infant can absorb these enteral nutrients is not known, although there is some evidence that calcium absorption continues to improve over time.[87]

In some fortunate cases, the surgeon may have had time to put in a mucous fistula to allow enteral access to the remainder of the gut. Once the distal bowel is healed, the refeeding of the stoma output to the mucous fistula can contribute to the nutrition of the infant, thus decreasing dependence on PN, and sometimes allows complete weaning from PN.[118] It also can make the next surgery easier by preventing mismatch in diameter when the distal bowel has not been used and is very small. There are now numerous reports documenting the advantage of this method that has been applied for years in the author's center.[119-121]

Controversy 6: What to Monitor and When?

A useful test for sodium sufficiency in infants and children with SBS is the spot urine sodium assay. Sodium depletion is common in infants without the colon in continuity. Growth can be affected when the urine sodium is <30 mmol/L. This is an easy

Sodium Supplementation Guideline

1. Deficit states:

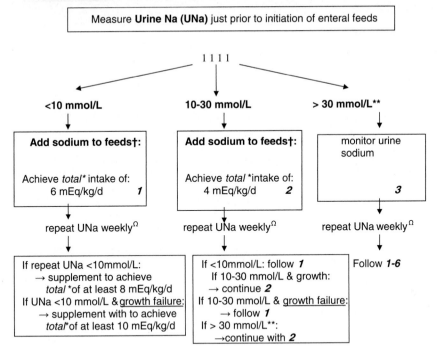

Fig. 8.1   Sodium supplementation guideline. (From: Butterworth SA, Lalari V, Dheensaw K: Evaluation of sodium deficit in infants undergoing intestinal surgery. *J Pediatr Surg.* 2014;40:736–740.)

test that can be used to determine improvement in growth; notable depletion in the urine value will occur long before the serum value indicates a problem.[122] An algorithm is depicted in Fig. 8.1 for management of care.

Most centers have routine monitoring of patients on PN, and this may be initially sufficient to guide the writing and monitoring of PN. Metabolic derangements are seen in these patients with micronutrient deficiencies or overloads a real possibility in these patients[123] (Table 8.1). As the infant transitions to more enteral feedings, there may be more malabsorption, and guidance is needed to maximize nutrition for these infants and children (Tables 8.2 and 8.3). Should enteral supplements be given? What form is better absorbed? Is there danger in supplementing a nutrient if there is competition and if it ultimately results in deficiency of another nutrient (e.g., zinc and copper)?

Trace mineral and vitamin levels need to be monitored, but there does not appear to be clear consensus as to what elements to monitor and when. Some nutrient values may be difficult to interpret in the presence of inflammation. In that case, does that involve obtaining and interpreting a C-reactive protein level, or is there a better marker of inflammation?

Deficiencies have been documented by Mziray-Andrew and Sentongo, and this topic has been discussed at many meetings.[124] The discussions also include deficiencies caused by medications given to infants with SBS or by some therapies, such as withholding copper in patients with cholestasis. Excesses can be caused by

Table 8.1 MICRONUTRIENT DEFICIENCY OR OVERLOAD SYNDROMES IN INTESTINAL FAILURE

Micronutrient	Pathophysiology	Clinical Deficiency Syndrome	Clinical Overload Syndrome	Laboratory Evaluation
Minerals and Trace Elements				
Calcium (Ca)	Fat malabsorption	Paresthesias, tetany, bone demineralization	*GI, genitourinary, bone complaints	Serum Ca, parathyroid hormone, dual-energy X-ray absorptiometry scan
Magnesium (Mg)	Fat malabsorption and high Gastrointestinal (GI) fluid losses	Weakness, cardiac, central nervous system	*Weakness, cardiac	Serum Mg
Zinc (Zn)	GI fluid losses	Poor growth, skin, hair, diarrhea	*Vomiting, headache, diarrhea, Cu deficiency	Serum Zn, low alkaline phosphatase
Copper (Cu)	Overload more common in cholestasis	*Hemolytic anemia, neutropenia	Hepatic overload, neuropsychiatric	Serum Cu
Manganese (Mn)	Overload more common in cholestasis	*Poor growth, ataxia, skeletal	Neurotoxicity	Serum Mn
Iron (Fe)	Absorbed proximally; not routinely in total parenteral nutrition	Microcytic anemia, irritability	Hepatotoxicity, GI bleeding, vomiting	Ferritin, total iron-binding capacity, hemoglobin, hematocrit, peripheral smear
Selenium (Se)	Absorbed throughout small bowel	Myopathy, cardiomyopathy	*Thyroid enlargement	Serum Se
Fat-soluble Vitamins				
A	Fat malabsorption, cholestasis	Xerophthalmia, blindness	Increased intracranial pressure (ICP), hepatitis, vomiting	Vitamin A: retinol binding protein ratio
D	Fat malabsorption, cholestasis	Hypocalcemia, hypophosphatemia, rickets	Emesis, renal impairment	25-OH vitamin D
E	Fat malabsorption, cholestasis	Myopathy, neuropathy, ataxia, hemolytic anemia	coagulopathy	Vitamin E: total serum lipid ratio
K	Fat malabsorption, cholestasis	Bleeding	Hemolytic anemia	Prothrombin time, PIVKA assay
Water-soluble Vitamins				
B12	Gastric or ileal resection	Megaloblastic anemia, central nervous system (CNS) including ataxia	None known	Serum B12, methylmalonic acid, homocysteine
Folate	Absorbed proxim	Anemia, thrombocytopenia, stomatitis, glossitis	None known	Serum Folate

Frymoyer A, Juul SE, Massaro AN, Bammler TK, Wu YW. High-Dose Erythropoietin Population Pharmacokinetics in Neonates with Hypoxic-Ischemic Encephalopathy Receiving Hypothermia. *Pediatr Res.* 2017.

Table 8.2 PROPOSED MONITORING OF INFANTS WITH SHORT BOWEL SYNDROME

Micronutrient	Pathophysiology	Clinical Deficiency Syndrome	Clinical Overload Syndrome	Laboratory Evaluation
Minerals and Trace Elements				
Calcium (Ca)	Fat malabsorption	Paresthesias, tetany, bone demineralization	GI, genitourinary (GU), bone complaints	Serum Ca, parathyroid hormone (PTH), dual-energy X-ray absorptiometry (DXA) scan
Magnesium (Mg)	Fat malabsorption and high Gastrointestinal (GI) fluid losses	Weakness, cardiac, central nervous system (CNS)	Weakness, cardiac	Serum Mg
Zinc (Zn)	GI fluid losses	Poor growth, skin, hair, diarrhea	Vomiting, headache, diarrhea, Cu deficiency	Serum Zn, low alkaline phosphatase
Copper (Cu)	Overload more common in cholestasis	Hemolytic anemia, neutropenia	Hepatic overload, neuropsychiatric	Serum Cu
Manganese (Mn)	Overload more common in cholestasis	Poor growth, ataxia, skeletal	Neurotoxicity	Serum Mn
Iron (Fe)	Absorbed proximally; not routinely in total parenteral nutrition (TPN)	Microcytic anemia, irritability	Hepatotoxicity, GI bleeding, vomiting	Ferritin, total Fe-binding capacity, hemoglobin, hematocrit, peripheral smear
Selenium (Se)	Absorbed throughout small intestine	Myopathy, cardiomyopathy	Thyroid enlargement	Serum Se

Table 8.3 LABORATORY MONITORING FOR INFANTS WITH SHORT BOWEL SYNDROME

Measurement	Comment	Initial Period	Long-Term Follow-Up
Weight		Daily	Three times per week
Length		Weekly	Every (Q) 2 weeks
HC		Weekly	Q 2 weeks
Electrolytes, calcium, phosphate, manganese, glucose	Patients on PN, also monitor when things change	Daily, then three to four times a week	Weekly, then Q 2 weeks
Hepatic transaminases, gamma-glutamyl transferase, direct bilirubin	Patients on PN	Twice a week	Weekly, Q 2 weeks
Total protein, prealbumin		Weekly	Q 2-4 weeks
Triglycerides		Twice a week	Weekly, Q 2 weeks
Urine sodium		Baseline	Weekly, Q 2 weeks
Urine specific gravity	Useful if no stoma and cannot determine	As needed	As needed
Prothrombin time, partial thromboplastin time, international normalized ratio		Baseline	As indicated
Complete blood count, reticulocyte count		As indicated or Q 2 weeks	As indicated or monthly if not obtained for other reasons

Continued

Table 8.3 LABORATORY MONITORING FOR INFANTS WITH SHORT BOWEL SYNDROME—cont'd

Measurement	Comment	Initial Period	Long-Term Follow-Up
Ferritin, Iron, total iron-binding capacity, transferrin	If anemic and on supplements	Q 3 months or as indicated	Q 3 months or as indicated
Vitamin D25-(OH)		Baseline 1 month	Q 3 months
Vitamins A, E, and K		Baseline 6 months	Q 6 months
Vitamin B_{12}, urine methylmalonic acid	Ileal resection, Macrocytic anemia		1 year off TPN; then 1 year after that
Vitamin B_1, whole blood	Inconsistent vitamins	At 2 weeks until normal	
Trace minerals copper, zinc, selenium, and manganese		Baseline at 3 months	Q 6 months
Serum copper, Ceruloplasmin	Persistent neutropenia and microcytic anemia	As indicated otherwise part of above monitoring	Q 6 months
Manganese	Cholestatic		If indicated Q 3 months
Selenium		Baseline 3 months	Q 3-6 months
Red blood cell folate	Extensive resection		Q 6 months
Dual-energy X-ray absorptiometry		1 year	Yearly
Triene/Tetraene ratio	If total fat intake is < 1 g/kg		
D-Lactate	Anion gap metabolic acidosis		
Body composition		Baseline	At discharge or as indicated; Q 6 months
Alphafetoprotein	Chronic liver disease		Q 12 months
Liver ultrasound	Chronic liver disease		Q 12 months
Iodine, urine thyroid-stimulating hormone, free T_4, thyroglobulin level	Patients on total parenteral nutrition (TPN)	>6 months of TPN	Q 6 months

Adapted from Cincinnati Children's Hospital Intestinal Rehabilitation Program Laboratory Monitoring of Patients with Intestinal Failure on Total Parenteral Nutrition and Enteral Feeding.

using trace mineral packages instead of individual nutrients, especially in the case of manganese. The cause of metabolic bone disease in this population appears to be multifactorial, but there are concerns about aluminum exposure as well as nutrient deficiencies caused by PN.[115] In a study by Pichler et al., the children underwent yearly dual-energy X-ray absorptiometry.[125] With newer technology, body composition measurements can go beyond traditional anthropometric measurements to get a better picture of the infant's lean body mass.[126] Currently, there are no guidelines, which are needed for what to measure and when to assess the infant or child with SBS.

Controversy 7: How Does One Predict Whether Full Intestinal Adaptation Will Occur?

The potential for the small bowel to adapt has been demonstrated to be a function of the remaining small bowel length (SBL), presence of the terminal ileum, ileocecal valve (ICV), ostomy closure, treatment of small bowel bacterial overgrowth, and a key element, the absence of intestinal dysmotility. An increased likelihood of intestinal adaptation has been associated with intestinal length of >35cm and an intact ICV.[127,128] However, adaptation can occur with SBL as short as 11 cm with the ICV intact, or 15 cm without the ICV.[129,130] Absence of the ICV has been associated with longer duration of PN.[127,131] Most infants will adapt within the first year, but some may take years but eventually attain enteral autonomy. Thoughtful surgical management is essential, especially for those not making progress in reaching enteral goals. A thorough discussion of surgical options is available elsewhere,[118] and these include minimizing, whenever possible, the time that the bowel is not in continuity.

A recent study has shown that infants with SBS as a result of NEC have a higher likelihood of reaching enteral autonomy compared with those without NEC in a review of 109 patients at a large intestinal rehabilitation program (overall 64.9% compared with 29.2%; $P = 0.001$).[132] A multicenter retrospective cohort study from the Pediatric Intestinal Failure Consortium found that underlying NEC, preservation of the ileocecal valve, and longer bowel length were predictors of ability to achieve enteral autonomy.[133]

Laboratory values have been examined for their utility in predicting intestinal adaptation. A 10-year review found that bilirubin, liver enzymes (aspartate transaminase, alanine transaminase), and platelet count were not reliable for predicting intestinal adaptation in patients younger than 5 months of age.[134] In patients older than 5 months of age, these parameters could be used reliably to distinguish between children at risk for death compared with children who will achieve enteral autonomy.[134]

The amino acid citrulline, which is synthesized exclusively in the intestine of humans, has been shown to be a marker of enterocyte mass and hence a surrogate marker of the absorptive function of the intestine. Citrulline is a nonprotein amino acid and is produced almost exclusively by enterocytes; thus patients with intestinal failure are expected to have low serum citrulline levels.[135] Rhoads et al. reported that serum citrulline levels correlated with remaining intestinal length and that levels of 19 μmol/L and higher were a sensitive predictor of the ability to be weaned off PN.[136] Others have suggested serum citrulline levels of 15 μmol/ and 10 μmol/ to predict likelihood of waning of parenteral nutrition.[132,137,138] Measurement of serial values of serum citrulline may be a simple method to assess the progression of intestinal adaptation.[135,138] These values are often very low before feeding and increase throughout the feeding process. Low serum citrulline values have been shown to correlate with catheter-related bloodstream infections.[138] Low citrulline levels have also been found in pediatric patients with bowel dysfunction but without resection.[139] Findings in a small study by Fjermestad et al. suggested that plasma citrulline is insufficiently discriminative as a biomarker in adults.[140] Although not a perfect marker, serum citrulline remains one of the biochemical methods of measuring intestinal adaptation.

Summary

Many questions remain with respect to how to optimally facilitate intestinal adaptation and thus survival in infants with SBS. Despite ambiguities and controversies, referral to specialized, multidisciplinary intestinal rehabilitation centers has been shown to be helpful in improving outcomes, with reduction in advanced liver disease and need for intestinal transplantation.[141,142] Outcomes have improved, even in patients with an ultrashort bowel.[143] A new simulation study shows improved survival as well as cost savings as a result of intestinal rehabilitation.[144] The work of individuals at these centers, along with the work of basic science and clinical researchers, has resulted in recent and continued advancement and progress in the management of SBS. Intestinal rehabilitation clinics can always boast of miraculous cures in babies who would not have been expected to survive if weaned off PN. These results signify the "blood, sweat, and tears" given by the team that contributes to their care and (last but not least) by the parents of these infants.

REFERENCES

1. Cole CR, Ziegler TR. Etiology and epidemiology of intestinal failure. In: Duggan C, Gura K, Jaksic T, eds. *Clinical Management of Intestinal Failure*. Boca Raton, FL: CRC Press; 2011:3–12.
2. Bark S, Holm I, Hakansson I, Wretlind A. Nitrogen-sparing effect of fat emulsion compared with glucose in the postoperative period. *Acta Chir Scand*. 1976;142:423–427.
3. Cavicchi M, Beau P, Crenn P, et al. Prevalence of liver disease and contributing factors in patients receiving home parenteral nutrition for permanent intestinal failure. *Ann Intern Med*. 2000;132:525–532.
4. Heyman MB, Storch S, Ament ME. The fat overload syndrome. Report of a case and literature review. *Am J Dis Child*. 1981;135:628–630.

5. Campbell AN, Freedman MH, Pencharz PB, Zlotkin SH. Bleeding disorder from the "fat overload" syndrome. *JPEN J Parenter Enteral Nutr*. 1984;8:447–449.

6. Bindl L, Lutjohann D, Buderus S, et al. High plasma levels of phytosterols in patients on parenteral nutrition: a marker of liver dysfunction. *J Pediatr Gastroenterol Nutr*. 2000;31:313–316.

7. Carter BA, Taylor OA, Prendergast DR, et al. Stigmasterol, a soy lipid-derived phytosterol, is an antagonist of the bile acid nuclear receptor FXR. *Pediatr Res*. 2007;62:301–306.

8. Cober MP, Killu G, Braitian A, et al. Intravenous fat emulsion reduction for patients with parenteral nutrition associated liver disease. *J Pediatr*. 2012;160:421–427.

9. Colomb V, Jobert-Giraud A, Lacaille F, et al. Role of lipid emulsions in cholestasis associated with long-term parenteral nutrition in children. *JPEN J Parenter Enteral Nutr*. 2000;24:345–350.

10. Rollins MD, Ward RM, Jackson WD, et al. Effect of decreased parenteral soybean lipid emulsion on hepatic function in infants at risk for parenteral nutrition-associated liver disease: a pilot study. *J Pediatr Surg*. 1013;48:1348–1356.

11. Sanchez SE, Braun LP, Mercer LD, et al. The effect of lipid restriction on the prevention of parenteral nutrition associated cholestasis in surgical infants. *J Pediatr Surg*. 2013;48:573–578.

12. Calkins KL, Havranek T, Kelley-Quon LI, et al. Low dose parenteral soybean oil for the prevention of parenteral nutrition associated liver disease in neonates with gastrointestinal disorders: a randomized controlled pilot study [published online May 29, 2015]. *JPEN J Parenter Enteral Nutr*. https://doi.org/10.1177/0148607115588334.

13. Ong MI, Purdy IB, Levit OL, et al. Two-year neurodevelopment and growth outcome for preterm neonates who received low-dose intravenous soybean oil [published online October 21, 2016]. *JPEN J Parenter Enteral Nutr*. https://doi.org/10.1177/0148607116674482.

14. Chesley PM, Sanchez SE, Melzer L, et al. Neurodevelopmental and cognitive outcomes in children with intestinal failure. *J Pediatr Gastroenterol Nutr*. 2016;63:41–45.

15. Morriss Jr FH, Saha S, Bell EF, et al. Surgery and neurodevelopmental outcome of very low birth weight infants. *JAMA Pediatr*. 2014;168:746–754.

16. Gura KM, Duggan CP, Collier SB, et al. Reversal of parenteral nutrition-associated liver disease in two infants with short bowel syndrome using parenteral fish oil: implications for future management. *Pediatrics*. 2006;118:e197–e201.

17. Gura KM, Lee S, Valim C, et al. Safety and efficacy of a fish-oil-based fat emulsion in the treatment of parenteral nutrition-associated liver disease. *Pediatrics*. 2008;121:e678–e686.

18. Diamond IR, Sterescu A, Pencharz PB, et al. Changing the paradigm: Omegaven for the treatment of liver failure in pediatric short bowel syndrome. *J Pediatr Gastroenterol Nutr*. 2009;48:209–215.

19. Chung PH, Wong KK, Wong RM, et al. Clinical experience in managing pediatric patients with ultra-short bowel syndrome using omega-3 fatty acid. *Eur J Pediatr Surg*. 2010;20:139–142.

20. Nandivada P, Baker MA, Mitchell PD, et al. Predictors of failure of fish oil therapy for intestinal failure associated liver disease in children. *Am J Clin Nutr*. 2016;104:663–670.

21. Soden JS, Lovell MA, Brown K, et al. Failure of resolution of portal fibrosis during omega-3 fatty acid lipid emulsion therapy in two patients with irreversible intestinal failure. *J Pediatr*. 2010;156:327–331.

22. Mercer DF, Hobson BD, Fischer RT, et al. Hepatic fibrosis persists and progresses despite biochemical improvement in children treated with intravenous fish oil emulsion. *J Pediatr Gastroenterol Nutr*. 2013;56:364–369.

23. US Food and Drug Administration. (n.d.) How to request Omegaven for Expanded Access Use. Retrieved from http://www.fda.gov/Drugs/DevelopmentApprovalProcess/HowDrugsareDeveloped andApproved/ApprovalApplications/InvestigationalNewDrugINDApplication/ucm368740.htm.

24. Rayyan M, Devlieger H, Jochum F, et al. Short term use of parenteral nutrition with a lipid emulsion containing a mixture of soybean oil, olive oil, medium-chain triglycerides, and fish oil: a randomized double-blind study in preterm infants. *JPEN J Parenter Enteral Nutr*. 2012;36(suppl 1):81S–94S.

25. Uthaya S, Liu X, Babalis D, et al. Nutritional Evaluation and Optimization in Neonates: a randomized, double blind comparison trial of amino acid regimen and intravenous lipid composition in preterm parenteral nutrition. *Am J Clin Nutr*. 2016;103:1443–1452.

26. Vanderhoof JA, Langnas AN. Short-bowel syndrome in children and adults. *Gastroenterology*. 1997;113:1767–1778.

27. Kelly DA. Intestinal failure-associated liver disease: what do we know today? *Gastroenterology*. 2006;130:S70–S77.

28. Marra AR, Opilla M, Edmond MB, Kirby DF. Epidemiology of bloodstream infections in patients receiving long-term total parenteral nutrition. *J Clin Gastroenterol*. 2007;41:19–28.

29. Duran B. The effects of long-term total parenteral nutrition on gut mucosal immunity in children with short bowel syndrome: a systematic review. *BMC Nurs*. 2005;4:2.

30. Niinikoski H, Stoll B, Guan X, et al. Onset of small intestinal atrophy is associated with reduced intestinal blood flow in TPN-fed neonatal piglets. *J Nutr*. 2004;134:1467–1474.

31. Burrin DG, Stoll B, Jiang R, et al. Minimal enteral nutrient requirements for intestinal growth in neonatal piglets: how much is enough? *Am J Clin Nutr*. 2000;71:1603–1610.

32. Deitch EA. Bacterial translocation of the gut flora. *J Trauma*. 1990;30:S184–S189.

33. MacFie J, O'Boyle C, Mitchell CJ, et al. Gut origin of sepsis: a prospective study investigating associations between bacterial translocation, gastric microflora, and septic morbidity. *Gut*. 1999;45:223–228.

34. Lichtman SM. Bacterial [correction of baterial] translocation in humans. *J Pediatr Gastroenterol Nutr*. 2001;33:1–10.

35. Garrouste-Org M, Marie O, Rouveau M, et al. Secondary carriage with multi-resistant Acinetobacter baumannii and Klebsiella pneumoniae in an adult ICU population: relationship with nosocomial infections and mortality. *J Hosp Infect*. 1996;34:279–289.
36. Lortholary O, Fagon JY, Hoi AB, et al. Nosocomial acquisition of multiresistant Acinetobacter baumannii: risk factors and prognosis. *Clin Infect Dis*. 1995;20:790–796.
37. Billiar TR, Maddaus MA, West MA, et al. Intestinal gram-negative bacterial overgrowth in vivo augments the in vitro response of Kupffer cells to endotoxin. *Ann Surg*. 1988;208:532–540.
38. O'Brien DP, Nelson LA, Kemp CJ, et al. Intestinal permeability and bacterial translocation are uncoupled after small bowel resection. *J Pediatr Surg*. 2002;37:390–394.
39. Wildhaber BE, Yang H, Spencer AU, et al. Lack of enteral nutrition–effects on the intestinal immune system. *J Surg Res*. 2005;123:8–16.
40. van Saene HK, Taylor N, Donnell SC, et al. Gut overgrowth with abnormal flora: the missing link in parenteral nutrition-related sepsis in surgical neonates. *Eur J Clin Nutr*. 2003;57:548–553.
41. Pierro A, van Saene HK, Jones MO, et al. Clinical impact of abnormal gut flora in infants receiving parenteral nutrition. *Ann Surg*. 1998;227:547–552.
42. Pichler J, Horn V, Macdonald S, Hill S. Sepsis and its etiology among hospitalized children less than 1 year of age with intestinal failure on parenteral nutrition. *Transplant Proc*. 2010;42:24–25.
43. Cole CR, Frem JC, Schmotzer B, et al. The rate of bloodstream infection is high in infants with short bowel syndrome: relationship with small bowel bacterial overgrowth, enteral feeding, and inflammatory and immune responses. *J Pediatr*. 2010;156:941–947.
44. Raphael BP, Mitchell PD, Finkton D, et al. Necrotizing enterocolitis and central line associated blood stream infection are predictors of growth outcomes in infants with Short Bowel Syndrome. *J Pediatr*. 2015;167:35–40.
45. Ardura MI, Lewis J, Tansmore JL, et al. Central catheter associated bloodstream infection reduction with ethanol lock prophylaxis in pediatric intestinal failure: broadening quality improvement initiatives from hospital to home. *JAMAPediatr*. 169:324:331.
46. Hadfield RJ, Sinclair DG, Houldsworth PE, Evans TW. Effects of enteral and parenteral nutrition on gut mucosal permeability in the critically ill. *Am J Respir Crit Care Med*. 1995;152:1545–1548.
47. Minard G, Kudsk KA. Effect of route of feeding on the incidence of septic complications in critically ill patients. *Semin Respir Infect*. 1994;9:228–231.
48. Mainous M, Xu DZ, Lu Q, et al. Oral-TPN-induced bacterial translocation and impaired immune defenses are reversed by refeeding. *Surgery*. 1991;110:277–283.
49. Shou J, Lappin J, Minnard EA, Daly JM. Total parenteral nutrition, bacterial translocation, and host immune function. *Am J Surg*. 1994;167:145–150.
50. Okada Y, Klein N, van Saene HK, Pierro A. Small volumes of enteral feedings normalise immune function in infants receiving parenteral nutrition. *J Pediatr Surg*. 1998;33:16–19.
51. Lilja H, Wefer H, Finkel Y, et al. Intestinal dysbiosis in children with sort bowel syndrome is associated with impaired outcome. *Microbiome*. 2015;3:18–24.
52. Piper HG, Fan D, Coughlin LA, et al. Severe gut microbiota dysbiosis is associated with poor growth in patients with short bowel syndrome. *JPEN J Parenter Enteral Nutr*. 2016;41(7):1202–1212.
53. Kles KA, Chang EB. Short chain fatty acids impact on intestinal adaptation, inflammation, carcinoma, and failure. *Gastroenterology*. 1006;130(suppl 1):S100–S105.
54. Davidovics ZH, Carter BA, Luna RA, et al. The fecal microbiome in pediatric patients with short bowel syndrome. *JPEN J Parenter Enteral Nutr*. 40:1106–1113.
55. Wang Y, Hoenig JD, Malin KJ, et al. 16S rRNA gene-based analysis of fecal microbiota from preterm infants with and without necrotizing enterocolitis. *ISME J*. 2009;3:944–954.
56. Mai V, Young CM, Ukhanova M, et al. Fecal microbiota in premature infants prior to necrotizing enterocolitis. *PLos One*. 2011;6:e20647.
57. Torrazza RM, Ukhanova M, Wang X, et al. Intestinal microbial ecology and environmental factors affecting necrotizing enterocolitis. *Plos One*. 2013;12:e83304.
58. Neu J, Pammi M. Pathogenesis of NEC: Impact of an altered microbiome. *Sem Perinatol*. 2017;41(1):29–35.
59. Joly F, Mayeur C, Bruneau A, et al. Drastic changes in fecal and mucosa-associated microbiota in adult patients with short bowel syndrome. *Biochimie*. 2010;92:753–761.
60. van Saene HK, Petros AJ, Ramsay G, Baxby D. All great truths are iconoclastic: selective decontamination of the digestive tract moves from heresy to level 1 truth. *Intensive Care Med*. 2003;29:677–690.
61. Caldarini MI, Pons S, D'Agostino D, et al. Abnormal fecal flora in a patient with short bowel syndrome. An in vitro study on effect of pH on D-lactic acid production. *Dig Dis Sci*. 1996;41:1649–1652.
62. Kaneko T, Bando Y, Kurihara H, et al. Fecal microflora in a patient with short-bowel syndrome and identification of dominant lactobacilli. *J Clin Microbiol*. 1997;35:3181–3185.
63. Bongaerts G, Bakkeren J, Severijnen R, et al. Lactobacilli and acidosis in children with short small bowel. *J Pediatr Gastroenterol Nutr*. 2000;30:288–293.
64. Halperin ML, Kamel KS. D-lactic acidosis: turning sugar into acids in the gastrointestinal tract. *Kidney Int*. 1996;49:1–8.
65. Hojo K, Bando Y, Itoh Y, et al. Abnormal fecal Lactobacillus flora and vitamin B12 deficiency in a patient with short bowel syndrome. *J Pediatr Gastroenterol Nutr*. 2008;46:342–345.
66. De Groote MA, Frank DN, Dowell E, et al. Lactobacillus rhamnosus GG bacteremia associated with probiotic use in a child with short gut syndrome. *Pediatr Infect Dis J*. 2005;24:278–280.

67. Kunz AN, Noel JM, Fairchok MP. Two cases of Lactobacillus bacteremia during probiotic treatment of short gut syndrome. *J Pediatr Gastroenterol Nutr*. 2004;38:457–458.

68. Moukarzel AA, Haddad I, Ament ME, et al. 230 Patient years of experience with home long-term parenteral nutrition in childhood: natural history and life of central venous catheters. *J Pediatr Surg*. 1994;29:1323–1327.

69. O'Keefe SJ, Burnes JU, Thompson RL. Recurrent sepsis in home parenteral nutrition patients: an analysis of risk factors. *JPEN J Parenter Enteral Nutr*. 1994;18:256–263.

70. Navarro F, Gleason W, Rhoads JM, Quiros-Tejeira RE. Short bowel syndrome: complications, treatment, and remaining questions. *NeoReviews*. 2009;10:e339–e350.

71. Weber TR. Enteral feeding increases sepsis in infants with short bowel syndrome. *J Pediatr Surg*. 1995;30:1086–1088.

72. Goulet OJ, Revillon Y, Jan D, et al. Neonatal short bowel syndrome. *J Pediatr*. 1991;119:18–23.

73. Lichtman SN, Sartor RB, Keku J, Schwab JH. Hepatic inflammation in rats with experimental small intestinal bacterial overgrowth. *Gastroenterology*. 1990;98:414–423.

74. Kaufman SS, Loseke CA, Lupo JV, et al. Influence of bacterial overgrowth and intestinal inflammation on duration of parenteral nutrition in children with short bowel syndrome. *J Pediatr*. 1997;131:356–361.

75. Ling PR, Khaodhiar L, Bistrian BR, et al. Inflammatory mediators in patients receiving long-term home parenteral nutrition. *Dig Dis Sci*. 2001;46:2484–2489.

76. Goulet O, Ruemmele F. Causes and management of intestinal failure in children. *Gastroenterology*. 2006;130:S16–S28.

77. Galloway DP, Troutt ML, Kocoshis SA, et al. Increased anti-flagellin and anti-liposaccharide immunoglobulins in pediatric intestinal failure: associations with fever and central line-associated bloodstream infections. *JPEN J Parenter Enteral Nutr*. 2015;39:562–568.

78. Reddy VS, Patole SK, Rao S. Role of probiotics in short bowel syndrome in infants and children – a systematic review. *Nutrients*. 2013;5:679–699.

79. Olieman JF, Penning C, Ijsselstijn H, et al. Enteral nutrition in children with short-bowel syndrome: current evidence and recommendations for the clinician. *J Am Diet Assoc*. 2010;110:420–426.

80. Tappenden KA. Mechanisms of enteral nutrient-enhanced intestinal adaptation. *Gastroenterology*. 2006;130:S93–S99.

81. Soondrum K, Hinds R. Management of intestinal failure. *Indian J Pediatr*. 2006;73:913–918.

82. Wilmore DW. Growth factors and nutrients in the short bowel syndrome. *JPEN J Parenter Enteral Nutr*. 1999;23:S117–S120.

83. Matarese LE, Steiger E. Dietary and medical management of short bowel syndrome in adult patients. *J Clin Gastroenterol*. 2006;40(suppl 2):S85–S93.

84. Ford WD, Boelhouwer RU, King WW, et al. Total parenteral nutrition inhibits intestinal adaptive hyperplasia in young rats: reversal by feeding. *Surgery*. 1984;96:527–534.

85. Dodge ME, Bertolo RF, Brunton JA. Enteral feeding induces early intestinal adaptation in a parenterally fed neonatal piglet model of short bowel syndrome. *J Parenter Enteral Nutr*. 2012;36(2):205–212. https://doi.org/10.1177/0148607111417447.

86. Feldman EJ, Dowling RH, McNaughton J, Peters TJ. Effects of oral versus intravenous nutrition on intestinal adaptation after small bowel resection in the dog. *Gastroenterology*. 1976;70:712–719.

87. DiBaise JK, Young RJ, Vanderhoof JA. Intestinal rehabilitation and the short bowel syndrome: part 1. *Am J Gastroenterol*. 2004;99:1386–1395.

88. Parker P, Stroop S, Greene H. A controlled comparison of continuous versus intermittent feeding in the treatment of infants with intestinal disease. *J Pediatr*. 1981;99:360–364.

89. Joly F, Dray X, Corcos O, et al. Tube feeding improves intestinal absorption in short bowel syndrome patients. *Gastroenterology*. 2009;136:824–831.

90. Vanderhoof JA. New and emerging therapies for short bowel syndrome in children. *J Pediatr Gastroenterol Nutr*. 2004;39(suppl 3):S769–S771.

91. Jawaheer G, Shaw NJ, Pierro A. Continuous enteral feeding impairs gallbladder emptying in infants. *J Pediatr*. 2001;138:822–825.

92. Bogue CO, Murphy AJ, Gerstle JT, et al. Risk factors, complications, and outcomes of gallstones in children: a single-center review. *J Pediatr Gastroenterol Nutr*. 2010;50:303–308.

93. Grant J, Denne SC. Effect of intermittent versus continuous enteral feeding on energy expenditure in premature infants. *J Pediatr*. 1991;118:928–932.

94. Rövekamp-Abels LW, Hogewind-Schoonenboom JE, de Wijs-Meijler DP, et al. Intermittent bolus or semicontinuous feeding for preterm infants? *J Pediatr Gastroenterol Nutr*. 2015;61:659–664.

95. Gosselin KB, Duggan C. Enteral nutrition in the management of pediatric intestinal failure. *J Pediatr*. 2014;165:1085–1090.

96. Cincinnati Children's Hospital Growing Through Knowing Note: Daily Food Guide for Infants 0-12 months with Intestinal Failure, KN-0505, Nutrition for Intestinal rehabilitation KN506.

97. ASPEN Pediatric Intestinal Rehabilitation Materials: Diet for Infants with Short bowel Syndrome.

98. American Academy of Pediatrics. Breastfeeding and the use of human milk. *Pediatrics*. 2012;129:e827–e841.

99. Andorsky DJ, Lund DP, Lillehei CW, et al. Nutritional and other postoperative management of neonates with short bowel syndrome correlates with clinical outcomes. *J Pediatr*. 2001;139:27–33.

100. Serrano MS, Schmidt-Sommerfeld E. Nutrition support of infants with short bowel syndrome. *Nutrition*. 2002;18:966–970.

101. Byrne TA, Wilmore DW, Iyer K, et al. Growth hormone, glutamine, and an optimal diet reduces parenteral nutrition in patients with short bowel syndrome: a prospective, randomized, placebo-controlled, double-blind clinical trial. *Ann Surg*. 2005;242:655–661.

102. Cummins AG, Thompson FM. Effect of breast milk and weaning on epithelial growth of the small intestine in humans. *Gut*. 2002;51:748–754.
103. Peila C, Moro E, Bertine E, et al. The effect of Holder pasteurization on nutrients and biologically-active components in donor human milk: a review. *Nutrients*. 2016;8:477.
104. Bines JE, Taylor RG, Justice F, et al. Influence of diet complexity on intestinal adaptation following massive small bowel resection in a preclinical model. *J Gastroenterol Hepatol*. 2002;17:1170–1179.
105. Squires RH, Dugan C, Teitelbaum DH, et al. Natural history of pediatric intestinal failure: initial report from the Pediatric Intestinal Failure Consortium. *J Pediatr*. 2012;161:723–728.
106. Nucci AM, Ellsworth K, Michalski A, et al. Survey of nutrition management practices in centers for pediatric intestinal rehabilitation. *Nutr Clin Pract*. 2017;1:884533617719670. https://doi.org/10.1177/0884533617719670.
107. Vanderhoof JA, Grandjean CJ, Burkley KT, Antonson DL. Effect of casein versus casein hydrolysate on mucosal adaptation following massive bowel resection in infant rats. *J Pediatr Gastroenterol Nutr*. 1984;3:262–267.
108. Playford RJ, Woodman AC, Clark P, et al. Effect of luminal growth factor preservation on intestinal growth. *Lancet*. 1993;341:843–848.
109. Lai HS, Chen WJ, Chen KM, Lee YN. Effects of monomeric and polymeric diets on small intestine following massive resection. *Taiwan Yi Xue Hui Za Zhi*. 1989;88:982–988.
110. Ksiazyk J, Piena M, Kierkus J, Lyszkowska M. Hydrolyzed versus nonhydrolyzed protein diet in short bowel syndrome in children. *J Pediatr Gastroenterol Nutr*. 2002;35:615–618.
111. Levy E, Frileux P, Sandrucci S, et al. Continuous enteral nutrition during the early adaptive stage of the short bowel syndrome. *Br J Surg*. 1988;75:549–553.
112. McIntyre PB, Fitchew M, Lennard-Jones JE. Patients with a high jejunostomy do not need a special diet. *Gastroenterology*. 1986;91:25–33.
113. Taylor SF, Sondheimer JM, Sokol RJ, et al. Noninfectious colitis associated with short gut syndrome in infants. *J Pediatr*. 1991;119:24–28.
114. Jeppesen PB, Mortensen PB. The influence of a preserved colon on the absorption of medium chain fat in patients with small bowel resection. *Gut*. 1998;43:478–483.
115. Malcolm WF, Lenfestey RW, Rice HE, et al. Dietary fat for infants with enterostomies. *J Pediatr Surg*. 2007;42:1811–1815.
116. Vanderhoof JA, Grandjean CJ, Kaufman SS, et al. Effect of high percentage medium-chain triglyceride diet on mucosal adaptation following massive bowel resection in rats. *JPEN J Parenter Enteral Nutr*. 1984;8:685–689.
117. Mu H, Porsgaard T. The metabolism of structured triacylglycerols. *Prog Lipid Res*. 2005;44:430–448.
118. Wessel JJ, Kotagal M, Helmrath MA. Management of pediatric intestinal failure. *Adv Pediatr*. 2017;64(1):253–267.
119. Lau EC, Fung AC, Wong KK, et al. Beneficial effects of mucous fistula refeeding in necrotizing enterocolitis with enterostomies. *J Pediatr Surg*. 2016;51:1914–1916.
120. Gause CD, Hayashi M, Haney C, et al. Mucous fistula refeeding decreases parenteral nutrition exposure in postsurgical premature infants. *J Pediatr Surg*. 2016;51:1759–1765.
121. Haddock CA, Stanger JD, Albersheim SG, et al. Mucous fistula refeeding in neonates with enterostomies. *J Pediatr Surg*. 50:779–782.
122. Butterworth SA, Lalari V, Dheensaw K. Evaluation of sodium deficit in infants undergoing intestinal surgery. *J Pediatr Surgery*. 2014;49:736–740.
123. Soden JS. Clinical assessment of the child with intestinal failure. *Sem Pediatr Surg*. 2010;19:10–19.
124. Mziray-Andrew CH, Sentongo TA. Nutritional deficiencies in intestinal failure. *Pediatr Clin N AM*. 2009;55:1185–1200.
125. Pichler J, Chomtho S, Fewtrell M, et al. Growth and bone health in pediatric intestinal failure receiving long term parenteral nutrition. *Am J Clin Nutr*. 013;97:1260–1269.
126. Rice MS, Valentine CJ. Neonatal body composition: measuring lean mass as a tool to guide nutrition management in the neonate. *Nutr Clin Prac*. 2015;30:625–632.
127. Goulet OJ, Revillon Y, Jan D, et al. Neonatal short bowel syndrome. *J Pediatr*. 1991;119:18–23.
128. Georgeson KE, Breaux Jr CW. Outcome and intestinal adaptation in neonatal short-bowel syndrome. *J Pediatr Surg*. 1992;27:344–348.
129. Vargas JH, Ament ME, Berquist WE. Long-term home parenteral nutrition in pediatrics: ten years of experience in 102 patients. *J Pediatr Gastroenterol Nutr*. 1987;6:24–32.
130. Quiros-Tejeira RE, Ament ME, Reyen L, et al. Long-term parenteral nutritional support and intestinal adaptation in children with short bowel syndrome: a 25-year experience. *J Pediatr*. 2004;145:157–163.
131. Chaet MS, Farrell MK, Ziegler MM, Warner BW. Intensive nutritional support and remedial surgical intervention for extreme short bowel syndrome. *J Pediatr Gastroenterol Nutr*. 1994;19:295–298.
132. Sparks EA, Khan FA, Fisher JG, et al. Necrotizing enterocolitis is associated with earlier achievement of enteral autonomy in children with short bowel syndrome. *J Pediatr Surg*. 2016;51:92–95.
133. Khan FA, Squires RH, Litman HJ, et al. Predictors of enteral autonomy in children with intestinal failure: a multicenter cohort study. *J Pediatr* 167:29–34.
134. Casey L, Lee KH, Rosychuk R, et al. Ten-year review of pediatric intestinal failure: clinical factors associated with outcome. *Nutr Clin Pract*. 2008;23:436–442.
135. Bailly-Botuha C, Colomb V, Thioulouse E, et al. Plasma citrulline concentration reflects enterocyte mass in children with short bowel syndrome. *Pediatr Res*. 2009;65:559–563.

136. Rhoads JM, Plunkett E, Galanko J, et al. Serum citrulline levels correlate with enteral tolerance and bowel length in infants with short bowel syndrome. *J Pediatr*. 2005;146:542–547.
137. Fitzgibbons S, Ching YA, Valim C, et al. Relationship between serum citrulline levels and progression to parenteral nutrition independence in children with short bowel syndrome. *J Pediatr Surg*. 2009;44:928–932.
138. Hull MA, Jones BA, Zurakowski D, et al. Low serum citrulline concentration correlates with catheter-related bloodstream infections in children with intestinal failure. *JPEN J Parenter Enteral Nutr*. 2011;35:181–197.
139. Stultz JS, Tillman EM, Helms RA. Plasma citrulline concentration as a biomarker for bowel loss and adaptation in hospitalized pediatric patients requiring parenteral nutrition. *Nutr Clin Pract*. 2011;26:681–687.
140. Fjermestad H, Hvistendahl M, Jeppesen PB. Fasting and postprandial plasma citrulline and the correlation to intestinal function evaluated by 72 hour metabolic balance studies in short bowel jejunostomy patients with intestinal failure [published online Jan 1, 2017]. *JPEN J Parenter Enteral Nutr*. https://doi.org/10.1177/0148607116687497.
141. Javid PJ, Malone FR, Reyes J, et al. The experience of a regional pediatric intestinal failure program: successful outcomes from intestinal rehabilitation. *Am J Surg*. 2010;199:676–679.
142. Torres C, Sudan D, Vanderhoof J, et al. Role of an intestinal rehabilitation program in the treatment of advanced intestinal failure. *J Pediatr Gastroenterol Nutr*. 2007;45:204–212.
143. Dore M, Junco PT, Moreno AA. Ultrashort bowel syndrome outcome in children treated in a multidisciplinary intestinal rehabilitation unit. *Eur J Pediatr Surg*. 2017;27:116–120.
144. Groen H, Neelis EG, Poley M, et al. Intestinal rehabilitation for children with intestinal failure is cost–effective: a simulation study. *Am J Clin Nutr*. 2017;105(2):417–425.

CHAPTER 9

New Lipid Strategies to Prevent/ Treat Neonatal Cholestasis

Kathleen M. Gura, PharmD, BCNSP, FASHP, FPPAG, FASPEN

Summary of Key Points

- Intestinal failure-associated liver disease (IFALD) is defined as liver disease that occurs as a result of management strategies for intestinal failure, such as prolonged courses of parenteral nutrition (PN) or repeated surgical interventions. Cholestasis associated with IFALD is typically defined as an elevated serum direct (i.e., conjugated) bilirubin ≥ 2 mg/dL (34.2 μmol/L).

- For infants requiring PN for more than 30 days, current best practice recommendation is that soybean oil-based intravenous lipid emulsions (ILEs) be given at a dose of no more than 1 g/kg/day. More severe restriction of soybean oil-based ILE strategies may increase the risk of essential fatty acid deficiency (EFAD). Because of the different compositions of essential fatty acids, alternative lipid emulsions, such as those derived from fish oil or other lipid blends (e.g., olive oil), which do not need restricted lipid dosing, can be used.

- For infants who do go on to develop cholestasis, fish oil-based ILE monotherapy rather than soybean oil-containing ILEs should be used. If fish oil is used as the exclusive source of lipids, at least 1 g/kg/day should be given, and the triene/tetraene ratio should be monitored to detect EFAD.

- In addition to dosage, other factors that may predispose infants receiving an ILE to cholestasis include exposure of the ILE to ambient light/phototherapy or infusing/storing the ILE in di(2-ethylhexyl) phthalate (DEHP) infusion sets or containers.

- When considering the optimal ILE for their patients, practitioners should consider the oil source, the inflammatory properties of that oil source, phytosterol content, and the amount of alpha-tocopherol present in the ILE formulation.

Introduction

Intestinal failure is a relatively rare condition and is associated with prolonged dependence on parenteral nutrition (PN). The term *intestinal failure*, first coined in 1981, is defined as "a reduction in the functioning gut mass below the minimal amount necessary for adequate digestion and absorption of nutrients."[1] In many instances, infants who are dependent on PN secondary to intestinal failure develop cholestatic liver disease, often referred to as intestinal failure–associated liver disease (IFALD).[2] IFALD is defined as hepatobiliary dysfunction as a result of medical and surgical strategies for IF, which can either progress to end-stage liver disease or can be stabilized or reversed if intestinal adaptation can occur. IFALD had been previously been referred to as *PN-associated liver disease/cholestasis* (PNALD/PNAC) and *PN liver disease* because of the association of PN in the pathogenesis of the disease. IFALD is a broader term, which is now preferred because of the inclusion of other patient- and treatment-associated factors.[3] It is more common in pediatric patients, particularly infants with a history of prematurity and/or bowel resection leading to short bowel syndrome and, until recently, has been a major cause of liver transplantation and death in this patient population.[4,5] In children with intestinal failure (IF), the diagnosis of IFALD is usually made on the basis of long-term PN dependence and cholestasis exclusive of any other causes of hepatic injury. Cholestasis associated with IFALD is commonly defined as an elevated serum conjugated bilirubin ≥2 mg/dL (34.2 μmol/L). IFALD is seen in 40% to 60% of children who receive long-term PN (i.e., >3 months) and 15% to 40% of adults on home parenteral nutrition.[2,6,7]

In neonates and infants with short bowel syndrome, IFALD tends to be more progressive and severe.[7,8] In the era before lipid-sparing strategies or the use of alternative lipid emulsions came into existence, one retrospective review of all neonates at a single health system receiving PN for at least 14 days noted that IFALD occurred in 14% of infants receiving PN for 2 to 4 weeks, 43% of those receiving PN for 4 to 8 weeks, 72% of those receiving PN for 8 to 14 weeks, and 85% of those receiving PN for >14 weeks.[9]

The mechanism of IFALD is still unknown but is probably multifactorial. Components of the PN could act as toxins, but sepsis and lack of enteral feeding are also thought to play major roles.[10] Risk factors for IFALD include prematurity, low birth weight, and intrauterine growth restriction, suggesting that hepatic immaturity is a predisposing factor.[3] Infants with IFALD will typically develop jaundice and elevated levels of conjugated bilirubin about 2 weeks after starting PN, but the onset may occur later. Clinical jaundice usually becomes evident when total bilirubin rises above 3 mg/dL (51.3 μmol/L).[11] The laboratory findings are not specific; in addition to conjugated bilirubin, aspartate aminotransferase, alanine aminotransferase (ALT), and gammaglutamyl transpeptidase (GGT) may be mildly elevated.[12,13] As part of making a diagnosis of IFALD, other major causes of cholestasis must first be excluded. Sepsis and infection are common causes of transient conjugated hyperbilirubinemia in neonates. In those infants with sustained conjugated hyperbilirubinemia, practitioners may wish to consider having the patient evaluated for biliary obstruction (e.g., biliary atresia), infection, and metabolic and genetic liver diseases that require specific therapy.

Histologic changes in IFALD range from steatosis to cirrhosis. Steatosis is often the first histologic change seen on liver biopsy and is more frequently seen in adults on PN.[14] With continued exposure to PN, progressive changes in hepatic histology can occur, including hepatocellular ballooning with steatosis, portal inflammation, canalicular and intracellular cholestasis (bile plugs), and bile duct proliferation that may mimic biliary obstruction.[15] The degree of fibrosis can range from minimal portal fibrosis to cirrhosis. Despite being progressive while PN is continued, the extent of liver disease may progress more slowly if oral feeds are advanced and total PN intake is decreased. The cholestasis and abnormalities shown by liver tests tend to improve after PN is discontinued but may continue to persist for months.[16-18] In one retrospective study, conjugated bilirubin normalized at a median of 13 weeks after weaning (95% confidence interval [CI] 8-14 weeks), and ALT levels normalized at a median of 35 weeks (95% CI 24-80 weeks).[16] Furthermore, 1 year after weaning from PN, despite all patients having normal conjugated bilirubin, 42% continued to have abnormal ALT. Until recently, it was often a "race against the clock" to wean the infant from PN and have bowel adaptation occur before the infant succumbed to IFALD-associated complications.

Role of Intravenous Lipid Emulsions

Mounting evidence suggests that specific components of PN solutions, and especially intravenous lipid emulsions (ILEs), are involved in the pathogenesis of IFALD. Interestingly, PN without the provision of any fat source results in a higher incidence of liver dysfunction compared with PN with fat, making it difficult to draw a correlation between the role of ILEs and IFALD as both the presence and absence of ILEs can predispose patients to developing IFALD.[19]

For more than 50 years, soybean oil-based ILE (SOLE) has been the most common form of ILE used throughout the world. This type of ILE is rich in omega-6 polyunsaturated fatty acids (PUFAs). Recent evidence, however, suggests that SOLE may be an important contributor to the pathogenesis of IFALD. Studies in animal models showed that SOLE is associated with liver injury compared with fish oil-based ILE (FOLE), which is rich in omega-3 PUFAs.[20,21] Moreover, studies in adults have shown that SOLE infusion of >1 g/kg is one of several risk factors for the development of cholestatic liver disease.[6] Excessive lipid provision is also thought to increase the incidence of IFALD.[22,23] Proposed mechanisms through which SOLE's excessive omega-6 PUFA content might cause liver injury include its proinflammatory effects and its ability to impair triglyceride export.[24] In contrast, omega-3 PUFAs tend to have anti-inflammatory and insulin-sensitizing effects, acting through the G-protein-coupled receptor (GPR)120.[25]

Inflammatory Characteristics of Oil Source

IFALD is considered by many to be a disease of inflammation. The presence of an underlying inflammatory source may be a key influence in the progression of PNALD in patients with IF.[26] C-reactive protein (CRP), an acute inflammatory marker, has been shown to reflect disease progression in nonalcoholic steatohepatitis, a disease that in many ways resembles IFALD.[27]

During episodes of acute inflammation, hepatocytes upregulate transcription and release of CRP, primarily in response to the cytokine interleukin-6 (IL-6). This response can be enhanced by a combination of IL-1β and tumor necrosis factor (TNF)-α. There is evidence from experimental animals that PN use, in comparison with enteral nutrition (EN), is associated with greater retention of TNF in the plasma compartment.[28] As an inflammatory marker, higher TNF levels could lead to a mild chronic inflammatory state and further amplify the CRP response in the case of IFALD.

PUFAs of the omega-6 and omega-3 family serve as substrates for eicosanoid synthesis, which directly influences an immune response. Eicosanoids are involved in modulating the intensity of an inflammatory reaction[29] (Fig. 9.1). SOLE is rich in omega-6 PUFA and linoleic acid (LA), which is the precursor of arachidonic acid (ARA), the structural backbone of proinflammatory eicosanoids (see Fig. 9.1; Fig. 9.2). In contrast, the omega-3 PUFAs found in fish oils but not in plant oils, such as docosahexaenoic acid (DHA) and eicosapentaenoic acid (EPA), are converted into

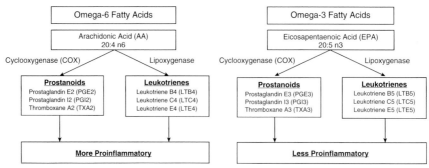

Fig. 9.1   Inflammatory properties of omega-3 and omega-6 fatty acids. (From: Lee S, Gura KM, Kim S, Arsenault DA, Bistrian BR, Puder M. Current clinical applications of omega-6 and omega-3 fatty acids. *Nutr Clin Pract.* 2006 Aug;21[4]:323–41.)

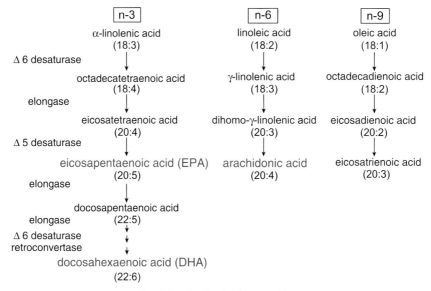

Fig. 9.2   Synthesis of fatty acids.

anti-inflammatory derivatives[30] (see Fig. 9.1, Fig. 9.2). Furthermore, ARA is a precursor of prostaglandin E2 and leukotriene B4, which have proinflammatory proprieties and influence cytokine synthesis. EPA from the omega-3 family serves as an alternative progenitor for cyclooxygenase and lipo-oxygenase pathways for eicosanoid synthesis with reduced inflammatory potencies. The balance between omega-6 and omega-3 PUFAs can affect eicosanoid synthesis, inflammatory response, and cytokine synthesis. PUFAs can influence proinflammatory gene expressions, such as peroxisome proliferator-activated receptor and nuclear factor-κB. PUFAs are necessary to prevent a deficiency of EFAs. However, when present in excess, they can have negative effects, leading to an unbalanced fatty acid pattern in cell membranes and the synthesis of eicosanoids. In a cohort of infants placed on ILEs within 48 hours of birth, Gawecka et al. showed that SOLE promoted an excess of IL-6 production compared with olive oil-containing ILEs.[22] Similarly, Raptis et al. demonstrated the anti-inflammatory role of omega-3 PUFAs via the GPR120 receptor using fish oil-based ILEs.[23] DHA has also been shown to inhibit palmitate-induced Toll-like receptor-4 (TLR4)–activated inflammation.[31,32] In addition to high omega-6 fatty acid content, SOLE also contains high levels of phytosterols, which impair bile secretion via antagonism of the nuclear receptor Farnesoid X receptor (FXR), which will be discussed in greater detail below.[32-34]

Table 9.1   COMPARISON OF LIPID EMULSIONS (10 G FAT/100 ML)

OIL	Intralipid	Omegaven	Clinolipid	SMOFlipid
Manufacturer	Fresenius Kabi (Uppsala, Sweden)	Fresenius Kabi (Bad Homburg, Germany)	Baxter (Deerfield, IL)	Fresenius Kabi (Uppsala, Sweden)
Lipid Source				
Soybean	100%		20%	30%
Medium-chain triglyceride				30%
Olive			80%	25%
Fish		100%		15%
Glycerol (% by weight)	2.25%	2.5%	2.5%	2.5%
Egg Phospholipid (% by weight)	1.2%	1.2%	1.2%	1.2%

Other Oil Sources

After the introduction of SOLE, a second-generation ILE was introduced in Europe, and it was a blend of 50% soybean oil and 50% medium-chain triglyceride (MCT) derived from coconut oil[35] (Table 9.1). These emulsions reduce the omega-6 PUFA content by 50%. MCTs are fatty acids that are 6 to 12 carbons long and include capric and caprylic acids.[36] Unlike long-chain triglycerides, MCTs are easily metabolized and lack proinflammatory properties, both characteristics unique to this fat source. Furthermore, MCTs are resistant to peroxidation. MCTs also do not accumulate in the liver and consequently do not impair hepatic function.[36] Despite these benefits, however, MCT oils are devoid of EFAs and thus cannot be used as a sole source of fat.

Since the 1980s, with the heightened awareness of the different inflammatory profiles of the available oil sources, there has been an evolution of ILE formulations. Emulsions have advanced from being solely made with soybean oil in the 1960s to being combined with MCTs in the 1980s, olive oil in the 1990s, and, more recently, with fish oil[37] (see Table 9.1).

As previously mentioned, in the 1990s, olive oil was introduced as an oil source in ILE. Olive oil is rich in omega-9 fatty acids, primarily as oleic acid, a type of monounsaturated fatty acid (MUFA), which is not considered essential because it is not a precursor of eicosanoids. Unlike soybean oil and fish oil, olive oil is considered immune neutral.[38] The relatively small amount of LA (approximately 5%) explains why this oil source requires blending with another oil source that contains EFA. In comparison with pure soybean oil, olive oil has a lower content of phytosterols and is naturally rich in alpha-tocopherol. Currently, the only available olive oil containing ILE is an 80% blend with 20% soybean oil (see Table 9.1). In this preparation, the mean concentration of LA is 35.8 mg/mL (range 27.6-44.0 mg/mL), and α-linolenic acid (ALA) is 4.7 mg/mL (range 1.0-8.4 mg/mL).[39] This product has 30% of the PUFA content of conventional SOLE. In comparison with soybean oil, olive oil is rich in MUFAs that possess less proinflammatory properties and are more resistant to oxidative stress injuries from free radicals. In many European countries, it is the preferred lipid source.[40] Although currently not approved in the United States for pediatric use, in a randomized controlled trial (RCT) from Australia, an olive oil-containing ILE used in preterm infants younger than 28 weeks' gestational age was found to be safe and well tolerated.[41]

Fish oil is the newest oil source to be used in ILE. Like olive oil, ILE containing fish oil is less proinflammatory than SOLE.[38] In comparison with those originating from omega-6 PUFAs in SOLE, the eicosanoids produced from omega-3 PUFAs in FOLE are generally less inflammatory. Unlike SOLE, FOLE has little LA and ALA but contains their downstream metabolites, ARA, EPA, and DHA.[35] The omega-3 PUFAs present in fish oil are also natural ligands to some receptors of the GPR family. Recent evidence demonstrates that the interaction with these receptors mediates some of the therapeutic benefits of omega-3 PUFAs in tissues, such as the liver.[23]

Le et al. assessed lipid and fatty acid profiles of 79 pediatric patients who developed IFALD while receiving standard PN with SOLE before and after being switched to FOLE.[42] Children who developed cholestasis while receiving PN with SOLE had their ILE administration discontinued and were treated with FOLE. FOLE was started at a dose of 1 g/kg/day infused over 12 to 24 hours. The serum fatty acid values at the end of the study were compared with baseline values that reflected the use of SOLE. The results showed a dramatic increase in omega-3 PUFAs, such as EPA and DHA. However, ALA, the precursor fatty acid to both EPA and DHA, decreased almost 60% from the baseline value. Switching from SOLE to FOLE also led to a decrease in all omega-6 PUFAs; in particular, gamma-linolenic acid, dihomo-gamma-linoleic acid, and ARA. The decrease in these fatty acids occurred concurrently with the decrease in omega-9 fatty acids (oleic acid and mead acid), which indicated that these patients did not produce extra nonessential fatty acids to compensate for the decrease in both ALA and LA concentrations. Lipid profiles of the 79 children showed decreases in low-density lipoprotein, very-low-density lipoprotein, cholesterol, and serum triglycerides. In addition to the improvement in lipid profiles, which are significant predictors of metabolic derangement, CRP also decreased significantly after treatment with FOLE.

Before being used as monotherapy, FOLE was blended with other oil sources. In a European retrospective study, the outcomes of 20 neonates with short bowel syndrome treated with an olive oil/soybean oil blend supplemented with FOLE was compared with the outcomes in a historical cohort of 18 patients with short bowel syndrome receiving SOLE alone.[43] The rationale for the use of this blend of oils was to provide an omega-6/omega-3 fatty acid ratio of 2:1 to 1:1. This was similar to a ratio that had been reported in a previous study using a 1:1 blend of soybean and fish oils.[44] This proportion is also within the optimal range for anti-inflammatory effects and is similar to that found in breast milk.[45] The researchers reported that in the olive oil/soybean oil/fish oil group, the direct bilirubin levels were reversed in all 14 survivors with cholestasis (direct bilirubin >50 μmol/L) with a median time to reversal of 2.9 months; two patients died as a result of liver failure (10%). In the SOLE controls, six patients (33%) died as a result of liver failure, and only two patients had normalization of bilirubin levels.[43]

Role of Phytosterols in the Pathogenesis of IFALD

Phytosterols are naturally occurring compounds found in plant cell membranes and are structurally similar cholesterol. In animal studies, phytosterols have been shown to interrupt hepatocyte FXR signaling and the expression of downstream bile acid transporters, thus decreasing bile flow.[46] In animal models, phytosterols have been shown to increase the risk of sepsis by altering the migratory and phagocytic functions of neutrophils, which can also contribute to IFALD.[33] Iyer et al. investigated the effect of intravenous plant sterols in piglets at doses equivalent to those used with commercial ILE preparations.[34] Although they did not demonstrate any clinical or histologic changes of cholestasis within the 14-day study period, serum bile acid levels were elevated in the sterol-treated piglets, suggesting early onset of cholestasis. As part of the same investigations, using a rat hepatocyte model, Iyer et al. showed that a commercial ILE enriched with plant sterols led to significant inhibition of hepatocyte secretory function. Similarly, El Kasmi et al. used mouse models to show that in comparison with FOLE, SOLE led to accumulation of stigmasterol in serum and in the liver and that it was associated with hepatic injury and cholestasis, along with reduced expression and function of the *Abcb11* and *Abcc2* genes, which play a critical role in bile transport.[47] On a molecular basis, they found that the expression of the canalicular exporter for stigmasterol, Abcg5/g8, was downregulated, resulting in hepatic accumulation of stigmasterol. This was associated with an inhibition in the expression of nuclear receptor FXR within the hepatocyte, which, in turn, reduced the expression of FXR-dependent genes, including bile salt export pumps that are responsible for driving bile flow.

Table 9.2 PHYTOSTEROL CONTENT OF COMMONLY USED INTRAVENOUS LIPID EMULSIONS

OIL	Intralipid	Omegaven	Clinolipid	SMOFlipid
Manufacturer	Fresenius Kabi (Uppsala, Sweden)	Fresenius Kabi (Bad Homburg, Germany)	Baxter (Deerfield, IL)	Fresenius Kabi (Uppsala, Sweden)
Lipid Source				
Soybean	100%		20%	30%
Medium-chain triglyceride				30%
Olive			80%	25%
Fish		100%		15%
Phytosterol Content (mg/L)	439 + 5.7	3.66	274 + 2.6	207

In neonates, phytosterols appear to accumulate rapidly. Nghiem-Rao et al. conducted a prospective cohort study in which 45 neonates (36 SOLE recipients versus 9 controls) underwent serial blood sample measurements of sitosterol, campesterol, and stigmasterol. They reported that very preterm infants receiving SOLE had higher sitosterol exposure and concluded that the poorly developed mechanisms of eliminating phytosterols might be a contributing factor for preterm infants being at greater risk for developing IFALD.[48]

The U.S. Food and Drug Administration (FDA), however, is concerned about the phytosterols content in ILEs. As part of the postmarketing process, manufacturers of several recently approved ILEs are now required to conduct studies in this area as a condition of the product's approval.[49,50] The requirements include developing and validating analytical methods for determining individual component phytosterol content and testing for individual component phytosterol content. On the basis of the results, data would be used to establish limits for individual phytosterol components. The FDA also requires manufacturers to develop and validate analytical methods for measuring phytosterol levels in plasma. Furthermore, FDA recommends that RCTs in pediatric patients (including neonates) be performed to compare an ILE product with a phytosterol-depleted formulation and a standard-of-care ILE to evaluate the incidence of liver injury, including IFALD.[50] Table 9.2 compares the phytosterol content of commonly used ILEs.

Not all animal models support the role of phytosterols as a causative factor in IFALD. In one study, premature piglets fed on an exclusively PN diet with different ILEs found that it was not the phytosterol content but, rather, the vitamin E or omega-3 PUFA content that was more hepatoprotective.[51] In fact, in subsequent studies using the same piglet model, the addition of phytosterols to 100% FOLE did not produce IFALD.[52] There is one major difference between the piglet model of IFALD and the murine model that may be responsible for some of the observed differences in results. It is customary to treat the piglets with broad-spectrum antibiotics, which may alter the intestinal microbiota, resulting in no intestinal injury or inflammation and thus no subsequent increase in intestinal permeability leading to IFALD.[46]

On the basis of this limited information, it would make sense to use an ILE with as little phytosterol content as possible. One means of reducing the phytosterol content in plant-based ILEs is to winterize the oil. This is a labor-intensive and somewhat expensive process and involves crystallization (or partial solidification) of the oil, followed by a separation of solids and fats.

Other Plant Toxins

Recent evidence also suggests that other plant toxins, such as isoflavonoids (i.e., biliatresone), may act to selectively destroy bile ducts outside the liver.[53] Interestingly, SOLE is rich in both phytosterols and isoflavonoids. In animal models, biliasterone was found to destroy bile ducts outside the liver, but not inside the liver, without toxic effects on other tissues. This suggests a toxin is responsible because of its affinity to large, extrahepatic bile ducts.

Table 9.3 ALPHA-TOCOPHEROL CONTENT OF REPRESENTATIVE LIPID EMULSIONS

OIL	Intralipid	Omegaven	Clinolipid	SMOFlipid
Manufacturer	Fresenius Kabi (Uppsala, Sweden)	Fresenius Kabi (Bad Homburg, Germany)	Baxter (Deerfield, IL)	Fresenius Kabi (Uppsala, Sweden)
Lipid Source				
Soybean	100%		20%	30%
Medium-chain triglyceride				30%
Olive			80%	25%
Fish		100%		15%
Vitamin E (mg/L)	38 mg	150-296 mg	32 mg	163-225 mg

Alpha-Tocopherol

Vitamin E is the major lipid-soluble antioxidant that protects unsaturated fatty acid acyl chains in the cell membranes from oxidative damage. It is added as alpha-tocopherol to ILE with high PUFA content to prevent peroxidation. Besides suppressing oxidant stress, vitamin E possesses diverse biologic functions, such as inducing bile acid activation and xenobiotic metabolism. The amount of vitamin E (as alpha-tocopherol) in ILEs may also play a role in IFALD. Alpha-tocopherol is abundant in pure fish oil and new-generation ILE blends. In humans, this form of vitamin E is preferentially absorbed and accumulated in tissues, whereas gamma-tocopherol, the principle form of vitamin E in SOLE, although easily metabolized in the liver, does not accumulate in plasma or tissues.[54] Gamma-tocopherol also has a much lower bioactivity compared with alpha-tocopherol. Moreover, patients who have received prolonged courses of SOLE have demonstrated reduced alpha-tocopherol concentrations in their plasma lipoproteins; this may further predispose patients to IFALD.[55] Table 9.3 summarizes the alpha-tocopherol content of representative ILEs.

In animal models, supplementation of SOLE with alpha-tocopherol has been shown to prevent hepatic damage, probably because of its antioxidant properties.[52] The hepatoprotective effects of vitamin E are thought to be mediated by activation of the *PXR* and *CAR* target genes involved in bile acid synthesis.[56] Others have shown, however, that in term neonatal piglets, supplemental ILE with alpha-tocopherol did not prevent cholestasis. Additional vitamin E was not associated with reduced inflammation or oxidative stress.[57] This suggests that the benefit of supplementing SOLE with vitamin E, rather than adding additional vitamin E to FOLE, to prevent early onset of IFALD is not applicable to all animal models of IFALD and requires further investigation. Clinically, results have also been mixed. In two large RCTs, treatment with vitamin E resulted in significant improvement in steatosis, ballooning, and inflammation in adults without diabetes or cirrhosis but did not offer any sustained benefit in children with nonalcoholic fatty liver disease.[58,59]

Impact of Lipid Dose on Predisposing Patients to IFALD

Regardless of type of substrate, macronutrient excess in PN has been shown to be harmful. Excessive lipid provision may be especially detrimental.[24,25] To date, data on the benefits of reducing lipid intake have been conflicting. SOLE dose reduction from 2 to 3 g/kg/day to 1 g/kg/day has not been proven to decrease the incidence of IFALD.[60,61] Low-dose SOLE may, however, slow the progression of hepatic disease, but when done to the extreme, it also carries the risk of predisposing patients to developing essential fatty acid deficiency (EFAD).[62]

As part of an analysis of factors contribution to IFALD in adults receiving home parenteral nutrition, Cavicchi et al. reported that SOLE doses of >1 g/kg/day were significantly associated with chronic cholestasis and liver disease.[6] Similarly, Cober et al. compared limiting doses of SOLE to 1 g/kg/day twice weekly in infants and compared total bilirubin levels with historical controls who received 3 g/kg/day of SOLE.[63] A marked reduction in SOLE intake was associated with a progressive decline in bilirubin levels in infants with IFALD, without a significant effect on growth, although there was a trend toward development of EFAD.

Impact of Lipid Dispensing/Infusion Practices

Even the method used to dispense or infuse ILEs may contribute to the development of IFALD. It has been well known for many years that photodegradation of amino acids may lead to IFALD.[64] Neuzil et al. hypothesized that ILE can be negatively affected by ambient light.[65] This is based on the premise that alpha-tocopherol could serve as a pro-oxidant in isolated lipoprotein suspensions, such as ILEs. Neuzil et al. exposed SOLE to a single spotlight, commonly used in the treatment of neonatal jaundice, and measured the formation of triglyceride hydroperoxides by using high-performance liquid chromatography. They observed that the concentrations of these hydroperoxides in different batches of SOLE increased by 60-fold after 24 hours of exposure to phototherapy lights. Triglyceride hydroperoxides were formed during phototherapy light exposure whether the SOLE was given via plastic intravenous administration sets used routinely for infusion or via glass containers. Although to a much lesser extent than observed with phototherapy, ambient light was also shown to cause significant peroxidation of ILEs. The authors concluded that phototherapy light-induced formation of triglyceride hydroperoxides could be prevented by covering SOLE with aluminum foil or supplementing it with sodium ascorbate before light exposure.

To further complicate matters, the type of oil in the ILE may also be important factor in determining the impact of photo-oxidation. Assuming that photo-oxidation of PN may result in production of 4-hydroxynonenal, which is suspected to be involved in the pathogenesis of IFALD, Miloudi et al. attempted to find a practical means to reduce 4-hydroxynonenal in PN and assessed the in vivo impact of PN containing low concentrations of 4-hydroxynonenal.[66] Using a newborn guinea pig model, hepatic markers of oxidative stress (glutathione, F[2α]-isoprostanes [GS-HNE]) and inflammation (messenger RNA [mRNA] of TNF-α and IL-1) were measured after the animals received infusions of PN compounded with either SOLE or FOLE over a 4-day period. Compared with SOLE, FOLE was found to reduce oxidative stress associated with PN and prevent hepatic inflammation.

Given the conflicting data and the lack of risk associated with protecting PN solutions from light, the choice remains one of risk to benefit, with many neonatal intensive care units (NICUs) opting to cover PN solutions and ILEs because this may confer some benefits and avoid the risk of undue harm.

A separate factor that has been suggested to play a role in the development of IFALD is use of tubing containing phthalates (di[2-ethylhexyl]phthalate [DEHP]) for administration of PN and ILEs. DEHP is a substance that can lead to an increase in oxidative stress and toxicity, especially in preterm infants and neonates who receive intensive care.[67] DEHP is a phthalic acid ester and is used as a plasticizer in polyvinylchloride (PVC) and other plastics. Most PVC infusion systems are plasticized with up to 60% of DEHP. Because DEHP is not covalently bound to the plastic matrix, DEHP is easily extracted from the tubing by PN solutions and has been shown to have toxic effects on various organ systems, including the livers of animals and humans. DEHP has the potential to reduce the canalicular excretion of bilirubin and, thus, to contribute to the development of cholestasis. The extent of DEHP leaching, however, is dependent on the type of fluid being infused. Crystalloids tend not to be problematic, but blood products and ILE are. Moreover, the type of ILE can also influence the amount of DEHP that can be extracted from the container and tubing. In a study assessing the potential role of the type of ILE on the quantity of DEHP leached, it was shown after 24 hours of exposure to PVC-based tubing that DEHP migration varied significantly ($P = 0.0000152$) according to lipid type. The olive oil-based ILE leached the most DEHP (65.8 μg/mL), followed by FOLE (37.8 μg/mL). SOLE showed comparable degrees of leaching (19.6-27.8 μg/mL).[68] Von Rettberg et al. assessed the effect of using DEHP-based tubing versus DEHP-free tubing in patients who had received PN containing ILEs for at least 14 days in pediatric intensive care units.[67] In the preintervention period, all intravenous infusion sets, including those for administering blood products, contained PVC. After 2001, all intravenous infusion sets were switched to non-PVC sets. Of the 30 patients in the PVC group, 15 developed signs of cholestasis, whereas of the 46 patients who were treated without using PVC infusion sets, only 6 did. This was equivalent to a reduction in the incidence of cholestasis from 50% to 13%. The authors concluded that the use of infusion systems that contained PVC lead to a 5.6-fold increase in risk for the development of hepatobiliary dysfunction.

Lipid Emulsion Strategies in the Treatment of IFALD

Soybean Oil–Based Lipid Emulsions

Several studies assessed the impact of minimizing exposure to SOLE for treatment of IFALD, as well as the concomitant risks of adverse effects on growth and EFAD. Cober et al. studied the effect of SOLE reduction to 1 g/kg/day two times per week in neonates diagnosed with IFALD.[63] Over a 2-year period, NICU surgical patients on chronic PN were enrolled if the following entry criteria were met: (1) ≥2 weeks of continuous PN, with SOLE typically administered at 3 g/kg/day; and (2) a serum direct bilirubin ≥2.5 mg/dL (or serum total bilirubin ≥5 mg/dL if serum direct bilirubin was not available). Members of the SOLE reduction group were matched with a historical control cohort of surgical patients who received PN between August 2003 and July 2005. Infants received SOLE at a dose of 1 g/kg/day given twice weekly. No other lipid emulsions were administered to these patients. Besides the amounts of SOLE, the compositions of the PN solution were essentially the same. To compensate for loss of calories as a result of lipid reduction, attention was given to increasing the patient's glucose infusion rate to ensure adequate growth and adequate energy delivery. In both groups, a target energy delivery of 100 to 125 kcal/kg/day was attempted using a combination of EN and PN. The control group was given SOLE to a maximum dose of 3 g/kg/day, regardless of the bilirubin level, as long as the serum triglyceride level remained less than 200 mg/dL. The primary study outcome measure was the change in serum bilirubin over time after beginning of the study. Two potential adverse outcomes were evaluated in the treatment group: (1) lack of adequate weight gain and (2) development of EFAD. The frequency of EFAD, as measured by the triene/tetraene ratio, and the absolute serum levels of LA and ALA were measured monthly in all patients with ILE reduction. Thirty-one infants were placed on the SOLE reduction protocol, and 31 matched controls were selected. The authors found a significant reduction in average bilirubin levels in the SOLE reduction group (estimated slope: −0.73 mg/dL/week; $P = 0.0097$) compared with a rise in levels in the control group across weeks (estimated slope: 0.29 mg/dL/week; $P = 0.0271$). A significant difference in the slopes was identified between the two groups ($P = 0.0017$). Thirteen of 31 infants in the SOLE reduction group had ≥1 EFA profile measured during the study period. Of these 13 infants, eight developed mild EFAD. None of the infants displayed physical manifestations of EFAD. The difference in rate of weight gain was not significantly different ($P = 0.937$). Overall, a marked reduction in SOLE administration was associated with a progressive decline in bilirubin levels in infants with IFALD. Use of the protocol did not affect overall growth; development of mild EFAD, however, emphasized the need for careful monitoring of EFA status.

Several other publications report findings with similar lipid minimization strategies. Colomb et al. demonstrated an association between decreases in lipid therapy and normalization of serum conjugated bilirubin.[69] Nusinovich et al. also described 32 patients with IFALD, of whom 31 had their hyperbilirubinemia normalized with aggressive intestinal rehabilitation that included restriction of SOLE to <1 g/kg/day, and Bianchi suggested improved outcomes with a "hepato-sparing regimen" with a SOLE dose <1.5 g/kg/day.[70,71]

Fish Oil–Based Lipid Emulsions

Because of the presumed role of SOLE in IFALD, much interest has been garnered around the use alternative ILE products, such as FOLE. Lam et al. performed the first prospective, double-blind RCT comparing SOLE with FOLE in the treatment of infants with pre-existing IFALD caused by SOLE.[72] Inclusion criteria were conjugated bilirubin ≥2 mg/dL (34 μmol/L) and expected PN requirement for >2 weeks.

The primary outcome was reversal of IFALD, defined as conjugated bilirubin level <2 mg/dL (<34 μmol/L) within 4 months after beginning of lipid treatment. The secondary outcomes were rate of change of weekly liver function tests, infant growth (i.e., head circumference, body weight), blood lipid profiles and number of episodes of late-onset sepsis. Eligible infants were randomly assigned to receive either FOLE or SOLE. Infants randomized to the FOLE arm received a starting dose of 0.5 g/kg/day and gradually advanced to the maximum of 1.5 at 0.5 g/kg/day increments every 2 days. Infants receiving SOLE had the dose of ILE decreased to 1.5 g/kg/day. A total of nine infants had been randomized to FOLE and seven to the SOLE group by the time the interim analysis was undertaken. With increasing public awareness of FOLE, parents were increasingly unwilling to consent to randomization. Therefore the authors decided to terminate the study prematurely. They found no difference in the primary outcome between groups because the median age of resolution of cholestasis was 110 (interquartile range [IQR] 82-158) versus 137 (IQR 106-150) days for FOLE and SOLE ($P = 0.74$), respectively. Three of the nine infants in the FOLE group recovered from IFALD while receiving PN, whereas none in the SOLE group did. All infants in the FOLE group survived and were subsequently discharged from hospital. There were two deaths in the SOLE group. In both instances, the infants died of hepatic failure and multiorgan failure secondary to sepsis. There was a significant increase in conjugated bilirubin of 0.79 mg/dL (13.5 μmol/L) per week in the SOLE group but not in the FOLE group (0.04 mg/dL [0.6 μmol/L] per week; $P = 0.90$). The rate of increase of conjugated bilirubin in the SOLE group was significantly greater than in the FOLE group ($P = 0.03$). Similarly, ALT significantly worsened, increasing by 9.1 IU/L per week in the SOLE group ($P <0.01$) but not in the FOLE group (1.1 IU/L per week; $P = 0.71$). After adjusting for baseline changes, increases in EN were associated with significant improvement of IFALD in infants receiving FOLE, with the conjugated bilirubin decreasing by 0.5 m/dL (8.5 μmol/L) per 10% increase in EN ($P < 0.01$). In contrast, infants receiving SOLE had no such improvement (conjugated bilirubin decreased by 0.09 mg/dL [1.6 μmol/L] per 10% increase in EN; $P = 0.96$). Although the primary outcome of IFALD at 4 months was not different between the two groups, there was a significant difference in the rates of change of conjugated bilirubin and liver function between them, and this study demonstrated that replacement of SOLE with FOLE ILE monotherapy could halt the progression of pre-existing IFALD.

Multiple nonrandomized studies using historical controls have been performed in infants with short bowel syndrome, suggesting that FOLE can reverse IFALD. Gura et al. assessed the safety and efficacy of fish oil-based lipid emulsion in IFALD.[73] Infants (n = 18) receiving PN with SOLE who developed cholestasis were treated with FOLE and prospectively followed up. They were compared with a historical cohort of 30 infants who had short bowel syndrome, were PN dependent for at least 90 days, and were treated at the same institution from 1986 to 1996. Outcomes of 21 eligible subjects were included. The primary study outcome was time to reversal of cholestasis, defined as time to the first of three consecutive serum direct bilirubin measurements of ≤2 mg/dL. Safety outcomes, including fatty acid and coagulation profiles, growth (weight-for-age z [WAZ] scores), and bloodstream infections, were systematically recorded. Patients were followed up from baseline to last observation date (at or before PN cessation) for a median time of 18.4 weeks (IQR 8.7-36.4 weeks). Two of the seven in the FOLE cohort died, whereas seven of fourteen in the historical cohort died; no patients in the FOLE cohort and six patients in the historical cohort died as a result of liver-related causes. Patients who did not die or undergo transplantation were followed up from baseline for a median time of 15.2 weeks (IQR 8.1-25.0 weeks). Among survivors, the median time to reverse cholestasis was 9.4 weeks (IQR 7.6-10.9 weeks) in the FOLE and 44.1 weeks (IQR 10.9-45.6 weeks) in the historical cohort ($P = 0.002$). Surviving patients in the FOLE cohort had a 3.8 (hazard ratio 4.8; 95% CI 1.6-14.1) times larger rate of reversing cholestasis than those in the historical cohort. The occurrence of undesirable safety outcomes in children receiving FOLE was comparable before and after treatment started, except for a single subject who briefly displayed biochemical evidence of

EFAD. No patients developed hypertriglyceridemia (triglyceride level 400 mg/dL) or coagulopathy (international normalized ratio >2) during therapy. Mean platelet counts were statistically significantly higher during the FOLE course ($P = 0.03$). New infection rates and WAZ scores were comparable across periods. The authors concluded that the use of FOLE in infants who depend on PN may reverse cholestasis and fatal liver disease. Importantly, they did not observe any deleterious adverse effects of treatment.

In the United States, use of FOLE is currently not FDA approved. Physicians can obtain permission to use FOLE for a single patient by submitting a Single Patient IND application to the FDA (see 21 CFR 312.3101 under the FDA Expanded Access Program, (https://www.fda.gov/drugs/developmentapprovalprocess/howdrugsarede velopedandapproved/approvalapplications/investigationalnewdrugindapplication/uc m368740.htm). If all the necessary patient data are provided, authorization to obtain the drug may be granted in <30 days but often is granted in <1 week. Once approval to obtain the drug is received, physicians can then request permission from the FDA to bill for FOLE. Because of its investigational status, however, some third parties may still not cover the costs of FOLE despite the prescriber receiving FDA approval to bill.

Concerns about Fish Oil Monotherapy

The use of FOLE has raised some concerns that are unique to this oil source. Toxicities attributed to FOLE, such as hypervitaminosis A and D and heavy metal toxicity, are, in fact, those seen with cod liver oil. Fish oil, unlike cod liver oil, is derived from the tissue of fish and is devoid of excessive levels of vitamins A and D. Both European and U.S. monographs have described limits on the amounts of heavy metals and other environmental contaminants that can be present in fish oil, and manufacturers are required to assay each batch of oil to ensure acceptable limits.[74]

Bleeding

The effects of EPA and DHA on platelet aggregation, coagulation, and other rheologic properties of blood have been extensively addressed in the literature. Eicosanoids and prostanoids derived from omega-3 PUFAs are anti-inflammatory mediators and are known to have important vascular and hemostatic effects.[75] Because of these properties, there are concerns that the hematologic attributes of fish oil may increase the risk of bleeding in patients administered omega-3 fatty acid–rich compounds. The hemostatic effects of omega-3 PUFAs are reflected in ex vivo platelet function tests. EPA and DHA can significantly reduce platelet aggregation and activation, as shown by results from aggregometry assays in humans[76] and thromboelastography platelet mapping in a neonatal piglet model.[77] Increased bleeding time has also been reported, although not consistently.[78]

The hemostatic effects of EPA and DHA are multifactorial. ARA is the most common precursor of prostaglandin synthesis. Omega-3 fatty acids inhibit platelet aggregation by decreasing the production of thromboxane A2, a proaggregatory derivative of ARA, and favor the formation of thromboxane A3, an antiaggregatory derivative of DHA.[78-80] Fish oil has also been shown to decrease platelet count, although a concomitant increase in platelet size seems to keep the platelet mass unchanged.[81] In endothelial cells, synthesis of prostaglandin I3, an inhibitor of platelet aggregation, is favored by the displacement of ARA by EPA.[82,83] Changes induced by omega-3 fatty acids at the membrane and intracellular levels also lead to inhibited platelet function through augmentation of the negative surface charge density, modulation of signal transduction molecules, and decreased adhesiveness and granule secretion.[78,84-86] The inhibitory effect of omega-3 fatty acids on procoagulant platelet- and monocyte-derived microparticles has also been described in specific situations.[87,88] Additionally, EPA and DHA can decrease platelet-mediated thrombin generation, thereby acting indirectly on the coagulation cascade.[89] Omega-3 PUFAs are also known to potentiate plasma fibrinolysis by increasing the levels of vascular plasminogen activator and reducing the levels of its inhibitors.[90] It is this combination of effects of omega-3 fatty acids that give them a role as cardioprotective molecules.

Nonetheless, a direct link has not been established between the theoretical risk and ex vivo studies and an increased bleeding risk in vivo with fish oil. Results from numerous RCTs and epidemiologic studies have failed to find an association between fish oil and bleeding.[78,91,92] Additionally, studies addressing the use of fish oil supplementation in different clinical settings have failed to show an increased risk of bleeding through assessment of secondary outcomes or adverse events.[78] This holds true even in studies in which patients received fish oil in addition to other antiplatelet agents or anticoagulants.[84,93] Regardless, because of the theoretical risk, surgeons and anesthesiologists still often recommend discontinuing fish oil therapy in preparation for invasive procedures.[94] Von Schacky et al. studied the incorporation and metabolism of EPA and DHA in humans supplemented with an omega-3 PUFA-rich diet.[95] They noted that the levels of DHA in erythrocyte membranes did not return to baseline even 20 weeks after stopping fish oil supplementation. As expected, platelet aggregation was persistently decreased while on fish oil, but returned to baseline at the end of the study period, nearly 20 weeks after stopping treatment. Based on these findings, the perioperative discontinuation of fish oil supplementation often recommended by surgeons and anesthesiologists should have minimal to no effect on the levels of fatty acids present and stored in cell membranes at the time of the procedure, and holding the supplements is therefore unwarranted. Similarly, studies using FOLE for treating IFALD have not reported instances of bleeding that were attributed to its use.[73]

Although omega-3 PUFAs are known to affect hemostatic pathways, clinical evidence supporting an increased bleeding risk is lacking. On the basis of an isolated case report, a retrospective chart review was performed to describe the incidence of clinically significant postprocedural bleeding (CSPPB) in children with IFALD receiving FOLE.[96] CSPPB was defined as bleeding leading to reoperation, transfer to the intensive care unit, readmission, or death, up to 1 month after any invasive procedure. Of the 244 patients treated with FOLE, 183 underwent ≥1 invasive procedures (n = 732). Five (0.68%; 95% CI 0.22-1.59) procedures resulted in CSPPB. FOLE therapy was never interrupted. No deaths resulted from bleeding. The authors concluded that FOLE therapy is safe, with a CSPPB risk no greater than that reported in the general population and that FOLE should not be withheld in preparation for procedures. These findings support those from prior studies showing that ex vivo hemostatic effects of omega-3 PUFA therapy do not necessarily translate into a clinically significant increased risk of bleeding.[78] Greenland Eskimos, for example, who base their diets on seafood products rich in omega-3 PUFAs, have prolonged bleeding times and mild bleeding tendencies that have never been described as clinically dangerous.[97]

The use of FOLE at a dose of 1 g/kg/day in patients with liver injury should be considered the extreme model of exposure to omega-3 PUFAs. To put this dosage in perspective, when used for cardioprotection, a typical dose of oral fish oil in a 70-kg male is 1 g/day or 3 to 5 g/day for the treatment of hypertriglyceridemia.[98] This translates to a dose of 14 to 71 mg/kg/day. When accounting the enteral bioavailability of enteral fish oil supplements, these numbers drop even further.[99]

Essential Fatty Acid Deficiency

The use of FOLE as the sole source of fat for patients receiving PN has raised concerns for the development of EFAD, hindering its adoption into clinical practice. Although relatively rare, EFAD can occur in as little as a few days in infants and within several weeks in older children and adults with chronic malnutrition and malabsorption. EFAD may also occur within weeks in patients receiving prolonged courses of PN with inadequate fat intake.[1] Because of their limited fat stores, premature infants may develop EFAD in <1 week when their intake of EFAs is <4% to 5% of their total caloric intake.[100] EFAD may lead to dermatitis, growth retardation, hair loss, infertility, impaired vision, coagulopathies, susceptibility to infections, as well as to hepatosteatosis induced by de novo lipogenesis.[1,101-103]

In a study of 10 patients completely dependent on PN and FOLE, the fatty acid profiles and growth data was reviewed for evidence of EFAD and growth failure.[104] After a median time of 3.8 months on exclusive PN and FOLE, none of the patients developed biochemical or clinical evidence of EFAD. Z-scores were not statistically different, indicating no growth impairment. Median direct bilirubin levels improved in 9 patients from 6.8 mg/dL to 0.9 mg/dL ($P = 0.009$). The authors concluded that when dosed appropriately, fish oil-based lipid emulsions contain sufficient amounts of EFAs to prevent EFAD and sustain growth in patients completely dependent on PN. In cases of pre-existing malnutrition, higher doses of FOLE may be necessary.

Introduction of low-fat or fat-free nutrition to severely malnourished patients, however, is not without risk. It may actually predispose patients to the development of EFAD. For example, biochemical signs of EFAD have been reported in malnourished adult patients upon initiation of PN and is believed to be the result of the synthetic activity of fatty acids being depressed in times of starvation and then elevated upon refeeding.[20,105,106] In another case series of severely malnourished adults with liver dysfunction, introduction of energy and other nutrients resulted in biochemical EFAD manifestations without evidence of dermatologic findings.[105] Baseline tissue stores of EFAs in this population were low and comparable with those of the control population when refeeding began. The authors suggested that short-term SOLE supplementation may not be able to reverse baseline EFAD and that more prolonged lipid supplementation may be necessary to replenish deficient stores.[105] Other data suggest that in severely malnourished infants being treated for IFALD, higher doses of FOLE may be required for adequate growth and to prevent EFAD. The provision of FOLE at 1 g/kg/day, typically used to treat IFALD, may simply be insufficient to replete EFA stores in malnourished patients and also treat IFALD.

Long-Term Use of Fish Oil Monotherapy

There are few data available on growth parameters in children with long-term PN dependence in general and none available for children receiving long-term FOLE instead of SOLE. Given the lack of previous long-term experience with FOLE monotherapy, concerns regarding its long-term use once cholestasis has been resolved have been raised.

A review of prospectively collected data was performed for children with IFALD who required at least 3 years of PN and FOLE secondary to chronic intestinal failure.[107] Of 215 patients with IFALD treated from 2004 to 2015, 30 required PN and FOLE for at least 3 years (median 4.6 years). To date, no patients have died, required transplantation, or developed EFAD. Biochemical markers of liver disease normalized within the first year of therapy with no recurrent elevations in the long term. WAZ and length-for-age Z (LAZ) scores improved and PN dependence decreased in the first year of therapy, with a stable rate of growth in the long term. Among the sickest cohort of infants with IFALD (i.e., those with cirrhosis), 76% experienced resolution of cholestasis with no mortality, need for transplantation, or recurrent liver disease. This improvement in patient survival marked a significant decrease from the 50% mortality and/or transplantation rate observed in the late 1990s and early 21st century.[108] Growth, however, remains a significant challenge in this population. Unfortunately, even in patients who undergo intestinal transplantation, gains in growth Z-scores are minimal. Venick et al. reported growth outcomes in 33 patients who underwent small bowel transplantation for chronic intestinal failure, with a mean follow-up of 3.8 years. Survival was high, with 85% alive at 5 years; WAZ and LAZ scores, however, did not change significantly over time after transplantation. In addition, five patients developed EFAD as a result of limitations in lipid provision in the setting of chylous ascites after transplantation.[109] Raphael et al. reported growth data for the first year of life in 51 PN-dependent infants with intestinal failure. A U-shaped growth curve was observed in their cohort, with median WAZ and LAZ scores decreasing until age 6 months and subsequently recovering by age 1 year. FOLE therapy was used for treatment of IFALD in 59% of these patients, but its use did not correlate with growth failure on regression analysis.[110] Pichler et al. reported growth data in 45 patients with intestinal failure receiving PN for a mean of 5 years. SOLE was used in 88% of the patients. PN-dependent patients had a mean WAZ of −0.8, LAZ of −1.8, and body mass index Z-score of 0.4, and 50% of their cohort had a LAZ <−2, consistent with growth failure. Dual-energy X-ray absorptiometry revealed that bone age was delayed by >2 standard deviations (SD) in 37% of the patients, highlighting the severity of growth failure in this population.[111] In the previously mentioned study by Nandivada et al., however, significant gains in growth Z-scores did occur during the first year of therapy, with stable rates of growth thereafter. These findings may reflect an early acceleration of growth in response to resolution of IFALD in the first year of FOLE therapy, with stable growth subsequently as bowel adaptation occurs. Importantly, there were no decelerations in growth Z-scores despite continued PN and FOLE dependence. Unfortunately, there are no other long-term age- and gender-adjusted growth data available for PN-dependent children for comparison.

Failure to Respond to Fish Oil Monotherapy

In PN-dependent patients in whom cholestasis is not resolved with FOLE, end-stage liver disease, requiring liver transplantation, or to death may ensue. To date, there are no tools for predicting which infants will fail to respond to FOLE. One study attempted to identify early patient factors associated with subsequent failure of FOLE so as to guide prognosis and patient referral to centers that offer this therapy.[112] Demographics, laboratory values, and medical history at the time of initiation of therapy of 182 patients treated with FOLE were compared between patients who achieved resolution of cholestasis and those in whom therapy failed. Among those patients treated with FOLE, 86% achieved resolution of cholestasis, and in 14% therapy failed. Patients in whom therapy failed had median (IQR) lower birth weight ($P = 0.03$) and were older at FOLE initiation ($P = 0.02$) than those whose cholestasis resolved. Patients in whom therapy failed also had more advanced liver disease at treatment initiation compared with those whose cholestasis resolved. A multivariate analysis revealed that a Pediatric End-Stage Liver Disease (PELD) score ≥15, history of gastrointestinal bleeding, IFALD ≥16 weeks, presence of other comorbidities, and mechanical ventilation at the time of FOLE initiation were independent predictors of treatment failure. Despite these limitations, this study demonstrated that most PN-dependent infants with IFALD will respond to FOLE with resolution of biochemical cholestasis and avoidance of liver transplantation. Critically ill patients with clinical and laboratory evidence of advanced liver disease, however, remain at a higher risk of FOLE therapy failure. Nonetheless, many patients with similarly advanced liver disease and a high acuity of general illness have responded to FOLE, suggesting that the likelihood of treatment failure cannot be reliably predicted. The authors suggest that early initiation of therapy with FOLE be initiated once cholestasis is detected because there are still no definitive tests or factors to identify which patients have irreversible liver disease.

Nandivada et al. sought to determine the need for liver and/or multivisceral organ transplantation and mortality in children with cirrhosis from IFALD after resolution of cholestasis with FOLE therapy.[113] In this retrospective analysis, medical records from 2004 to 2012 of all patients younger than 12 years treated with FOLE monotherapy at a dose of 1 g/kg/day were reviewed. The primary endpoints of this study were the incidence of multivisceral or hepatic transplantation and/or mortality in children who had cirrhosis caused by IFALD and who experienced resolution of cholestasis after treatment with FOLE. Secondary endpoints included recurrent cholestasis, hepatic injury, hepatic synthetic function, growth, and presence of symptomatic cirrhosis caused by IFALD requiring medical or surgical therapy. A total of 178 patients treated with FOLE for IFALD from January 1, 2004, to January 1, 2012, were identified. Fifty-one of the 178 (29%) patients had a concurrent diagnosis of cirrhosis from IFALD. Of the 51 patients with cirrhosis, 39 (76%) experienced resolution of cholestasis after initiation of FOLE. Median time to resolution of cholestasis was 74 days (IQR 39-123 days). The duration of PN dependence ranged from 1 month to 9 years, with a median of 2.7 years. Thirty-nine patients with cirrhosis caused by IFALD had resolution of biochemical cholestasis with FOLE therapy; none required liver or multivisceral transplantation, and the follow-up range was 1 to 9 years. Two of the 39 patients died after initiation of FOLE. One patient died 3 months after initiation of FOLE secondary to complications associated with severe pulmonary stenosis and heart failure. Another patient died 3 months after initiation of FOLE from sepsis with multiorgan failure after surgery for a small bowel obstruction. Neither death was related to liver failure or central line–associated bloodstream infection. In the patients who remained PN-dependent, the direct bilirubin remained at <2 mg/dL for the remainder of the follow-up period after resolution of cholestasis. The PELD score in the study population decreased from 16 ± 4.6 at initiation of FOLE to -1.2 ± 4.6, 12 months after resolution of cholestasis ($P < 0.001$). For the small number of patients with persistent PN dependence, the PELD score remained in the normal range for the remainder of the follow-up period after resolution of cholestasis. Transaminases also decreased after resolution of cholestasis and remained at low levels. These results suggest that children with cirrhosis from IFALD who experience resolution of cholestasis with FOLE therapy have preserved liver function and do not require subsequent liver transplantation.

Soy–Fish Oil Blends

Diamond et al. studied a retrospective cohort of 12 children with IFALD who had been treated with a 1:1 mixture of SOLE and FOLE.[44] At the time that FOLE was initiated, all had either been listed for liver and/or intestinal transplantation or were undergoing assessment by the transplantation program. One patient had undergone an isolated liver transplantation and had developed recurrent IFALD in the grafted liver. Of the 12 subjects, nine had complete resolution of hyperbilirubinemia; three patients received liver-intestine allografts while being treated. There were no complications or alterations in coagulation parameters associated with FOLE. Four achieved complete resolution of hyperbilirubinemia while receiving the 1:1 blend of SOLE and FOLE, whereas in five cases, resolution of cholestasis occurred only after discontinuation of the SOLE and the initiation of FOLE monotherapy. In addition to resolution of hyperbilirubinemia, there was also evidence of reduction in serum transaminases and a statistically significant increase in serum albumin.

Alternative Lipid Emulsions

Other lipid emulsions have also been studied for treating IFALD. SMOFlipid (Fresenius Kabi, Uppsala, Sweden) is a composite ILE that contains soybean oil (30%), medium MCT (30%), olive oil (25%), and fish oil (15%). The product has an omega-6 PUFA/omega-3 PUFA ratio of 2.5:1. In comparison with SOLE, the lipid composition of SMOFlipid more closely approximates that of human milk. Approved by the FDA in 2016 for use in adults as a noninferior lipid source in comparison with pure soybean lipid emulsions, several pediatric postmarketing studies are currently ongoing in the United States.[50] In a double-blind, parallel-group study conducted in Athens, Greece, Skouroliakou et al. demonstrated reduced oxidative stress with SMOFlipid relative to SOLE in a cohort of 38 preterm infants.[114] After 14 days of treatment, however, there was no difference in serum bilirubin levels. When Tomsits et al. compared SMOFlipid to SOLE in 60 premature neonates treated at Semmelweis University, Budapest, Hungary, they demonstrated improvements in serum GGT with those receiving SMOFlipid.[115]

An Australian study compared SMOFlipid to olive oil-based and soybean oil-based emulsions in a group of very preterm neonates (23-30 weeks) for 7 days.[41] Both emulsions were well tolerated without any adverse events. DHA levels in both groups were similar despite the higher contents of DHA in SMOFlipid product. As expected, EPA and vitamin E concentrations were significantly increased in the SMOFlipid group. No differences in direct bilirubin or hepatic enzymes were observed, but given the short duration of the study (7 days), this was not considered unusual. The authors concluded that SMOFlipid, in comparison with soybean oil/olive oil ILEs, exhibited beneficial effects in terms of reduction of oxidative stress by reducing lipid peroxidation levels in high-risk preterm neonates.

A recent Canadian multicenter, blinded pilot RCT compared SMOFlipid with SOLE in a cohort of infants with the early stages of IFALD.[116] A total of 24 infants (mean age 6 weeks) participated in the trial (13 SOLE, 11 SMOFlipid). They were similar in gestational age (34.5 weeks in the SMOFlipid group, 35.2 weeks in the SOLE group), although the SMOFlipid group had a higher preponderance of small bowel atresia (46% versus 23%) and necrotizing enterocolitis (18% versus 8%) in comparison with the SOLE group. Conversely, the SOLE-treated infants had a higher incidence of gastroschisis (31%) in comparison with 18% in the SMOFlipid group. The trial duration was up to 12 weeks, unless the infant achieved full enteral tolerance sooner. At the end of the study, infants who received SMOFlipid had a lower conjugated bilirubin compared with those who received SOLE (mean difference −59 µmol/L; $P = 0.03$). Moreover, infants receiving SMOFlipid were also more likely to have a decrease in conjugated bilirubin to 0 mg/dL than those in the SOLE group ($P = 0.03$). The time to achievement of full enteral tolerance did not differ statistically ($P = 0.59$) between the groups. There was no statistical difference in immunologic parameters or triglyceride levels. The authors concluded that compared with SOLE, SMOFlipid was found to reduce the risk of progressive IFALD in children with intestinal failure; the study design did not allow for determining whether initiating SMOFlpid from day 1 of PN in extremely premature at risk infants would prevent or reduce the incidence of IFALD.

Similar to what was seen with the 1:1 ratio of SOLE/FOLE experience, patients treated with SMOFlipid for IFALD may still require rescue with FOLE monotherapy before clinical improvement in cholestasis is seen.[117] In one case series, two infants developed IFALD while receiving SMOFlipid 2 to 3 g/kg/day, over 24 hours that was later reversed by switching from blended-oil ILE to FOLE monotherapy.

Role of Lipid Emulsions in the Prevention of IFALD

The etiology of IFALD appears to be multifactorial, with some combination of disease-related risk factors plus environmental triggers leading to its development. In light of the mixed success of various treatment modalities, prevention of IFALD has become increasingly important. Various treatments discussed previously have been studied for preventive purposes, again with mixed results. The major role of PN in the development of IFALD clearly points to maximization of EN as the key preventive measure. The more enteral intake that a patient can tolerate and the more quickly they can be weaned off PN while maintaining their nutritional status, the better would be their likely outcome.

Soybean Oil

In centers where access to FOLE is limited, restricting SOLE intake in hopes of preventing IFALD is a common management strategy. In one pilot trial, reduced dose SOLE was compared with a standard dose of SOLE in neonates at risk for IFALD.[62] This prospective RCT was performed from 2009 to 2011 and involved surgical patients ≥26 weeks' gestation anticipated to require >50% of daily caloric intake from PN for at least 4 weeks. Infants (n = 28) were randomized to either reduced (1 g/kg/day) or standard (3 g/kg/day) groups. Groups had similar PN calories and protein intake throughout the study with average treatment duration of 5.4 weeks. Total direct bilirubin increase from baseline was smaller in the reduced versus standard groups ($P = -0.04$). WAZ scores increased more in the standard group, and no patient experienced EFAD. The authors concluded that the markers of cholestasis rose at a slower rate using reduced lipid doses, suggesting it may delay the onset of IFALD and possibly prevent it if the infant could be weaned off PN.

Prophylactic SOLE restriction was also used in a study involving surgical infants at risk for developing IFALD.[118] An experimental group comprising 82 surgical infants was treated with lipid restriction (i.e., SOLE 1 g/kg/day), from 2009 to 2011, and was retrospectively compared with a control cohort of 132 infants who received standard ILE dosing (i.e., SOLE 2 g/kg/day), from 2005 to 2008. A significant reduction in the incidence of IFALD was demonstrated in the lipid restricted group compared with the control group (22% versus 43%; $P = 0.003$). Patients treated with standard lipid provisions were 1.77 times more likely to develop IFALD than those who had been lipid restricted.

Others have found no benefit in lipid restriction. Levit et al. compared lower doses of SOLE to standard dosing but maintained daily administration.[61] When the lower dose group was compared with the control group, there was no difference in cholestasis rates. Although the low dose group received less SOLE and total calories over time compared with the control group, weight, length, and head circumference at 28 days of life, discharge, and over time were not different. The authors concluded that compared with the control dose, low-dose SOLE was not associated with a reduction in cholestasis or growth.

This same research group subsequently conducted a follow-up study involving neonates with gastrointestinal disorders at risk for IFALD.[119] The objective of this multicenter RCT was to determine whether a lower dose of SOLE (1 g/kg/day) compared with a higher dose (i.e., 3 g/kg/day) prevented cholestasis without compromising growth. A total of 36 neonates diagnosed with gastrointestinal disease ≤5 days of age were randomized to SOLE 1 g/kg/day or control dose, 3 g/kg/day. The primary outcome was cholestasis after the first 7 days of age with secondary outcomes of growth, duration of PN and episodes of sepsis. When the 1 g/kg/day group was compared with the 3 g/kg/day group, there was no difference in cholestasis (30% versus 38%; $P = 0.7$). Similar to the study by Rollins et al., however, the mean direct bilirubin rate of change over the first 8 weeks and the entire study period was lower in the 1 g/kg/day group compared with the 3 g/kg/day group (0.07 ± 0.04 versus 0.3 ± 0.09 mg/dL/week; $P = 0.01$). Growth was comparable between the groups.

Fish Oil

Given its role in the treatment of IFALD, it seems logical to consider the use of FOLE in the prevention of IFALD in at-risk patients. One pilot study did attempt to assess the safety and efficacy of FOLE in reducing the incidence of cholestasis in neonates in comparison with SOLE.[120] This was a double-blind RCT, in which 19 infants were randomized to either 1 g/kg/day SOLE (n = 10) or 1 g/kg/day FOLE (n = 9). Nutrition assessments and laboratory studies were serially obtained for the duration of PN use or until 6 months' corrected gestational age. Neurodevelopmental outcomes were assessed at 6 and 24 months' corrected age. There were no differences between groups in demographic characteristics; nor were there were any differences between groups in baseline laboratory values, the duration of PN, amount of enteral intake, or the number of operative procedures. Because of the tight inclusion/exclusion criteria, the majority of patients were not critically ill. As the study protocol did not allow for prior exposure to any form of ILE, no patients with necrotizing enterocolitis were included because the study took place in a center that was not a birthing hospital and those patients were transferred in already on an ILE. As a result, the incidence of cholestasis among enrolled patients was significantly lower than expected. The study was terminated early because of inability to assess for differences in the incidence of cholestasis. The use of FOLE was not associated with growth impairment, EFAD, coagulopathy, infectious complications, hypertriglyceridemia, or adverse neurodevelopmental outcomes.

Conclusion

Current opinion in the United States is that there is insufficient evidence to support the use of alternative lipid emulsions in the prevention of IFALD. This was summarized in the "Nutrition Support Clinical Guideline Recommendations in Pediatric Patients with Intestinal Failure" of the American Society for Parenteral and Enteral Nutrition.[121] Using the Grading of Recommendations Assessment, Development and Evaluation (GRADE) strategy, the group attempted to answer the question: "What fat emulsion strategies can be used in pediatric patients with intestinal failure to reduce the risk of or treat PNALD?" On the basis of the quality of evidence and currently available products, the only recommendation the group could make (and it was a weak one at that) was to consider using low-dose SOLE at <1 g/kg/day. With regard to the use of alternative lipid emulsions, such as fish oil and olive oil, the group could not make any recommendations.

Despite the use of different dosing schema and alternative lipid emulsions, the most effective therapy remains discontinuation of PN entirely and transitioning to full enteral feedings.[122] In patients who cannot be weaned off PN, the use of lipid restriction if SOLE is used or the combining of SOLE with other oil sources, such as FOLE, has been shown to be somewhat effective in reducing the risk of IFALD or delaying its progression. FOLE monotherapy, when introduced early in the course of IFALD, in comparison with SOLE, appears to be more effective in the treatment of IFALD. To date, there is still no ideal ILE that has been identified for use in this vulnerable population.

REFERENCES

1. Fleming CR. Intestinal failure. In: GL Hill, ed. *Nutrition and the Surgical Patient*. Edinburgh: Churchill Livingstone; 1981:219–235.
2. Kelly DA. Liver complications of pediatric parenteral nutrition—epidemiology. *Nutrition*. 1998;14(1):153–157.
3. Lacaille F, Gupte G, Colomb V, et al. ESPGHAN Working Group of Intestinal Failure and Intestinal Transplantation. Intestinal failure-associated liver disease: a position paper of the ESPGHAN Working Group of Intestinal Failure and Intestinal Transplantation. *J Pediatr Gastroenterol Nutr*. 2015;60(2):272–283.
4. Beath SV, Kelly D. Total parenteral nutrition-induced cholestasis: prevention and management. *Clin Liver Dis*. 2016;20(1):159–176.
5. Sondheimer JM, Asturias E, Cadnapaphornchai M. Infection and cholestasis in neonates with intestinal resection and long-term parenteral nutrition. *J Pediatr Gastroenterol Nutr*. 1998;27(2):131–137.
6. Cavicchi M, Beau P, Crenn P, et al. Prevalence of liver disease and contributing factors in patients receiving home parenteral nutrition for permanent intestinal failure. *Ann Intern Med*. 2000;132(7):525.
7. Kelly DA. Intestinal failure-associated liver disease: what do we know today? *Gastroenterology*. 2006;130(2 suppl 1):S70.
8. Cooper A, Floyd TF, Ross 3rd AJ, et al. Morbidity and mortality of short-bowel syndrome acquired in infancy: an update. *J Pediatr Surg*. 1984;19(6):711.
9. Christensen RD, Henry E, Wiedmeier SE, et al. Identifying patients, on the first day of life, at high-risk of developing parenteral nutrition-associated liver disease. *J Perinatol*. 2007;27(5):284.
10. Moss RL, Amii LA. New approaches to understanding the etiology and treatment of total parenteral nutrition-associated cholestasis. *Semin Pediatr Surg*. 1999;8(3):140.
11. Klein CJ, Revenis M, Ravenis M, et al. Parenteral nutrition-associated conjugated hyperbilirubinemia in hospitalized infants. *J Am Diet Assoc*. 2010;110(11):1684–1695.
12. Teitelbaum DH. Parenteral nutrition-associated cholestasis. *Curr Opin Pediatr*. 1997;9(3):270.
13. Hofmann AF. Defective biliary secretion during total parenteral nutrition: probable mechanisms and possible solutions. *J Pediatr Gastroenterol Nutr*. 1995;20(4):376.
14. Nightingale JM. Hepatobiliary, renal and bone complications of intestinal failure. *Best Pract Res Clin Gastroenterol*. 2003;17(6):907.
15. Zambrano E, El-Hennawy M, Ehrenkranz RA, et al. Total parenteral nutrition induced liver pathology: an autopsy series of 24 newborn cases. *Pediatr Dev Pathol*. 2004;7(5):425.
16. Yang CF, Lee M, Valim C, et al. Persistent alanine aminotransferase elevations in children with parenteral nutrition-associated liver disease. *J Pediatr Surg*. 2009;44(6):1084.
17. Forchielli ML, Walker WA. Nutritional factors contributing to the development of cholestasis during total parenteral nutrition. *Adv Pediatr*. 2003;50:245.
18. Javid PJ, Collier S, Richardson D, et al. The role of enteral nutrition in the reversal of parenteral nutrition-associated liver dysfunction in infants. *J Pediatr Surg*. 2005;40(6):1015.
19. Sheldon GF, Peterson SR, Sanders R. Hepatic dysfunction during hyperalimentation. *Arch Surg*. 1978;113(4):504–548.
20. Alwayn IP, Gura K, Nosé V, et al. Omega-3 fatty acid supplementation prevents hepatic steatosis in a murine model of nonalcoholic fatty liver disease. *Pediatr Res*. 2005;57(3):445.
21. Van Aerde JE, Duerksen DR, Gramlich L, et al. Intravenous fish oil emulsion attenuates total parenteral nutrition-induced cholestasis in newborn piglets. *Pediatr Res*. 1999;45(2):202.
22. Gawecka A, Michalkiewicz J, Kornacka MK, et al. Immunologic properties differ in preterm infants fed olive oil vs soy-based lipid emulsions during parenteral nutrition. *JPEN J Parenter Enteral Nutr*. 2008;32(4):448.
23. Raptis DA, Limani P, Jang JH, et al. GPR120 on Kupffer cells mediates hepatoprotective effects of ω3-fatty acids. *J Hepatol*. 2014;60(3):625–632.
24. Chen WJ, Yeh SL, Huang PC. Effects of fat emulsions with different fatty acid composition on plasma and hepatic lipids in rats receiving total parenteral nutrition. *Clin Nutr*. 1996;15(1):24–28.
25. Aksnes J, Eide TJ, Nordstrand K. Lipid entrapment and cellular changes in the rat myocard, lung and liver after long-term parenteral nutrition with lipid emulsion. A light microscopic and ultrastructural study. *APMIS*. 104(7-8):515–522.
26. Chan S. Incidence, prognosis, and etiology of end-stage liver disease in patients receiving home total parenteral nutrition. *Surgery*. 1999;126:28–34.

27. Putchakayala K, Polensky S, Fitzhugh J, et al. An evaluation of the model for end-stage liver disease and serum C-reactive protein as prognostic markers in intestinal failure patients on parenteral nutrition. *JPEN J Parenter Enteral Nutr*. 2009;33(1):55–61.

28. Matsui J. Nutritional, hepatic and metabolic effects of cachectin/tumor necrosis factor in rats receiving TPN. *Gastroenterology*. 1993;104:235–243.

29. Goulet O, Ruemmele F. Causes and management of intestinal failure in children. *Gastroenterology*. 2006;130(2 suppl 1):16–28.

30. Blau J, Sridhar S, Mathieson S, Chawla A. Effects of protein/nonprotein caloric intake on parenteral nutrition associated cholestasis in premature infants weighing 600-1000 grams. *JPEN J Parenter Enteral Nutr*. 2007;31(6):487–490.

31. Huuang S, Rutkowsky JM, Snodgrass RG, et al. Saturated fatty acids activate TLR-mediated proinflammatory signaling pathways. *J Lipid Res*. 2012;53(9):2002–2013.

32. Carter BA, Taylor OA, Prendergast DR, et al. Stigmasterol, a soy lipid-derived phytosterol, is an antagonist of the bile acid nuclear receptor FXR. *Pediatr Res*. 2007;62(3):301–306.

33. Clayton PT, Whitfield P, Iyer K. The role of phytosterols in the pathogenesis of liver complications of pediatric parenteral nutrition. *Nutrition*. 1998;14(1):158–164.

34. Iyer KR, Spitz L, Clayton P. BAPS prize lecture: New insight into mechanisms of parenteral nutrition-associated cholestasis: role of plant sterols. British Association of Paediatric Surgeons. *J Pediatr Surg*. 1998;33(1):1–6.

35. Waitzberg DL, Torrinhas RS, Jacintho TM. New parenteral lipid emulsions for clinical use. *JPEN J Parenter Enteral Nutr*. 2006;30(4):351–367.

36. Ulrich H, Pastores SM, Katz DP, Kvetan V. Parenteral use of medium-chain triglycerides: a reappraisal. *Nutrition*. 1996;12(4):231–238.

37. Vanek VW, Seidner DL, Allen P, et al. A.S.P.E.N. position paper: clinical role for alternative intravenous fat emulsions. *Nutr Clin Pract*. 2012;27(2):150–192.

38. Kalish BT, Fallon EM, Puder M. A tutorial on fatty acid biology. *JPEN J Parenter Enteral Nutr*. 2012;36(4):380–388.

39. *Clinolipid [package insert]*. Deerfield, IL: Baxter Healthcare Corporation; 2014.

40. Sala-Vila A, Barbosa VM, Calder PC. Olive oil in parenteral nutrition. *Curr Opin Clin Nutr Metab Care*. 2007;10(2):165–174.

41. Deshpande G, Simmer K, Deshmukh M, Mori TA, Croft KD. Kristensen J Fish Oil (SMOFlipid) and olive oil lipid (Clinoleic) in very preterm neonates. *J Pediatr Gastroenterol Nutr*. 2014;58(2):177–182.

42. Le HD, de Meijer VE, Robinson EM, et al. Parenteral fish-oil-based lipid emulsion improves fatty acid profiles and lipids in parenteral nutrition-dependent children. *Am J Clin Nutr*. 2011;94(3):749–758.

43. Angsten G, Finkel Y, Lucas S, et al. Improved outcome in neonatal short bowel syndrome using parenteral fish oil in combination with ω-6/9 lipid emulsions. *JPEN J Parenter Enteral Nutr*. 2012;36(5):587–595.

44. Diamond IR, Sterescu A, Pencharz PB, et al. Changing the paradigm: Omegaven for the treatment of liver failure in pediatric short bowel syndrome. *J Pediatr Gastroenterol Nutr*. 2009;48:209–215.

45. Goulet O, Joly F, Corriol O, Colomb-Jung V. Some new insights in intestinal failure-associated liver disease. *Curr Opin Organ Transplant*. 2009;14:256–261.

46. Lee WS, Sokol RJ. Intestinal microbiota, lipids, and the pathogenesis of intestinal failure-associated liver disease. *J Pediatr*. 2015;167(3):519–526.

47. El Kasmi KC, Anderson AL, Devereaux MW, et al. Phytosterols promote liver injury and Kupffer cell activation in parenteral nutrition-associated liver disease. *Sci Transl Med*. 2013;5(206):206ra137.

48. Nghiem-Rao TH, Tunc I, Mavis AM, Cao Y, Polzin EM, Firary MF, et al. Kinetics of phytosterol metabolism in neonates receiving parenteral nutrition. *Pediatr Res*. 2015;78(2):181–189.

49. Center for Drug Evaluation and Research. Application Number:204508Orig1s000, Summary Review. http://www.accessdata.fda.gov/drugsatfda_docs/nda/2013/204508Orig1s000SumR.pdf. Accessed January 2, 2017.

50. SMOFLIPID (lipid injectable emulsion). – FDA http://www.accessdata.fda.gov/drugsatfda_docs/appletter/2016/207648Orig1s000ltr.pdf. Accessed January 2, 2017.

51. Vlaardingerbroek H, Ng K, Stoll B, et al. New generation lipid emulsions prevent PNALD in chronic parenterally fed preterm pigs. *J Lipid Res*. 2014;55(3):466–477.

52. Ng K, Stoll B, Chacko S, et al. Vitamin E in new-generation lipid emulsions protects against parenteral nutrition-associated liver disease in parenteral nutrition-fed preterm pigs. *JPEN J Parenter Enteral Nutr*. 2016;40(5):656–671.

53. Lorent K, Gong W, Koo KA, et al. Identification of a plant isoflavonoid that causes biliary atresia. *Sci Transl Med*. 2015;7(286):286ra67.

54. Shin H, Eo H, Lim Y. Similarities and differences between alpha-tocopherol and gamma-tocopherol in amelioration of inflammation, oxidative stress and pre-fibrosis in hyperglycemia induced acute kidney inflammation. *Nutr Res Pract*. 2016;10(1):33–41.

55. Carpentier YA, Simoens C, Siderova V, et al. Recent developments in lipid emulsions: relevance to intensive care. *Nutrition*. 1997;13(suppl 9):S73–S78.

56. Burrin DG, Ng K, Stoll B, et al. Impact of new-generation lipid emulsions on cellular mechanisms of parenteral nutrition-associated liver disease. *Adv Nutr*. 2014;5(1):82–91.

57. Muto M, Lim D, Soukvilay A, et al. Supplemental parenteral vitamin E into conventional soybean lipid emulsion does not prevent parenteral nutrition-associated liver disease in full-term neonatal piglets. *JPEN J Parenter Enteral Nutr*. 2015.

58. Pacana T, Sanyal AJ. Vitamin E and nonalcoholic fatty liver disease. *Curr Opin Clin Nutr Metab Care*. 2012;15(6):641–648.

59. Lavine JE, Schwimmer JB, Van Natta ML, et al. Nonalcoholic Steatohepatitis Clinical Research Network. Effect of vitamin E or metformin for treatment of nonalcoholic fatty liver disease in children and adolescents: the TONIC randomized controlled trial. *JAMA*. 2011;305(16):1659–1668.

60. Nehra D, Fallon EM, Carlson SJ, et al. Provision of a soy-based intravenous lipid emulsion at 1 g/kg/d does not prevent cholestasis in neonates. *JPEN J Parenter Enteral Nutr*. 2013;37(4):498–505.

61. Levit OL, Calkins KL, Gibson LC, et al. Low-dose intravenous soybean oil emulsion for prevention of cholestasis in preterm neonates. *JPEN J Parenter Enteral Nutr*. 2016;40(3):374–382.

62. Rollins MD, Ward RM, Jackson WD, et al. Effect of decreased parenteral soybean lipid emulsion on hepatic function in infants at risk for parenteral nutrition-associated liver disease: a pilot study. *J Pediatr Surg*. 2013;48(6):1348–1356.

63. Cober MP, Killu G, Brattain A, et al. Intravenous fat emulsions reduction for patients with parenteral nutrition-associated liver disease. *J Pediatr*. 2012;160(3):421–427.

64. Shattuck KE, Bhatia J, Grinnell C, Rassin DK. The effects of light exposure on the in vitro hepatic response to an amino acid-vitamin solution. *JPEN J Parenter Enteral Nutr*. 1995; 19(5):398–402.

65. Neuzil J, Darlow BA, Inder TE, et al. Oxidation of parenteral lipid emulsion by ambient and phototherapy lights: potential toxicity of routine parenteral feeding. *J Pediatr*. 1995;126(5 Pt 1): 785–790.

66. Miloudi K, Comte B, Rouleau T, et al. The mode of administration of total parenteral nutrition and nature of lipid content influence the generation of peroxides and aldehydes. *Clin Nutr*. 2012;31(4):526–534.

67. von Rettberg H, Hannman T, Subotic U, et al. Use of di(2-ethylhexyl)phthalate-containing infusion systems increases the risk for cholestasis. *Pediatrics*. 2009;124(2):710–716.

68. Bagel S, Dessaigne B, Bourdeaux D, et al. Influence of lipid type on bis (2-ethylhexyl)phthalate (DEHP) leaching from infusion line sets in parenteral nutrition. *JPEN J Parenter Enteral Nutr*. 2011;35(6):770–775.

69. Colomb V, Jobert-Giraud A, Lacaille F, et al. Role of lipid emulsions in cholestasis associated with long-term parenteral nutrition in children. *JPEN J Parenter Enteral Nutr*. 2000;24(6):345–350.

70. Nusinovich Y, Revenis M, Torres C. Long-term outcomes for infants with intestinal atresia studied at Children's National Medical Center. *J Pediatr Gastroenterol Nutr*. 2013;57(3):324–329.

71. Bianchi A. From the cradle to enteral autonomy: the role of autologous gastrointestinal reconstruction. *Gastroenterology*. 2006;130(2 suppl 1):S138–S146.

72. Lam HS, Tam YH, Poon TC, et al. A double-blind randomised controlled trial of fish oil-based versus soy-based lipid preparations in the treatment of infants with parenteral nutrition-associated cholestasis. *Neonatology*. 2014;105(4):290–296.

73. Gura KM, Lee S, Valim C, et al. Safety and efficacy of a fish-oil-based fat emulsion in the treatment of parenteral nutrition-associated liver disease. *Pediatrics*. 2008;121(3):e678–e686.

74. European Directorate for the Quality of Medicines. Council of Europe. Fish oil, rich in omega-3 fatty acid. In: *European Pharmacopeia*. Supplement 6.0. Monograph no. 1912. Strasbourg, France: European Directorate for the Quality of Medicines; 2008:1893–1895.

75. Leaf A, Weber PC. Cardiovascular effects of n-3 fatty acids. *N Engl J Med*. 1988;318(9):549–557.

76. Gao LG, Cao J, Mao QX, et al. Influence of omega-3 polyunsaturated fatty acid-supplementation on platelet aggregation in humans: a meta-analysis of randomized controlled trials. *Atherosclerosis*. 2013;226(2):328–334.

77. Dicken BJ, Bruce A, Samuel TM, et al. Bedside to bench: the risk of bleeding with parenteral omega-3 lipid emulsion therapy. *J Pediatr*. 2014;164(3):652–654.

78. Wachira JK, Larson MK, Harris WS. n-3 Fatty acids affect haemostasis but do not increase the risk of bleeding: clinical observations and mechanistic insights. *Br J Nutr*. 2014;111(9):1652–1662.

79. Dyerberg J. Eicosapentaenoic acid and prevention of thrombosis and atherosclerosis? *Lancet*. 1978;2(8081):117–119.

80. Thorngren M, Gustafson A. Effects of 11-week increase in dietary eicosapentaenoic acid on bleeding time, lipids, and platelet aggregation. *Lancet*. 1981;2(8257):1190–1193.

81. Simopoulos AP. Omega-3 fatty acids in health and disease and in growth and development. *Am J Clin Nutr*. 1991;54(3):438–463.

82. Moncada S, Gryglewski R, Bunting S, Vane JR. An enzyme isolated from arteries transforms prostaglandin endoperoxides to an unstable substance that inhibits platelet aggregation. *Nature*. 1976;263(5579):663–665.

83. Goodnight Jr SH, Harris WS, Connor WE. The effects of dietary omega 3 fatty acids on platelet composition and function in man: a prospective, controlled study. *Blood*. 1981;58(5):880–885.

84. Li XL, Steiner M. Fish oil: a potent inhibitor of platelet adhesiveness. *Blood*. 1990;76(5):938–945.

85. Cohen MG, Rossi JS, Garbarino J, et al. Insights into the inhibition of platelet activation by omega-3 polyunsaturated fatty acids: beyond aspirin and clopidogrel. *Thromb Res*. 2011;128(4):335–340.

86. Larson MK, Shearer GC, Ashmore JH, et al. Omega-3 fatty acids modulate collagen signaling in human platelets. *Prostaglandins Leukot Essent Fatty Acids*. 84(3–4):93–98.

87. Del Turco S, Basta G, Lazzerini G, et al. Effect of the administration of n-3 polyunsaturated fatty acids on circulating levels of microparticles in patients with a previous myocardial infarction. *Haematologica*. 2008;93(6):892–899.

88. Phang M, Lincz L, Seldon M, Garg ML. Acute supplementation with eicosapentaenoic acid reduces platelet microparticle activity in healthy subjects. *J Nutr Biochem.* 2012;23(9):1128–1133.

89. Larson MK, Tormoen GW, Weaver LJ, et al. Exogenous modification of platelet membranes with the omega-3 fatty acids EPA and DHA reduces platelet procoagulant activity and thrombus formation. *Am J Physiol Cell Physiol.* 2013;304(3):C273–C279.

90. Barcelli U, Glas-Greenwalt P, Pollak VE. Enhancing effect of dietary supplementation with omega-3 fatty acids on plasma fibrinolysis in normal subjects. *Thromb Res.* 1985;39(3):307–312.

91. Bays HE. Safety considerations with omega-3 fatty acid therapy. *Am J Cardiol.* 2007;99(6A):35C–43C. Epub 2006 Nov 28.

92. Harris WS. Expert opinion: omega-3 fatty acids and bleeding–cause for concern? *Am J Cardiol.* 2007;99(6A):44C–46C.

93. Gajos G, Rostoff P, Undas A, Piwowarska W. Effects of polyunsaturated omega-3 fatty acids on responsiveness to dual antiplatelet therapy in patients undergoing percutaneous coronary intervention: the OMEGA-PCI (OMEGA-3 fatty acids after pci to modify responsiveness to dual antiplatelet therapy) study. *J Am Coll Cardiol.* 55(16):1671–1678.

94. Cairns JA, Gill J, Morton B, et al. Fish oils and low-molecular-weight heparin for the reduction of restenosis after percutaneous transluminal coronary angioplasty. The EMPAR Study. *Circulation.* 1996;94(7):1553–1560.

95. von Schacky C, Fischer S, Weber PC. Long-term effects of dietary marine omega-3 fatty acids upon plasma and cellular lipids, platelet function, and eicosanoid formation in humans. *J Clin Invest.* 1985;76(4):1626–1631.

96. Nandivada P, Anez-Bustillos L, O'Loughlin AA, Mitchell PD, Baker MA, Dao DT, et al. Risk of post-procedural bleeding in children on intravenous fish oil. *Am J Surg.* 2017;214(4):733–737.

97. Simopoulos AP. Summary of the conference on the health effects of polyunsaturated fatty acids in seafoods. *J Nutr.* 1986;116(12):2350–2354.

98. Kris-Etherton PM. Fish consumption, fish oil, omega-3 fatty acids, and cardiovascular disease. *Arterioscler Thromb Vasc Biol.* 2003;23(2):e20–e30.

99. Lawson LD, Hughes BG. Human absorption of fish oil fatty acids as triacylglycerols, free acids, or ethyl esters. *Biochem Biophys Res Commun.* 1988;152(1):328–335.

100. Friedman Z, Danon A, Stahlman MT, et al. Rapid onset of essential fatty acid deficiency in the newborn. *Pediatrics.* 1976;58:640–649.

101. Holman RT. The ratio of trienoic: tetraenoic acids in tissue lipids as a measure of essential fatty acid requirement. *J Nutr.* 1960;70:405–410.

102. Cunnane SC, Belza K, Anderson MJ, Ryan MA. Substantial carbon recycling from linoleate into products of de novo lipogenesis occurs in rat liver even under conditions of extreme dietary linoleate deficiency. *J Lipid Res.* 1998;39(11):2271–2276.

103. Alfin-Slater RB, Aftergood L. Essential fatty acids reinvestigated. *Physiol Rev.* 1968;48:758–784.

104. de Meijer VE, Le HD, Meisel JA, Gura KM, Puder M. Parenteral fish oil as monotherapy prevents essential fatty acid deficiency in parenteral nutrition-dependent patients. *J Pediatr Gastroenterol Nutr.* 2010;50(2):212–218.

105. Duerksen DR, Nehra V, Palombo JD, et al. Essential fatty acid deficiencies in patients with chronic liver disease are not reversed by short-term intravenous lipid supplementation. *Dig Dis Sci.* 1999;44(7):1342–1348.

106. Duerksen D, McCurdy K. Essential fatty acid deficiency in a severely malnourished patient receiving parenteral nutrition. *Dig Dis Sci.* 2005;50(12):2386–2388.

107. Nandivada P, Fell GL, Mitchell PD, et al. Long-term fish oil lipid emulsion use in children with intestinal failure-associated liver disease. *JPEN J Parenter Enteral Nutr.* 2017;41(6):930–937.

108. Squires RH, Duggan C, Teitelbaum DH, et al. Natural history of pediatric intestinal failure: initial report from the Pediatric Intestinal Failure Consortium. *J Pediatr.* 2012;161(4):723–728.e2.

109. Venick RS, Wozniak LJ, Colangelo J. Long-term nutrition and predictors of growth and weight gain following pediatric intestinal transplantation. *Transplantation.* 2011;92(9):1058–1062.

110. Raphael BP, Mitchell PD, Finkton D, et al. Necrotizing enterocolitis and central line associated blood stream infection are predictors of growth outcomes in infants with short bowel syndrome. *J Pediatr.* 2015;167(1):35–40.e1.

111. Pichler J, Chomtho S, Fewtrell M, et al. Growth and bone health in pediatric intestinal failure patients receiving long-term parenteral nutrition. *Am J Clin Nutr.* 2013;97(6):1260–1269.

112. Nandivada P, Baker MA, Mitchell PD, et al. Predictors of failure of fish-oil therapy for intestinal failure-associated liver disease in children. *Am J Clin Nutr.* 2016;104(3):663–670.

113. Nandivada P, Chang MI, Potemkin AK, et al. The natural history of cirrhosis from parenteral nutrition-associated liver disease after resolution of cholestasis with parenteral fish oil therapy. *Ann Surg.* 2015;261(1):172–179.

114. Skouroliakou M, Konstantinou D, Koutri K, et al. A double-blind, randomized clinical trial of the effect of omega-3 fatty acids on the oxidative stress of preterm neonates fed through parenteral nutrition. *Eur J Clin Nutr.* 2010;64(9):940–947.

115. Tomsits E, Pataki M, Tölgyesi A, et al. Safety and efficacy of a lipid emulsion containing a mixture of soybean oil, medium-chain triglycerides, olive oil, and fish oil: a randomised, double-blind clinical trial in premature infants requiring parenteral nutrition. *J Pediatr Gastroenterol Nutr.* 2010;51(4):514–521.

116. Diamond IR, Grant RC, Pencharz PB, et al. Preventing the progression of intestinal failure-associated liver disease in infants using a composite lipid emulsion: a pilot randomized controlled trial of SMOFlipid. *JPEN J Parenter Enteral Nutr.* 2017;41(5):866–877.

117. Lee S, Park HJ, Yoon J, et al. Reversal of intestinal failure-associated liver disease by switching from a combination lipid emulsion containing fish oil to fish oil monotherapy. *JPEN J Parenter Enteral Nutr*. 2016;40(3):437–440.
118. Sanchez SE, Braun LP, Mercer LD, et al. The effect of lipid restriction on the prevention of parenteral nutrition-associated cholestasis in surgical infants. *J Pediatr Surg*. 2013;48(3):573–578.
119. Calkins KL, Havranek T, Kelley-Quon LI, et al. Low-dose parenteral soybean oil for the prevention of parenteral nutrition-associated liver disease in neonates with gastrointestinal disorders: a multicenter randomized controlled pilot study. *JPEN J Parenter Enteral Nutr*. 2017;41(3):404–411.
120. Nehra D, Fallon EM, Potemkin AK, et al. A comparison of 2 intravenous lipid emulsions: interim analysis of a randomized controlled trial. *JPEN J Parenter Enteral Nutr*. 2014;38(6):693–701.
121. Wales PW, Allen N, Worthington P, George D, Compher C, American Society for Parenteral and Enteral Nutrition, Teitelbaum D. A.S.P.E.N. clinical guidelines: support of pediatric patients with intestinal failure at risk of parenteral nutrition-associated liver disease. *JPEN J Parenter Enteral Nutr*. 2014;38(5):538–557.
122. Javid PJ, Collier S, Richardson D, et al. The role of enteral nutrition in the reversal of parenteral nutrition-associated liver dysfunction in infants. *J Pediatr Surg*. 2005;40(6):1015–1018.

9

CHAPTER 10

Neonatal Gastrointestinal Tract as a Conduit to Systemic Inflammation

Mary W. Lenfestey, MD, Josef Neu, MD

Overview

The primary role of the gastrointestinal (GI) tract is to facilitate digestion and absorption of nutrients, but the intestines also engage in a multitude of other biologic functions, including significant immunologic and neuroendocrine activities. The intestinal surface is composed of a layer of epithelial cells that comprise villi, which provide a sizeable surface area to facilitate exposures to a vast array of food antigens, bacteria flora, and microbial metabolites.

The neonatal intestine functions during a period of major transition, including alterations in luminal and surface enzyme activities, changes in both the innate and adaptive immune systems, and major shifts in the microbiome, depending on environmental factors, such as diet and other exposures. In addition, premature infants may be still completing basic morphogenesis and development in addition to coping with the changes in their environments. There is new recognition that the neonatal intestine is exposed to microbes in utero and that this likely plays a major role in intestinal development, even before birth and subsequent exposure to the extrauterine milieu. This chapter will provide an overview of the intestinal mechanism that relates to systemic inflammation, the relationship and interactions between the intestinal microbiota and the intestinal mucosa, as well as the resultant effects on the developing nervous system.

Components and Functions of the Gastrointestinal Epithelium

The GI surface is composed of several types of cells. The epithelial layer originates from the endoderm and throughout gestation changes and differentiates through recanalization of the intestinal lumen and, later, through the development of villi and crypts.[1] The adult-type crypt epithelium architecture is present by 30 weeks' gestational age. Many genes that are necessary for cellular differentiation and migration have been identified (Table 10.1, Fig. 10.1). The cell types present in the epithelium include enterocytes, goblet cells, enteroendocrine cells, Paneth cells, microfold cells, lymphocytes, and tuft cells (Table 10.2).

The intestinal epithelium contains several types of cell junctions that are important for normal functioning. These junctions appear at the 10th week of gestation and

157

Table 10.1 DIFFERENT GENES INVOLVED IN DIFFERENTIATION OF
GASTROINTESTINAL EPITHELIUM

Gene	Function
Hox	Gut patterning along the anterior–posterior axis
Hoxd13	Controls final epithelial phenotype
Hoxa13	Controls final epithelial phenotype
Cdx2	Provides positional information for specification of midgut endoderm
Parahox	Anterior-posterior gut development
Hedgehog	Directs organogenesis
BMP	Controls gut muscular development, Epithelial homeostasis
FGF	Establishing gut tube domains along the A-P axis
WNT	Epithelial proliferation and development

From Santa Barbara P, Van Den Brink GR, Roberts DJ. Development and differentiation of the intestinal epithelium. *Cell Mol Life Sci.* 2003;60(7):1322–1332; and Dessimoz J, Opoka R, Kordich JJ, Grapin-Botton A, Wels JM, et al. FGF Signaling is necessary for establishing gut tube domains along the anterior-posterior axis in vivo. *Mech Dev.* 2006;123(1):42–55.

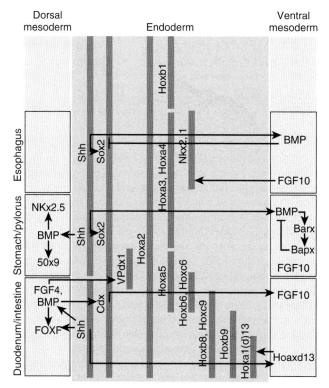

Fig. 10.1 Genes involved with differentiation of gastrointestinal epithelium. (From Wyllie R, Hyams J. *Pediatric Gastrointestinal and Liver Disease*, 5th ed. Philadelphia, PA: Elsevier, 2016.)

continue to develop from that point on. There are four types of junctions, and their primary purpose is to maintain the mechanical and chemical barriers of the GI lumen (Fig. 10.2). *Desmosomes* are complexes derived from cadherin and are located on the lateral sides of the enterocyte. They function to provide mechanical strength by linking adjacent cells by the cytoskeleton. *Adherens* junctions are multiprotein complexes that assist with epithelial cohesion, polarity, and cell migration. *Gap* junctions primarily allow for intercellular chemical communication via molecules, ions, and electrical impulses. Finally, *tight* junctions are composed of nearly 40 different proteins and are quite possibly the most important type of junction. The tight junction protein components form a continuous ribbon around the cells near the borders of the lateral and apical membranes and serve as a barrier between the GI lumen and the subepithelial environment by preventing the passage of a certain luminal antigens,

Table 10.2 DESCRIPTION OF EPITHELIAL CELL TYPES AND FUNCTION

Cell Type	Function
Enterocytes	Most numerous cell type Nutrient absorption • Express many catabolic and hydrolytic enzymes on their exterior luminal surface to break down molecules to sizes appropriate for transport into the cell • Examples of molecules taken up by enterocytes are ions, water, simple sugars, vitamins, lipids, peptides and amino acids
Goblet cells	Secrete the mucus layer that protects the epithelium from the luminal contents
Enteroendocrine cells	Secrete various gastrointestinal hormones • Secretin • Pancreozymin • Enteroglucagon
Paneth Cells	Produce antimicrobial peptides • Human beta defensin
Lymphocytes • B cells • T cells	Found in lymphoid follicles (Peyer patches) • Primarily in the ileum
Microfold cells • M cells	Sample antigens from the lumen and present them to the gut-associated lymphoid tissue (GALT) • Found in Peyer patches in the small intestine
Cup cells	No known function
Tuft cells	Involved in immune response
Intraepithelial lymphocytes	Located beneath the tight junctions, in between epithelial cells • Involved in immune response

From Santa Barbara P, Van Den Brink GR, Roberts DJ. Development and differentiation of the intestinal epithelium. *Cell Mol Life Sci.* 2003;60(7):1322–1332; Merchant J. Hedgehog signaling in gut development, physiology and cancer. *J Physiol.* 2012;590(Pt 3):421–32; and Dessimoz J, Opoka R, Kordich JJ, Grapin-Botton A, Wels JM, et al. FGF Signaling is necessary for establishing gut tube domains along the anterior-posterior axis in vivo. *Mech Dev.* 2006;123(1):42–55.

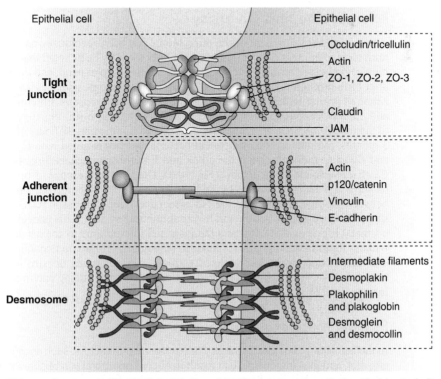

Fig. 10.2 There are four types of intercellular junctions found in the gastrointestinal epithelium, including desmosomes, adherens junctions, gap junctions, and tight junctions. (From Neunlist M, Van Landeghem L, Mahe MM, et al. The digestive neuronal-glial-epithelial unit: a new actor in gut health and disease. *Nat Rev Gastroenterol Hepatol.* 2013;10:90–100.)

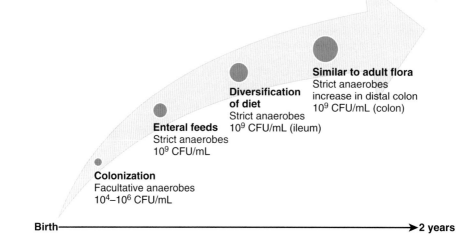

Fig. 10.3 The neonatal microbiome evolves over the course of the first 1 to 2 years of life. There are several major shifts in the gut flora, at birth, with introduction of enteral feeds (breast milk, formula), and later with diversification of the diet. The microbiota is comparable to the adult flora profile by 2 years of life. (From Wyllie R, Hyams J. *Pediatric Gastrointestinal and Liver Disease*, 5th ed. Philadelphia, PA: Elsevier, 2016; and Langhendries JP. Early bacterial colonisation of the intestine: why it matters. *Arch Pediatr*. 2006;13:1526–34.)

microorganisms, and toxins. The intercellular components also interact with different scaffold proteins, adapter proteins, and signaling complexes that regulate the cytoskeleton and the polarity of the cell and are involved in cell signaling and trafficking and serve to provide selective paracellular transport of solutes. These tight junctions are dynamic and can adapt to different physiochemical properties in the intestinal lumen. Disruption in the integrity of the tight junction has been associated with many disease processes, including inflammatory bowel disease, celiac disease, and type 1 diabetes.[2]

Microbiome and Diversity

Although the development of the microbiome has been recognized as critical to the normal development of the GI tract, it has only recently been noted that colonization may begin before birth.[3,4] The microbiome continues to expand, and does so shortly after birth through the first 2 years of life.[5,6] Typical progression begins with colonization of primarily facultative anaerobes, such as *Streptococcus*, Enterobacteriaceae, and *Staphylococcus* species within the hours following birth; this quickly expands to include *Bifidobacterium* and *Lactobacillus* within the first 48 hours of life. By age 3 months, regionalization of different bacterial species is noted with *Fusobacterium* and *Eubacterium* colonizing the colon and Enterobacteriaceae, *Streptococcus*, and *Clostridium* found in the ileum[7] (Fig. 10.3). Despite the presence of tight junctions, bacteria and their metabolic byproducts penetrate the submucosa; the interaction between the microbiome and the gut-associated lymphoid tissue (GALT) serves to shape the development of the gut mucosal immune system. This coevolution during postnatal life allows the host and the intestinal microbiome to coexist as symbionts, without limiting the immune response to pathogens.[8] Failure to maintain this symbiotic relationship has been associated with diseases, including obesity, inflammatory bowel disease, atopic conditions, celiac disease, and necrotizing enterocolitis (NEC) in neonates.[9-15]

Special Neonatal Challenges

In the neonatal population, a variety of environmental factors, such as mode of delivery, diet, and gestational age, can result in altered microbial establishment within the GI tract (Fig. 10.4).[16-18] Preterm neonates are more at risk for an altered microbiome

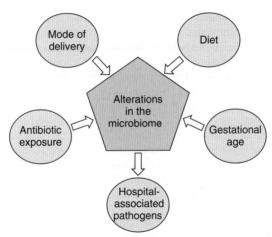

Fig. 10.4   The preterm neonate has many unique exposures that serve to alter the gastrointestinal microbiome.

because of their medicalized environment; these infants are exposed to pathogenic bacteria more frequently as a result of prolonged hospitalization within the neonatal intensive care unit (NICU). In addition, certain therapies, such as antibiotics, compound the issue by reducing species diversity so that preterm infants are often colonized by a less diverse quotient of bacteria.[19] These environmental challenges often produce a microbiome with less beneficial bacteria (bifidobacteria, lactobacilli) and larger populations of potential pathogens (*Klebsiella*, enterococci, staphylococci, *Bacteroides*, and *Enterobacteria*).[20] Clinically, this may have both short- and long-term effects; a growing number of studies have correlated prolonged courses of antibiotic therapy with increased incidence of NEC, sepsis, and death.[21-23]

In addition to environmental challenges, the preterm neonate has less efficient immune function and abnormal mucosal barriers within the gut that allow for translocation of pathogenic bacteria and initiation of a systemic inflammatory response. Under normal circumstances, the intestinal epithelium serves a challenging role of facilitating transport of nutrients while maintaining a barrier against microorganisms. The physical barrier is composed of the epithelial cells and their tight junctions, as previously described. The intestinal epithelial cells are active members of this barrier; Paneth cells respond to certain signals and respond with antimicrobial peptides. Intestinal epithelial cells also express certain receptors that allow recognition of ligands produced by both commensal and pathogenic bacteria; the recognition of these ligands triggers a cytokine interaction between the intraepithelial lymphocyte and the underlying GALT.[24] The immune response of the GI mucosa comprises both adaptive immune cells, such as effector T and B lymphocytes found in the GALT, as well as innate cells, such as dendritic cells, monocytes/macrophages, and the recently identified heterogeneous group of innate lymphoid cells.[25] The preterm neonate has qualitatively or quantitatively less of these immune cells present.[26,27]

There are many signaling pathways between the involved cells types; intestinal signaling through Toll-like receptors (TLRs) has been particularly well studied. Rakoff-Nahoum et al. were the first to demonstrate that intestinal signaling through TLRs stimulated by the intestinal microbiome is necessary for homeostasis.[28] The intestinal immune cells must find a balance between mounting appropriate defenses against pathogenic organisms and developing tolerance toward commensal organisms. Excessive activation of the immune response would cause excessive production of inflammatory cytokines, resulting in local cell death and an inflammatory response. The TLR helps maintain balance through cell signaling in response to byproducts, such as lipopolysaccharides (LPSs) produced by commensal bacteria; this pathway ultimately enhances the ability of the epithelial cells to withstand chemical and inflammatory injuries. Significant differences have been identified in the degree of TLR function and TLR subtype activity in preterm infants and full-term infants. TLR4 activity has been noted to be highest in the preterm infant. This pathway is associated with epithelial apoptosis, mucosal barrier disruption, bacterial translocation, and reduced ability to recover from injury (Fig. 10.5).[29-33] Paneth cells also serve a role in tolerance of intestinal bacteria by producing antimicrobial proteins and peptides; cathelicidin (LL-37) is one such amyloid precursor protein, which functions to decrease inflammatory cytokine response to LPSs.[34] Preterm infants appear to have a shift in balance, from an anti-inflammatory cytokine and protein environment to one that is more proinflammatory. Preterm infants have a higher expression of TLR4 activity, as well as interleukin-8 (IL-8) and IL-1. Protective LL-37 levels have been noted to drop off around 2 weeks after birth in mice models.[34-36] Prenatal steroids increase intestinal maturation and reduce IL-8 production (via reduction in nuclear factor-κB nuclear translocation), which may help to explain, in part, why this prenatal therapy is associated with reduction in NEC.[37] Overall, the immature innate immune system of the preterm neonate is often insufficient to adequately protect against the numerous challenges faced by it.[38]

There are several basic physiologic mechanisms that are not fully functional in the preterm population, compared with those in full-term infants; these include peristalsis, gastric acidity, presence of proteolytic activity, intestinal mucus, cell-surface glycoconjugates, and intercellular tight junctions.[2] There are immunologic differences, including decreased secretory immunoglobulin A (IgA) production and less antimicrobial peptides (specifically defensin) secretion by Paneth cells. These anatomic, physiologic, and immunologic discrepancies compound each other, resulting in a less capable intestinal mucosa that is more susceptible to damage, less able to heal itself, and more at risk for bacterial translocation.[31,39-42] Clinically, this is thought to contribute to bacterial overgrowth, dysbiosis, and NEC.[43] In summary, the initial development of a symbiotic relationship between the intestinal mucosa and the microbiome is critical to a neonate's health. In preterm infants, several mechanisms, such as innate immune function and mucosal integrity, function either suboptimally or with a proinflammatory shift compared with their full-term counterparts, which increases the risk of sepsis, systemic inflammatory responses, and NEC.[44]

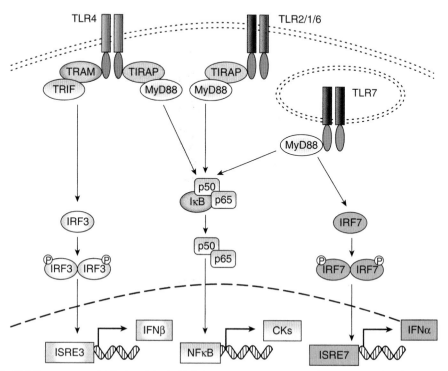

Fig. 10.5 Toll-like receptor (TLR)-4 activity is high in preterm neonates and is associated with activation of the inflammatory response with epithelial apoptosis, mucosal barrier disruption, bacterial translocation, and reduced ability to recover. (From Thomson CA, McColl A, Cavanagh J, Graham GJ. Peripheral inflammation is associated with remote global gene expression changes in the brain. *J Neuroinflamm*. 2014;11:73.)

Total Parenteral Nutrition

Many of the common interventions that are necessary for the care of preterm infants compound their innate challenges of establishing a healthy intestinal microbial relationship. Total parenteral nutrition (TPN) and lack of enteral feeds is one such factor. It is not uncommon for the preterm neonate, particularly the very low–birth weight (VLBW) and extremely low–birth weight infant, to require parenteral nutrition. Depending on the patient's clinical status, enteral nutrition may be withheld for days to weeks. The lack of enteral stimulation by ingested nutrients ultimately alters normal gut physiology. Many of the gastric hormones are stimulated by the presence of intraluminal peptides, fatty acids, and glucose. Hormones, such as gastrin, cholecystokinin, motilin, and vasoactive intestinal polypeptide, help regulate normal intestinal function and are critical for trophic effects on the gastric mucosa, growth and function of the exocrine pancreas, intestinal motility, and pancreatic and intestinal secretions, respectively. With lack of enteral nutritional stimulation, there is an imbalance of normal neuroendocrine hormones, with subsequent malfunction of the GI tract.[1,45] This has also been correlated with decreased secretory IgA and mucosal atrophy, with increased translocation of intestinal microbes and increased likelihood of systemic inflammatory response syndrome and sepsis.[46] Given the degree of development of the neonatal GI tract, with crypt epithelium not fully developed until 30 weeks' gestation, the lack of enteral stimulation may be even more detrimental to this population than in adults or older children. In addition to the immature epithelium, there is typically hypomobility of the peristaltic movements in the small bowel, and this may increase bacterial adherence and overgrowth.[2] Several randomized controlled trials have shown that rapid advancement of enteral feeds is associated with a shorter time to full feeds and more rapid attainment of birth weight without increased incidence of NEC.[47,48] Logistically, parenteral nutrition requires central venous access—with prolonged use being associated with late-onset sepsis.[49] In addition to increased risks of inflammation and infection, differences in growth related to enteral nutrition versus parenteral nutrition have been demonstrated. Stoddart and Widdowson were among the first to note that suckling pigs gain 42% of their weight in the first 24 hours and that it did not occur in the nonsuckling animals.[50] Other researchers have expanded on these findings to demonstrate differences in intestinal mucosal growth, hepatic and superior mesenteric artery (SMA) blood flow, intestinal motility, IgA secretion, and decreased permeability in infants receiving enteral feeds.[51-54] Given the need for different nutritional components (amino acids, fatty acids, glucose) to stimulate various GI hormones, it is not surprising that the substrate chosen for enteral feeds also effects the intestinal mucosa. Breast milk has epithelial growth factor, erythropoietin, insulin-like growth factor, and anti-inflammatory IL-10—all of which may provide protective benefits, such as tissue growth and development while limiting inflammation.[55,56] The use of standardized feeding protocols and enteral nutrition, as opposed to relying primarily on TPN, when possible, is recommended because it has been shown to be protective.[57]

Antibiotic Use and the Microbiome

In a retrospective review, Clark et al. found that antibiotics are the most commonly used class of medications in neonates in the NICU. Four of the 10 most commonly used mediations noted in a large national data set were antibiotics, with the top two medications (ampicillin and gentamicin) having been used twice as often as the remainder of medications.[58] The decision to administer antibiotics to the premature neonatal population is a challenging one. Ambiguous clinical signs of infection often overlap with noninfectious, typical behaviors in the VLBW preterm population. Significant limitations in the accuracy of adjunctive diagnostic laboratory tests for sepsis may, in part, explain why so many VLBW infants receive prolonged antibiotic courses.[59] Interestingly, the true incidence of culture-proven early-onset bacteremia and sepsis may be lower than initially thought. A study by Stoll et al. showed that blood culture–proven early-onset sepsis was relatively uncommon—only present in approximately 1% to 2% of VLBW infants.[60] The use of antibiotics has been associated with alterations in the gut microbiome, which may have several unintended consequences. Infants who receive >5 days of antibiotic therapy have lower bacterial diversity in subsequent weeks of life and a higher abundance of *Enterobacter* species.[19] Preterm infants are often exposed to more pathogenic microbes as a result of their prolonged stay in the hospital environment. The use of broad-spectrum antibiotics may select a population of resistant organisms that can exacerbate lack of biodiversity and predilection toward a pathogenic microbiome. Several studies have correlated early antibiotic courses and longer duration of antibiotic exposure with increased incidence of NEC, sepsis, and death.[19,21-23] Although it is not suggested here that antibiotic therapy not be used in preterm neonates, it is an area that deserves further investigation in the future because evidence suggests that antibiotic therapy is not wholly benign. It is important to balance the suspicion of a true infection with the possible negative short- and long-term effects of antibiotic use in this population.

Gastrointestinal Impact on Systemic Inflammation

The effects of environmental stressors on the gut epithelium and subsequent alterations in the intestinal microbiome are not solely confined to the GI tract. Instead, there is a dynamic relationship between the GI integrity and systemic inflammation. When the epithelial tight junctions are compromised, translocation of bacteria occurs; this can trigger a gut-derived inflammatory response, with production of toxic mediators that drive systemic inflammation, which, then, feeds back and promotes increased intestinal permeability and further local immune activation. This cyclic inflammatory cascade ultimately can drive the body to systemic inflammatory response syndrome (SIRS), sepsis, septic shock with multiorgan failure, and even death.[61-65] Several mechanisms are thought to contribute to this gut–body inflammatory relationship (Fig. 10.6).

Systemic stress can serve as an inciting factor for GI derangements, such as denudation of villi, impairments in the gut barrier, and translocation of luminal contents.[66] Major shifts to pathogenic species have coincided with reduced microbial diversity that occurs in neonates with SIRS and sepsis.[67] Commensal microflora are vital to the digestion of dietary substrates, prevent colonization of pathogens, encourage enterocyte differentiation and proliferation, and help prime the mucosal and systemic immune systems.[68] They are also involved with fermentation of complex carbohydrates, which results in the production of short-chain fatty acids; this has demonstrated beneficial effects on immune cells and also mediates anti-inflammatory effects through G-protein coupled receptors 41 and 43 (GPR41, GPR43).[69] One could conclude that potential shifts in the microflora may alter this normal homeostatic function. Although there are, as yet, no routinely used means to measure bowel function in clinical practice, one potential means to do so is citrulline. Plasma citrulline

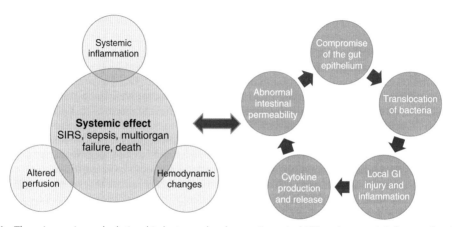

Fig. 10.6   There is a reciprocal relationship between local gastrointestinal (GI) and systemic inflammation, in which the GI tract may serve as an initiating trigger for systemic inflammation and vice versa.

levels are representative of enterocyte function and mass, and decreased levels may be associated with loss of gut barrier integrity.[67,70-72] Low citrulline levels in adult patients have been associated with elevated C-reactive protein levels, indicating systemic inflammation, as well as with higher mortality.[73]

Although inflammation may begin with an insult to the intestine, resulting from microbiota changes or ischemic injury, it is not necessarily contained there. The portal vein is composed of tributaries that drain the majority of GI blood products from the lower third of the esophagus to halfway down the anal canal and to the spleen, pancreas, and gallbladder. The portal vein flows into the liver, providing approximately 70% of the organ's blood flow—which makes the liver an important filter for clearing systemic bacterial infections derived from gut barrier dysfunction and for maintaining gut homeostasis. The hepatic sinusoids are lined with Kupffer cells, which are macrophages that are often the first immune cells to encounter pathogens that translocated from the gut lumen.[74] Dysbiosis of the microbiome has been found to trigger local inflammation within the liver and in patients with underlying liver disease (nonalcoholic fatty liver disease) may prompt progression from moderate disease to steatohepatitis.[75] A study in rat models noted that microbiota-dependent activation of the chemokine receptor (CX3CR1) in intestinal macrophages (which affects guts barrier integrity) regulates progression to steatohepatitis.[76] This is a good example of how damage to the GI barrier subsequently leads to inflammation within the liver, which, in turn, can result in circulatory changes that then worsen intestinal damage.[77] The relationship between gut microflora and the immune response within the liver has been further explored in recent studies; Balmer et al. found that although the liver remains sterile during periods of intestinal health, during times of translocation, the liver becomes a "secondary firewall" for mesenteric circulation.[78] Microbial products, such as LPS or bacterial DNA, can also breach the intestine and affect the liver; these events have been associated with activation of the inflammasome complex and systemic inflammatory responses.[79-81] The recognition of microbial antigens activating TLRs on hepatic cells (Kupffer cells, stellate cells, hepatocytes, lymphocytes, and endothelial cells) results in production of proinflammatory cytokines.[82,83] As in the intestines, the TLR plays a role in liver homeostasis. Although stimulation of TLRs on Kupffer cells is generally proinflammatory, continuous low levels of LPS stimulation, in fact, induces LPS tolerance in the liver and secretion of antiinflammatory cytokine IL-10.[84] This interplay between the GI microbiota and the liver may serve as one pathway and explains GI changes being a trigger for systemic inflammatory processes.

The lymphatic system offers another venue through which the gut and systemic circulation are connected. Mesenteric lymph containing lipophilic macromolecules drains from the intestinal villi into the mesenteric lymph nodes and ultimately into systemic circulation via the thoracic duct. Within the lymph nodes, antigen presentation occurs and can spur activation of the adaptive immune system. The mesenteric lymph does not go into portal circulation, thus avoiding the "secondary firewall" established by the liver. Lymph may also contain luminal byproducts, such as endotoxins and locally produced cytokines. These cytotoxic factors, in addition to activated immune cells that exit the mesenteric lymph node, are able to merge into systemic circulation, where the pulmonary circulation sees them initially. There have been adult studies correlating this "gut–lung–lymph" axis, with direct toxic pulmonary effects on the pulmonary endothelium and subsequent lung injury and even acute respiratory distress syndrome.[85] Interestingly, in animal models, this has not been demonstrated to be associated to microbial products but, instead, was related to various acute-phase proteins, possibly generated at the intestinal epithelium[86,87] (Fig. 10.7). Paneth cells are a key source of multiple proinflammatory products that may serve to influence the initiation of a systemic inflammatory response. Paneth cells are found to secrete both α-defensin[88] and phospholipase A2, which is an enzyme that generates lipids mediators, such as prostaglandins [89,90]; the levels of both these products have been found to be increased in toxic mesenteric lymph. When activated, they also produce IL-17A, which is a proinflammatory cytokine that serves to activate neutrophils.[91] In mouse models, Vandenbroucke et al. found that mice that are deficient in matrix

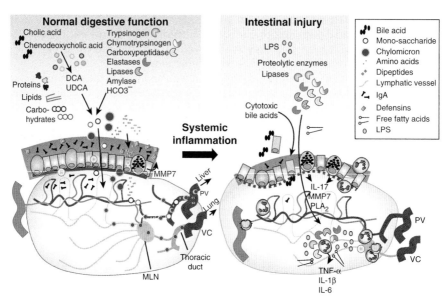

Fig. 10.7 The gastrointestinal tract has several mechanisms in which it may trigger a systemic inflammatory response. (From De Jong PR, Gonzalez-Navajas JM, Jansen NJ. The digestive tract as the origin of systemic inflammation. *Crit Care.* 2016;20:279.)

metalloproteinase 7 (MMP7), which is an enzyme required for posttranslational activation of Paneth cells, were protected against LPS-inducted lethality. [92] A study by Lee et al. found increased levels of IL-17A in the small intestine, liver and plasma after mice were subjected to SMA ischemia (ischemia/reperfusion insults), resulting in small bowel, hepatic, and renal injuries; however, they noted that genetic knock-out mice for IL-17A were protected against both intestinal damage and subsequent hepatic and renal effects.[93]

More data are becoming available from studies on animal models demonstrating the active role that the GI tract plays in systemic inflammation. In the preterm infant, local changes, such as the microbiome alterations caused by medical interventions (e.g., antibiotics), underlying host factors affected by prematurity, and source of nutrition that certainly affects the local GI inflammatory response, are involved. The GI tract itself was once thought only to act as a sieve through which translocation occurs, but current data suggest a much more dynamic relationship. It seems that there is significant interplay through which the GI system serves as an initiation point and a promoter of systemic inflammation during times of stress, even outside of NEC and local bacterial translocation.

Developmental Sequelae of Inflammation

In preterm infants there are unique pathologies, such as chorioamnionitis, sepsis, and NEC, all of which generate significant systemic inflammation.[94] The neonatal mortality following severe inflammatory and infectious insults, such as NEC and septic shock, has been reported to be as high as 30% to 40%.[95,96] There is often significant neurodevelopmental morbidity in patients who do survive.[96,97] Multiple studies have described the association between poor neurodevelopmental outcomes in preterm infants surviving after clinical conditions associated with severe neonatal inflammatory insults.[98] Stoll et al. noted an increased risk for impairment in vision, hearing, and mental and psychomotor developmental indices, as well as reduction in brain size, in patients with sepsis and NEC.[99] Preterm infants are more susceptible to ischemia, inflammation, and resultant free radical attacks, which predispose them to loss of premyelinating oligodendrocytes and white matter injury.[100] Sepsis, NEC, and recurrent infection-mediated neurodevelopmental impairment are associated with systemic upregulation of inflammatory cytokines and diffuse activated

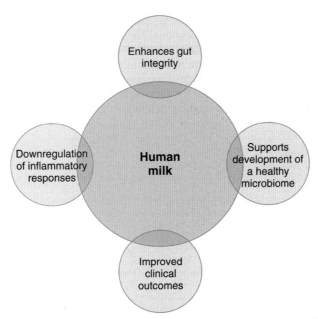

Fig. 10.8   Human milk provides protection for the preterm gastrointestinal tract through several mechanisms.

microgliosis, as well as glutamate receptor–mediated oligodendrocyte injury leading to maturation-dependent cell death and loss of cellular processes (excitotoxicity). Each of these factors contributes to white matter injury seen on brain magnetic resonance imaging.[100-102] The involvement of many mechanisms in the relationship between long-term neurodevelopmental outcomes and systemic inflammation is an area that requires further research.

Preventive Measures

Early initiation of enteral feeds is of the utmost importance to reduce gut-driven pathology in preterm neonates. In the past several decades, significant data have consistently demonstrated the beneficial priming effects of enteral nutrition; this is especially true of human milk consumption. Human milk feeding of preterm infants (mother's milk or donor milk) is associated with a significant reduction in the risk of developing many devastating clinical sequelae, including sepsis, NEC, and retinopathy of prematurity.[103-105] It has also been correlated with improved developmental outcomes.[106,107] In the intestine, human milk downregulates inflammatory responses and provides multiple cellular and noncellular immune constituents that enhance gut integrity and helps establish the intestinal microbiome.[108-110] Preterm milk contains a higher concentration of immunologic factors, such as lactoferrin, lysozyme, and secretory IgA, which may help counter developmental deficiencies in the preterm intestine (Fig. 10.8).[111] Because human milk contains many factors that can reduce damage to the gut in critical illness, human milk may also provide benefit to older infants with gut-derived sepsis and inflammation.[112] There has also been discussion regarding the usefulness of polyunsaturated fatty acids (metabolites of omega-3 and -6 fatty acids), bovine lactoferrin, gangliosides, and pre- and probiotics as immunomodulators of the GI tract.[113-116] Means of enhancing gut integrity and function continue to be investigated.

Summary

It is clear that the neonatal GI tract plays a dynamic role in the overall health of the preterm neonate. There are many unique challenges, both internal and external, that the preterm neonate faces. The innate immaturity of the preterm GI tract is easily damaged, and throughout their course in the NICU, preterm infants are often exposed to more pathogenic organisms, microbiome-altering antibiotics, and other possibly detrimental interventions. These combined risk factors increase the risk of systemic inflammation and infection, which can have long-term effects on both morbidity and mortality. There are data to suggest that the GI tract itself is a driving force in the systemic inflammatory cascade. Fortunately, modifiable risk factors are beginning to be identified. Further research and progress in this area is important to continue to improve neonatal outcomes.

REFERENCES

1. Hurtado CW, Li BUK. *The NASPGHAN Fellows Concise Review of Pediatric Gastroenterology, Hepatology and Nutrition.* 2nd ed. NASPGHAN; 2017.
2. Wyllie R, Hyams J. *Pediatric Gastrointestinal and Liver Disease.* 5th ed. Philadelphia, PA: Elsevier; 2016.
3. Mshvildadze M, Neu J, Shuster J, et al. Intestinal microbial ecology in premature infants assessed with non-culture based techniques. *J Pediatr.* 2010;156:20–25.
4. Eggesbo M, Moen B, Peddada S, et al. Development of gut microbiota in infants not exposed to medical interventions. *APMIS.* 2011;119:17–35.
5. Gerritsen J, Smidt H, Rijkers GT, et al. Intestinal microbiota in human health and disease: the impact of probiotics. *Genes Nutr.* 2011;6:209–240.
6. Langhendries JP. Early bacterial colonisation of the intestine: why it matters? *Arch Pediatr.* 2006;13:1526–1534.
7. Furet JP, Kong LC, Tap J, et al. Differential adaptation of human gut microbiota to bariatric surgery-induced weight loss: links with metabolic and low-grade inflammation markers. *Diabetes.* 2010;59:3049–3057.
8. Garrett WS, Gordon JI, Glimcher LH. Homeostasis and inflammation in the intestine. *Cell.* 2010;140(6):859–870.
9. Round JL, Lee SM, Li J, et al. The Toll-like receptor 2 pathway establishes colonization by a commensal of the human microbiota. *Science.* 2011;332:974–977.
10. Elinav E, Strowig T, Kau AL, et al. NLRP6 inflammasome regulates colonic microbial ecology and risk for colitis. *Cell.* 2011;145:745–757.
11. Dicksved J, Halfvarson J, Rosenquist M, et al. Molecular analysis of the gut microbiota of identical twins with Crohn's disease. *ISME J.* 2008;2:716–727.
12. Daniel H, Moghaddas Gholami A, Berry D, et al. High-fat diet alters gut microbiota physiology in mice. *ISME J.* 2014;8:295–308.
13. Martinez I, Perdicaro DJ, Brown AW, et al. Diet-induced alterations of host cholesterol metabolism are likely to affect the gut microbiota composition in hamsters. *Appl Environ Microbiol.* 2013;79:516–524.
14. Wang Y, Hoenig JD, Malin KJ, et al. 16S rRNA gene-based analysis of fecal microbiota from preterm infants with and without necrotizing enterocolitis. *ISME J.* 2009;3:944–954.
15. Penders J, Thijs C, van den Brandt PA, et al. Gut microbiota composition and development of atopic manifestations in infancy: the KOALA birth cohort study. *Gut.* 2007;56:661–667.
16. Dominguez-Bello MG, Costello EK, Contreras M, et al. Delivery mode shapes the acquisition and structure of the initial microbiota across multiple body habitats in newborns. *Proc Natl Acad Sci USA.* 2010;107:11971–11975.
17. Orrhage K, Nord CE. Factors controlling the bacterial colonization of the intestine in breastfed infants. *Acta Paediatr Suppl.* 1999;28:19–25.
18. Bjorkstrom MV, Hall L, Sodelund S, et al. Intestinal flora in very low-birth weight infants. *Acta Paediatr.* 2009;98:1762–1767.
19. Greenwood C, Morrow AL, Lagomarcino AJ, et al. Early empiric antibiotic use in preterm infants is associated with lower bacterial diversity and higher relative abundance of enterobacter. *J Pediatr.* 2014.
20. Westerbeek EA, van den Berg A, Lafeber HN, et al. The intestinal bacterial colonisation in preterm infants: a review of the literature. *Clin Nutr.* 2006;25:361–368.
21. Cotten CM, Taylor S, Stoll B, et al. Prolonged duration of initial empirical antibiotic treatment is associated with increased rates of necrotizing enterocolitis and death for extremely low birth weight infants. *Pediatrics.* 2009;123:58–66.
22. Alexander VN, Northrup V, Bizzarro MJ. Antibiotic exposure in the newborn intensive care unit and the risk of necrotizing enterocolitis. *J Pediatr.* 2011;159:392–397.
23. Kuppala VS, Meinzen-Derr J, Morrow AL, Schibler KR. Prolonged initial empirical antibiotic treatment is associated with adverse outcomes in premature infants. *J Pediatr.* 2011;159:720–725.
24. Tomasello E, Bedoui S. Intestinal innate immune cells in gut homeostasis and immunosurveillance. *Immunol Cell Biol.* 2013;91:201–203.
25. Maynard CL, Elson CO, Hatton RD, Weaver CT. Reciprocal interactions of the intestinal microbiota and immune system. *Nature.* 2012;489:231–241.
26. Russell GJ, Winter HS, Fox VL, et al. Lymphocytes bearing the gamma delta T-cell receptor in normal human intestine and celiac disease. *Hum Patho.* 1991;22:690–694.
27. Lundell AC, Rabe H, Quiding-Jarbrink M, et al. Development of gut-homing receptors on circulating B cells during infancy. *Clin Immunol.* 2011;138:97–106.

28. Rakoff-Nahoum S, Paglino J, Eslami-Varzaneh F, et al. Recognition of commensal microflora by toll-like receptors is required for intestinal homeostasis. *Cell.* 2004;118:229–241.
29. Leaphart CL, Cavallo J, Gribar SC, et al. A critical role for TLR4 in the pathogenesis of necrotizing enterocolitis by modulating intestinal injury and repair. *J Immunol.* 2007;179:4808–4820.
30. Neal MD, Leaphart C, Levy R, et al. Enterocyte TLR4 mediates phagocytosis and translocation of bacteria across the intestinal barrier. *J Immunol.* 2006;176:3070–3079.
31. Sodhi CP, Shi XH, Richardson WM, et al. Toll-like receptor 4 inhibits enterocyte proliferation via impaired beta-catenin signaling in necrotizing enterocolitis. *Gastroenterology.* 2010;138:185–196.
32. Sodhi C, Levy RM, Gill R, et al. DNA attenuates enterocyte Toll-like receptor 4 mediated intestinal mucosal injury after remote trauma. *Am J Physiol Gastrointest Liver Physiol.* 2011;300:G862–G873.
33. Neu J, Walker WA. Necrotizing enterocolitis. *N Engl J Med.* 2011;364:255–264.
34. Mookherjee N, Brown KL, Bowdish DM, et al. Modulation of the TLR-mediated inflammatory response by the endogenous human host defense peptide LL-37. *J Immuno.* 2006;176:2455–2464.
35. Menard S, Forster V, Lotz M, et al. Developmental switch of intestinal antimicrobial peptide expression. *J Exp Med.* 2008;205:183–193.
36. Nathakumar NN, Fusunyan RD, Sanderson I, et al. Inflammation in the developing human intestine: a possible pathophysiologic contribution to necrotizing enterocolitis. *Proc Natl Acad Sci USA.* 2000;97:6043–6048.
37. Nathakumar NN, Young C, Ko JS, et al. Glucocorticoid responsiveness in developing human intestine: possible role in prevention of necrotizing enterocolitis. *Am J Physiol Gastrointest Liver Physiol.* 2005;288:G85–G92.
38. Wynn JL, Levy O. Role of innate host defenses in susceptibility to early-onset neonatal sepsis. *Clin Perinatol.* 2010;37:307–337.
39. Claud EC. Neonatal necrotizing enterocolitis—inflammation and intestinal immaturity. *Antiinflamm Antiallergy Agents Med Chem.* 2009;8:248–259.
40. Martin CR, Walker WA. Intestinal immune defenses and the inflammatory response in necrotizing enterocolitis. *Semin Fetal Neonatal Med.* 2006;11:369–377.
41. Wolfs TG, Buurman WA, Zoer B, et al. Endotoxin induced chorioamnionitis prevents intestinal development during gestation in fetal sheep. *PloS One.* 2009;4:e5837.
42. Udall Jr JN. Gastrointestinal host defense and necrotizing enterocolitis. *J Pediatr.* 1990;117:S33–S43.
43. Salzman NH, Polin RA, Harris MC, et al. Enteric defensin expression in necrotizing enterocolitis. *Pediatr Res.* 1998;44:20–26.
44. Wynn JL, Wong HR. Pathophysiology and treatment of septic shock in neonates. *Clin Perinatol.* 2010;37:439–479.
45. Johnson L. The trophic action of gastrointestinal hormones. *Gastroenterology.* 1976;70:278–288.
46. Hermsen JL, San Y, Kudsk KA. Food fight!: parenteral nutrition, enteral stimulation and gut-derived mucosal immunity. *Langenbecks Arch Surg.* 2009;394:17–30.
47. Karagol BS, Zencirogly A, Okumus N, et al. Randomized controlled trial of slow vs. rapid enteral feeding advancements on the clinical outcomes of preterm infants with birth weight 750-1250 g. *JPEN J Parenter Enteral Nutr.* 2013;37(2):223–228.
48. Caple J, Armentrout D, Huseby V, et al. Randomized, controlled trial of slow versus rapid feeding volume advancement in preterm infants. *Pediatrics.* 2004;114(6):1597–1600.
49. Benjamin Jr DK, Stoll BJ, Fanaroff AA, et al. Neonatal candidiasis among extremely low birth weight infants: risk factors, mortality rates, and neurodevelopmental outcomes at 18 to 22 months. *Pediatrics.* 200;117:84–92.
50. Stoddart RW, Widdowson EM. Changes in the organs of pigs in response to feeding for the first 24h after birth. III. Fluorescence histochemistry of the carbohydrates of the intestine. *Biol Neonate.* 1976;29:18–27.
51. Niinikoski H, Stoll B, Guan X, et al. Onset of small intestinal atrophy is associated with reduced intestinal blood flow in TPN-fed neonatal piglets. *J Nutr.* 2004;134:1467–1474.
52. Owens L, Burrin DG, Berseth CL. Minimal enteral feeding induces maturation of intestinal motor function but not mucosal growth in neonatal dogs. *J Nutr.* 2002;132:2717–2722.
53. Kang W, Kudsk KA. Is there evidence that the gut contributes to mucosal immunity in humans? *JPEN J Parenter Enteral Nutr.* 2007;31:246–258.
54. Shulman RJ, Schanler RJ, Lau C, et al. Early feeding, antenatal glucocorticoids, and human milk decrease intestinal permeability in preterm infants. *Pediatr Res.* 1998;44:519–523.
55. Meizen-Derr J, Poindexter B, Wrage L, et al. Role of human milk in extremely low birth weight infants' risk of necrotizing enterocolitis or death. *J Perinatol.* 2009;29(1):57–62.
56. Berseth CL, Bisquera JA, Paje VU, et al. Prolonging small feedings early in life decreases the incidence of necrotizing enterocolitis in very low birthweight infants. *Pediatrics.* 2003;111(3):529–534.
57. Patole SK, de Klerk N. Impact of standardized feeding regimens on incidence of neonatal necrotizing enterocolitis: a systematic review and meta-analysis of observational studies. *Arch Dis Child Fetal Neonatal Ed.* 2005;90(2):F147–F151.
58. Clark RH, Bloom BT, Spitzer AR, Gerstmann DR. Reported medication use in the neonatal intensive care unit: data from a large national data set. *Pediatrics.* 2006;117:1979–1987.
59. Benitz WE. Adjunct laboratory tests in the diagnosis of early-onset neonatal sepsis. *Clin Perinatol.* 2010;37:412–438.
60. Stoll BJ, Gordon T, Korones SB, et al. Early-onset sepsis in very low birth weight neonates: a report from the National Institute of Child Health and Human Development Neonatal Research Network. *J Pediatr.* 1996;129:72–80.

61. Nieuwenhuijzen GA, Goris RJ. The gut: the "motor" of multiple organ dysfunction syndrome? *Curr Opin Clin Nutr Metab Care*. 1999;2:399–404.

62. Buchholz BM, Bauer AJ. Membrane TLR signaling mechanisms in the gastrointestinal tract during sepsis. *Neurogastroenterol Motil*. 2010;22:232–245.

63. Abt MC, Artis D. The intestinal microbiota in health and disease: the influence of microbial products on immune cell homeostasis.

64. Hietbrink F, Besselink MG, Renooij W, et al. Systemic inflammation increases intestinal permeability during experimental human endotoxemia. *Shock*. 2009;32:374–378.

65. Taylor DE. Revving the motor of multiple organ dysfunction syndrome. Gut dysfunction in ARDS and multiorgan failure. *Respir Care Clin N Am*. 1998;4:611–631, vii-viii.

66. Clark JA, Coopersmith CM. Intestinal crosstalk: a new paradigm for understanding the gut as the "motor" of critical illness. *Shock*. 2007;28(4):384–393.

67. Madan JC, Salari RC, Saxena D, et al. Gut microbial colonization in premature neonates predicts neonatal sepsis. *Arch Dis Child Fetal Neonatal Ed*. 2012;97(6):F456–F462.

68. Tremaroli V, Backhed F. Functional interactions between the gut microbiota and host metabolism. *Nature*. 2012;489(7415):242–249.

69. Maslowski KM, Vieira AT, Ng A, et al. Regulation of inflammatory responses by gut microbiota and chemoattractant receptor GPR43. *Nature*. 2009;461(7268):1282–1286.

70. Piton G, Manzon C, Cypriani B, Carbonnel F, Capellier G. Acute intestinal failure in critically ill patients: is plasma citrulline the right marker? *Intensive Care Med*. 2011;37(6):911–917.

71. Derikx JP, Blijlevens NM, Donnelly JP, et al. Loss of enterocyte mass is accompanied by diminished turnover of enterocytes after myeloablative therapy in hematopoietic stem-cell transplant recipients. *Ann Oncol*. 2009;20(2):337–342.

72. Typpo KV, Larmonier CB, Deschenes J, Redford D, Kiela PR, Ghishan FK. Clinical characteristics associated with postoperative intestinal epithelial barrier dysfunction in children with congenital heart disease. *Pediatr Crit Care Med*. 2015;16(1):37–44.

73. Piton G, Manzon C, Monnet E, et al. Plasma citrulline kinetics and prognostic value in critically ill patients. *Intensive Care Med*. 2010;36(4):702–706.

74. De Jong PR, Gonzalez-Navajas JM, Jansen NJ. The digestive tract as the origin of systemic inflammation. *Crit Care*. 2016;20:279.

75. Henao-Mejia J, Elinav E, Jin C, et al. Inflammasome-mediated dysbiosis regulates progression of NAFLD and obesity. *Nature*. 2012;482(7384):179–185.

76. Schneider KM, Bieghs V, Heymann F, et al. CX3CR1 is a gatekeeper for intestinal barrier integrity in mice: limiting steatohepatitis by maintaining intestinal homeostasis. *Hepatology*. 2015;62(5):1405–1416.

77. Prin M, Bakker J, Wagener G. Hepatosplanchnic circulation in cirrhosis and sepsis. *World J Gastroenterol*. 2015;21(9):2582–2592.

78. Balmer ML, Slack E, de Gottardi A, et al. The liver may act as a firewall mediating mutualism between the host and its gut commensal microbiota. *Sci Transl Med*. 2014;6(237): 237ra66.

79. Lozano-Ruiz B, Bachiller V, Garcia-Martinez I, et al. Absent in melanoma 2 triggers a heightened inflammasome response in ascitic fluid macrophages of patients with cirrhosis. *J Hepatol*. 2015;62(1):64–71.

80. Frances R, Zapater P, Gonzalez-Navajas JM, et al. Bacterial DNA in patients with cirrhosis and noninfected ascites mimics the soluble immune response established in patients with spontaneous bacterial peritonitis. *Hepatology*. 2008;47(3):978–985.

81. Gonzalez-Navajas JM, Bellot P, Frances R, et al. Presence of bacterial-DNA in cirrhosis identifies a subgroup of patients with marked inflammatory response not related to endotoxin. *J Hepatol*. 2008;48(1):61–67.

82. Nakamoto N, Kanai T. Role of toll-like receptors in immune activation and tolerance in the liver. *Front Immunol*. 2014;5:221.

83. Paik YH, Schwabe RF, Bataller R, Russo MP, Jobin C, Brenner DA. Toll-like receptor 4 mediates inflammatory signaling by bacterial lipopolysaccharide in human hepatic stellate cells. *Hepatology*. 2003;37(5):1043–1055.

84. Knolle P, Schlaak J, Uhrig A, Kempf P. Meyer zum Buschenfelde KH, Gerken G. Human Kupffer cells secrete IL-10 in response to lipopolysaccharide (LPS) challenge. *J Hepatol*. 1995;22(2):226–229.

85. Deitch EA. Gut lymph and lymphatics: a source of factors leading to organ injury and dysfunction. *Ann N Y Acad Sci*. 2010;1207(suppl 1):E103–E111.

86. Adams Jr CA, Xu DZ, Lu Q, Deitch EA. Factors larger than 100 kd in posthemorrhagic shock mesenteric lymph are toxic for endothelial cells. *Surgery*. 2001;129(3):351–363.

87. Fang JF, Shih LY, Yuan KC, Fang KY, Hwang TL, Hsieh SY. Proteomic analysis of post-hemorrhagic shock mesenteric lymph. *Shock*. 2010;34(3):291–298.

88. Atkins JL, Hammamieh R, Jett M, Gorbunov NV, Asher LV, Kiang JG. Alpha-defensin-like product and asymmetric dimethylarginine increase in mesenteric lymph after hemorrhage in anesthetized rat. *Shock*. 2008;30(4):411–416.

89. Gonzalez RJ, Moore EE, Ciesla DJ, Biffl WL, Offner PJ, Silliman CC. Phospholipase A(2)–derived neutral lipids from posthemorrhagic shock mesenteric lymph prime the neutrophil oxidative burst. *Surgery*. 2001;130(2):198–203.

90. Keshav S. Paneth cells: leukocyte-like mediators of innate immunity in the intestine. *J Leukoc Biol*. 2006;80(3):500–508.

91. Park SW, Kim M, Kim JY, et al. Paneth cell-mediated multiorgan dysfunction after acute kidney injury. *J Immunol*. 2012;189(11):5421–5433.

92. Vandenbroucke RE, Vanlaere I, Van Hauwermeiren F, Van Wonterghem E, Wilson C, Libert C. Pro-inflammatory effects of matrix metalloproteinase 7 in acute inflammation. *Mucosal Immunol.* 2014;7(3):579–588.

93. Lee HT, Kim M, Kim JY, et al. Critical role of interleukin-17A in murine intestinal ischemia-reperfusion injury. *Am J Physiol Gastrointest Liver Physiol.* 2013;304(1):G12–G25.

94. Ng PC, Li K, Wong RP, et al. Proinflammatory and anti-inflammatory cytokine responses in preterm infants with systemic infections. *Arch Dis Child Fetal Neonatal Ed.* 2003;88:F209–F213.

95. Ftizgibbons SC, Ching Y, Yu D, et al. Mortality of necrotizing enterocolitis expressed by birth weight categories. *J Pediatr Surg.* 2009;44:1072–1075; discussion 5–6.

96. Kermorvant-Duchemin E, Laborie S, Rabilloud M, et al. Outcome and prognostic factors in neonates with septic shock. *Pediatr Crit Care Med.* 2008;9:186–191.

97. Henry MC, Moss RL. Necrotizing enterocolitis. *Annu Rev Med.* 2009;60:111–124.

98. Adams-Chapman I, Stoll BJ. Neonatal infection and long-term neurodevelopmental outcome in the preterm infant. *Curr Opin Infect Dis.* 2006;19:290–297.

99. Stoll BJ, Hansen NI, Adams-Chapman I, et al. Neurodevelopmental and growth impairment among extremely low-birth weight infants with neonatal infection. *JAMA.* 2004;292:2357–2365.

100. Kjwaha O, Volpe JJ. Pathogenesis of cerebral white matter injury of prematurity. *Arch Dis Child Retal Neonatal Ed.* 2008;93:F153–F161.

101. Shah DK, Doyle LW, Anderson PJ, et al. Adverse neurodevelopment in preterm infants with postnatal sepsis or necrotizing enterocolitis is mediated by white matter abnormalities on magnetic resonance imaging at term. *J Pediatr.* 2008;153:170–175, e1.

102. Glass HC, Bonifacio SL, Chau V, et al. Recurrent postnatal infections are associated with progressive white matter injury in premature infants. *Pediatrics.* 2008;122:299–305.

103. Howie PW, Forsyth JS, Ogston SA, et al. Protective effect of breast feeding against infection. *BMJ.* 1990;300:11–16.

104. Lucas A, Cole TJ. Breast milk and neonatal necrotising enterocolitis. *Lancet.* 1990;336:1519–1523.

105. Heller CD, O'Shea M, Yao Q, et al. Human milk intake and retinopathy of prematurity in extremely low birth weight infants. *Pediatrics.* 2007;120:1–9.

106. Isaacs EB, Fischl BR, Quinn BT, et al. Impact of breast milk on IQ, brain size, and white matter development. *Pediatr Res.* 2010;67:357–362.

107. Vohr BR, Poindexter BB, Dusick AM, et al. Persistent beneficial effects of breast milk ingested in the neonatal intensive care unit on outcomes of extremely low birth weight infants at 30 months of age. *Pediatrics.* 2007;120:e953–e959.

108. LeBouder E, Rey-Nores JE, Raby AC, et al. Modulation of neonatal microbial recognition: TLR-mediated innate immune responses are specifically and differentially modulated by human milk. *J Immunol.* 2006;176:3742–3752.

109. Walker A. Breast milk as the gold standard for protective nutrients. *J Pediatr.* 2010;156:S3–S7.

110. Liedel JL, Guo Y, Yu Y, et al. Mother's milk induced Hsp70 expression preserves intestinal epithelial barrier function in an immature rat pup model. *Pediatr Res.* 2011;69(5 Pt 1):395–400.

111. Bauer J, Gerss J. Longitudinal analysis of macronutrients and minerals in human milk produced by mothers of preterm infants. *Clin Nutr.* 2010;30(2):215–220.

112. Dominguez JA, Coopersmith CM. Can we protect the gut in critical illness? The role of growth factors and other novel approaches.

113. Indrio F, Neu J. The intestinal microbiome of infants and the use of probiotics. *Curr Opin Pediatr.* 2011;23:145–150.

114. Caplan MS, Russell T, Xiao Y, et al. Effect of polyunsaturated fatty acid (PUFA) supplementation of intestinal inflammation and necrotizing enterocolitis (NEC) in neonatal rat model. *Pediatr Res.* 2001;49:647–652.

115. Manzoni P, Decembrino L, Stolfi I, et al. Lactoferrin and prevention of late-onset sepsis in the preterm neonates. *Early Hum Dev.* 2010;86(suppl 1):59–61.

116. Schnabl KL, Larsen B, Van Aerde Je, et al. Gangliosides protect bowel in an infant model of necrotizing enterocolitis by suppressing proinflammatory signals. *J Pediatr Gastroenterol Nutr.* 2009;49:382–392.

117. Spits H, Cupedo T. Innate lymphoid cells: emerging insights in development, lineage relationships, and function. *Annu Rev Immunol.* 2012;30:647–675.

118. Sanos SL, Diefenbach A, Innate lymphoid cells: from border protection to the initiation of inflammatory diseases. *Immunol Cell Biol.* 2013;91:215–224.

119. Martin CR, Dammann O, Allred EN, et al. Neurodevelopment of extremely preterm infants who had necrotizing enterocolitis with or without late bacteremia. *J Pediatr.* 2010;157:751–756. e1.

CHAPTER 11

Adult Consequences of Neonatal and Fetal Nutrition: Mechanisms

Lisa A. Joss-Moore, PhD, Cheri Bantilan, MS, Kjersti Aagaard-Tillery, MD, PhD, FACOG, Nicole Mitchell, MD, Clotilde desRoberts, MD, Robert H. Lane, MD

11

Early Nutrition and Adult Phenotype

An infant's early nutrition affects the adult phenotype (Table 11.1). As old and intuitive as this concept may be, it has re-entered the consciousness of the research community only in the last 20 years. As a result, the overall interest in the specific experiences and mechanisms through which different perinatal nutritional environments lead to adult-onset diseases has grown exponentially. This interest is an important research priority because it is an avenue for preventing adult diseases, such as diabetes, obesity, and hypertension, before they exact a direct toll.

The continuum of early nutrition experienced by humans varies greatly within a single population, let alone between different populations. As a result, the majority of epidemiologic studies interested in understanding the adult consequences of fetal and neonatal nutrition have used poor growth, both in utero and in the early postnatal period, as a marker of poor nutrition. Therefore an important assumption of this chapter is that poor nutrition leads to poor growth in both the fetus and the neonate. Epidemiologic studies on this subject have historically been limited to infants who are small for gestational age (SGA), which is typically defined as weight <10th percentile. Infants included in this group may be small for multiple reasons, including normal genetic variation. Furthermore, these studies that focus only on SGA infants miss infants who are smaller than they should be but are still >10th percentile. More recently, epidemiologic studies have separated those infants who fail to grow to their genetic potential, that is, those who suffer intrauterine growth restriction (IUGR), from those who are SGA, but do not have IUGR. Generally, these studies include maternal and fetal parameters that contribute to poor growth, such as maternal uteroplacental insufficiency.

Despite these limitations, the epidemiology in this field has been vitally important and often elegant, which is certainly true of the three cohorts (and their respective studies) that have set the standard for understanding the adult consequences of neonatal and fetal nutrition. These cohorts involve the (1) Dutch famine of 1944 to

Table 11.1   ADULT PHENOTYPES ASSOCIATED WITH GROWTH RESTRICTIONS

Attention deficit disorder	Insulin resistance
Chronic lung disease	Neurodevelopmental delay
Divorce	Neuroendocrine reprogramming
Dyslipidemia	Poor postnatal growth
Hypertension	Renal insufficiency
Immunodeficiency	Schizophrenia

1945; (2) the early studies by Barker et al., hence the "Barker Hypothesis"; and (3) the more recent Nurses' Health Study.

The first of these cohorts involves the Dutch famine of 1944 to 1945. This famine occurred as a result of German reprisal for a general railway strike intended to disrupt the transport of German reinforcements against Allied liberation movements.[1,2] The famine lasted approximately 5 months. Daily rations in Amsterdam dropped from 1800 kcal/day in December 1943 to 400 to 800 kcal/day in April 1945. Although a goal was set for children under age 1 year and for pregnant or lactating women to receive supplemental rations, this was not possible at the height of the famine. After liberation in May 1945, caloric intake increased to >2000 kcal/day. The effects of the famine on the Dutch population have been examined via multiple sources, including population-based cohorts, military induction records, psychiatric registries, and self-reports. One of the more comprehensive studies is the Dutch famine birth cohort study, through which the investigators interviewed 912 individuals who were born at term between November 1, 1943, and February 28, 1947, and assessed socioeconomic factors, lifestyles, and medical histories.[3] Babies exposed to famine conditions early in gestation were not smaller or lighter than nonexposed infants; however, they suffered from an increased incidence of coronary heart disease, hypertension, dyslipidemia, and obesity later in life. Although not quite statistically significant, the adults with coronary heart disease were also more likely to have had lower birth weights and smaller head circumferences. Similarly, a cohort born in the Wilhelmina Gasthuis of Amsterdam between November 1943 and February 1947 revealed an association between maternal experience of famine early in pregnancy and an atherogenic lipid profile (higher low-density lipoprotein/high-density lipoprotein [LDL/HDL] cholesterol ratios).[4] Famine experienced early in gestation also altered the perceptions of affected individuals in that the proportion of people reporting self-perceived poor health was significantly higher in the group of famine exposure early during gestation compared with those who had not experienced the famine conditions in utero.[5]

Babies exposed to the famine during gestation suffered from an increased incidence of obstructive airway disease as well as an increased incidence of microalbuminuria.[6,7] Interestingly, both these findings were independent of size at birth. Babies exposed to the famine in late gestation were also more likely to exhibit impaired glucose tolerance compared with those who had not experienced the famine conditions in utero.[8] Furthermore, affective disorders occurred more often in those individuals exposed to famine conditions in utero in mid-to-late gestation.[9] Other findings from the Dutch famine cohort that are intriguing, and somewhat frightening, include the associations between experiencing the famine in utero and increased rates of schizophrenia, schizophrenia spectrum disorders, and antisocial personality disorder.[10]

For all three groups of infants with early, mid-, or late gestation exposure to the Dutch famine, the rate of mortality at age 50 years was higher. Group-specific mortality at age 50 years for early, mid-, or late gestation exposure was 11.5%, 11.2%, and 15.2%, respectively. In contrast, mortality at age 50 years among those born after the famine was 7.2%.[11]

The second set of studies is the work by Barker, who, along with his research group, pioneered the epidemiology of the adult consequences of neonatal and fetal nutrition, also known as the Developmental Origins of Health and Disease. As early as 1986, Barker and Osmond noted, in an article in the *Lancet*, a geographic association between ischemic heart disease in 1968 to 1978 and infant mortality in 1921 to 1925.[12] These authors astutely speculated that "poor nutrition in early life increases susceptibility to the effects of an affluent diet."

The observation linking infant mortality and adult disease was continued by the Hertfordshire studies, which are still the standard in this area. An initial focus of these studies was a cohort of 5654 men born between 1911 and 1930 in Hertfordshire, England.[13] The 1989 manuscript revealed that men who had the lowest weights at birth and at age 1 year had the highest death rates from cardiovascular disease. A subset of these men was further used to evaluate the relationship between insulin sensitivity and birth weight. Specifically, 468 men born, raised, and living in east Hertfordshire were studied after ingesting a 75-g glucose drink.[14] Men with impaired glucose sensitivity and non-insulin-dependent diabetes were characterized by lower weight at birth and at age 1 year. Furthermore, the percentage of men with impaired insulin sensitivity decreased as weight increased at age 1 year; this progression was statistically significant and independent of the adult body mass. This concept—that reduced growth in early life leads to impaired glucose tolerance—has impacted the way numerous clinicians and investigators now approach perinatal metabolism and nutrition.

Barker's study and the findings on the people of Hertfordshire continue to contribute significantly to our understanding of the relationship between early nutrition and growth and adult diseases. By 2005, the cohort included 37,615 men and women born in Hertfordshire.[15] Low birth weight in men from this population increases the risk of cardiovascular disease, whereas low birth weight in women predisposes the affected adults to cardiovascular and musculoskeletal disease, as well as pneumonia and diabetes. Although there are gender differences, data suggest that an increase in birth weight by 1 standard deviation (SD) would reduce mortality by 0.86% in both genders at age 75 years.

The third historically significant cohort was the Nurses' Health Study cohort.[16,17] This study was established in 1976 when approximately 122,000 married female registered nurses, ages 30 to 55 years, responded to a mailed questionnaire about their life histories. The study has continued through follow-up questionnaires every 2 years, thus eliciting updated histories and medical information. The validity of self-reported birth weights was assessed via the Nurses' Health Study II, which compared weights recorded on birth certificates to the reported weights.[18] The Spearman correlation coefficient between the two weights was 0.74. This study added weight to the observations of Barker et al. by noting a significantly increased relative risk for non-insulin-dependent diabetes in women who had low birth weight (<5.5 lb) compared with those women of median birth weight (7.1-8.5 lb).[17] The relative risk for women whose birthweight was <5.5 lb and 5.5 lb was 1.88 (1.59-2.21) and 1.55 (1.32-1.83), respectively. Adjusting for age, body mass index (BMI), and maternal history of diabetes strengthened the association between low birth weight and non-insulin-dependent diabetes. No significant effects on relative risk were noted after adjustment for prematurity, multiple births, maternal age at birth, participant breastfeeding, ethnicity, parental occupation at age 16 years, paternal diabetes, participant height, parity, cigarette smoking, and physical activity.

The Nurses' Health Study findings have also been used to investigate the relationship between birth weight and cardiovascular disease in women.[19] Nonfatal myocardial infarctions were included as an endpoint of the study if the criteria of the World Health Organization were met. Nonfatal strokes were included as another endpoint if the criteria of the national survey of stroke were met. For every 454-g increase in birth weight, a 5% decrease in the risk of nonfatal myocardial infarction was noted, as was an 11% decrease in the risk of nonfatal stroke. As with the Nurses' Health Study focusing on insulin resistance, these findings were largely independent of other key factors, such as adult body weight, hypertension, diabetes, lifestyle, and childhood socioeconomic class.

The investigations involving these three cohorts have provided important and seminal insights into the relationship between early growth and nutrition and adult diseases. They have provided an impetus to further studies that identify possible physiologic and molecular mechanisms, which may lead to either in utero interventions or postnatal therapies to moderate the impending risks. The following section will focus on recently identified important biologic targets.

Developmental Biology of the Adult Consequences of Neonatal and Fetal Nutrition

This section is presented in two parts. The first part discusses recent insights into how fetal growth restriction affects phenotype in humans, and animal studies used to investigate possible mechanisms. The discussion is not meant to be all inclusive but focuses on some of the most recent and thought-provoking observations. The second part discusses recent insights into how growth restriction in the premature infant potentially leads to later morbidities and how dietary interventions may either contribute to or moderate these effects.

Fetus/Intrauterine Growth Restriction

Multiple studies from different regions of the world containing racially distinct cohorts have associated fetal growth restriction with adult morbidities, as previously discussed. One of the more recent trends is the realization that the lasting effects of fetal growth restriction are evident in both early life and adulthood. Furthermore, weight gain and nutrition modify the effect of IUGR on these early results. These findings pertain to issues involving glucose homeostasis, lipid biology, and hypertension; however, an important central theme to this literature, as well as the literature focusing on adult phenotype, is that cohorts differ, whether as a result of fetal growth restriction or postnatal consequences. Consequently, the findings of these studies differ slightly, which has led to the conundrum that multiple mechanisms may be involved. For example, Mericq et al. followed up SGA and appropriate for gestational age (AGA) infants through the first 3 years of life.[20] This group measured infants' weights and lengths at 1, 2, and 3 years. At 48 hours of life, glucose and insulin levels were measured in these infants, and at 1 and 3 years of life an intravenous glucose tolerance test was administered after an overnight fast. A calculation of insulin resistance was determined by using the homeostasis model. At 48 hours of life, SGA infants had lower insulin levels compared with AGA infants. At 1 and 3 years of age, SGA children exhibited higher fasting insulin levels and lower insulin sensitivity compared with AGA children.

Growth restriction also appears to affect cellular energy homeostasis. Chessex et al. compared 6 SGA and 13 AGA newborns, in terms of energy expenditure.[21] Energy expenditure in SGA infants was 4.8 kcal/kg/day greater than in AGA infants, primarily via increased fat oxidation. In contrast, when infant oral glucose disposal was studied in prepubertal and early pubertal children (ages 8-14 years) with a history of IUGR, and compared with that of healthy age- and weight-matched control children, lower glucose oxidation characterized the IUGR subjects, although no decrease in overall energy expenditure was noted. Interestingly, lipid oxidation was increased nearly twofold, although not significantly based on variation.[22]

The study by Arends et al.[22a] also noted other differences between SGA and AGA counterparts, similar to the large epidemiologic studies discussed above. First, systolic blood pressure was significantly increased in the SGA children. Second, although fasting serum free fatty acids, triglycerides, total cholesterol, HDL, and LDL levels were not significantly different between groups, 6 of the 28 children in the SGA group had serum free fatty acids above the normal range. In terms of lipid biology, much of the focus has been on leptin and adiponectin. For example, in a population of 1-year-old SGA infants from Santiago, Chile, SGA infants were characterized by decreased leptin levels (0.29 ± 0.19 nM versus 0.40 versus 0.07 nM; $P < 0.05$), as well as a trend toward increased triglycerides ($P = 0.053$).[23]

Table 11.2   HORMONES LINKED TO THE FETAL ORIGINS OF ADULT DISEASE

Adiponectin	Leptin
Androgens	Glucocorticoids
Angiotensin	Insulin and its binding proteins

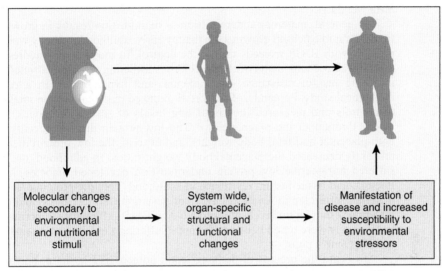

Fig. 11.1   Early life insults associated with the environment and nutrition stimulate molecular alterations. The resulting molecular alterations cause changes in the structure and function of various organs. As age and additional stressors interact, disease results.

The next sections will delve into specific mechanisms through which IUGR induces many of these phenotypic changes involving glucose metabolism, lipid homeostasis, and other cardiovascular risk factors. The list is neither exhaustive nor exclusive, and, in fact, evidence continues to accumulate that IUGR adult phenotype is a result of many moderate adjustments that are complementary and probably interdependent (Table 11.2). One theme that becomes evident when looking at the whole body of IUGR physiologic studies is that many of the adjustments that are implemented early not only provide short-term advantages in terms of survival but also lead to adult morbidities, such as diabetes, dyslipidemia, and cardiovascular disease, with the passage of time (Fig. 11.1).

Metabolism

Leptin

Leptin is a 167–amino-acid protein that is produced by adipocytes, which performs multiple functions. Among the most important functions of leptin is the regulation of hypothalamic centers that determine, at least in part, whole-body energy expenditure and fat mass.[24] In general, leptin increases energy expenditure and reduces food intake. As a result, humans and rodents lacking either leptin or the leptin receptor develop severe obesity and hyperphagia. In practical terms, increased serum levels of leptin characterize most obese conditions, and in fact, leptin levels typically correlate directly with body fat mass and BMI. The failure of increased levels of leptin in regulating weight loss suggests a potential state of leptin resistance in many cases of obesity.

Within the context of IUGR, maternal serum leptin levels are generally noted to be increased, whereas fetal IUGR serum leptin levels are generally noted to be decreased. For example, Pighetti et al. measured maternal and fetal serum leptin levels in 43 "normal" term pregnancies and 27 pregnancies complicated by asymmetric IUGR.[25] Women from both groups had normal pregravid BMIs (20-27 kg/m^2); pregnancies complicated by diabetes or hypertension were excluded. In utero ultrasonography identified fetal growth restriction by an abdominal circumference below the 10th percentile, which was confirmed at birth if the birth weight was similarly below the 10th percentile. IUGR correlated with increased serum leptin levels in the mothers (45 ng/mL versus 29 ng/mL; $P < 0.01$) and decreased umbilical cord serum levels in the infants (8.4 ng/mL versus 13.1 ng/mL; $P < 0.01$). No significant differences were noted between male and female infants in either group. As expected, umbilical cord serum leptin levels correlated with neonatal birth weight.

In general, maternal undernutrition or malnutrition results in growth restriction and rapid catch-up growth such that by early adulthood the body weight of the progeny with IUGR exceeds that of the control. In most animal studies, the animals develop components of the morbidities afflicting growth-restricted humans, including insulin resistance, dyslipidemia, and hypertension. In a remarkable methodical study, Fernandez-Twinn et al. reduced maternal protein intake to 50% of controls and measured the circulating levels of several hormones, including leptin, throughout the pregnancies.[26] The low-protein diet significantly reduced both placental and fetal body weights, and at term, the low-protein diet also significantly decreased the placental/body weight ratios. In adulthood, the pups that suffered intrauterine low-protein undernutrition developed diabetes, hyperinsulinemia, and tissue insulin resistance in adulthood. The low-protein diet increased maternal serum leptin levels at day 17 of gestation (term 21 days) and decreased maternal serum leptin levels at term. No significant differences in perinatal serum leptin levels were noted between the pups suffering the low-protein maternal diet and the control pups.

To begin the process of defining leptin homeostasis in the postnatal growth-restricted rat, Krechowec et al. used a similar model of maternal food restriction, in which dams received 30% of ad libitum food intake versus the controls.[27] This study demonstrated that prenatal malnutrition may lead to the developmental of leptin resistance, particularly in adult female rats. Mechanisms responsible for this phenomenon may include cross-talk between the insulin and leptin receptors, as well as hepatic insulin resistance leading to hypertriglyceridemia and subsequent impairment of leptin transport across the blood–brain barrier. Regardless, such studies suggest that leptin biology plays a significant role in the effects of early nutrition on the adult phenotype. Future studies will delve further into "chicken and egg" issues to more clearly differentiate the relative importance of leptin and other molecules produced by adipocytes.

Adiponectin

Adiponectin is also produced by adipocytes, and its receptors adiponectin receptor-1 and adiponectin receptor-2 are found in skeletal muscle and liver, respectively.[28] A 244–amino-acid protein is translated from the most abundant messenger RNA (mRNA; apM1) found in human adipocytes.[29] In mice, administration of adiponectin reduces insulin resistance and serum glucose levels. In humans, serum levels of adiponectin correlate directly with insulin sensitivity, but not with serum lipid profiles or obesity.

In growth-restricted humans, the impact of the early malnutrition appears to vary with age. Iniguez et al. measured leptin levels in 1- and 2-year-old SGA and AGA infants.[30] The SGA infants experienced catch-up growth such that at 2 years of age, only moderate differences existed between the two groups. Although no significant differences existed between SGA infants and control infants in absolute serum adiponectin levels, differences in adiponectin levels were inversely related to weight gain between 1 and 2 years of age. In contrast to leptin, adiponectin levels were unrelated to insulin levels, and multiple regression analysis found that adiponectin related only to postnatal age. If postnatal age was excluded from the analysis, then determinants of adiponectin levels included lower postnatal body weight ($P < 0.001$) and male gender ($P < 0.03$). Although the findings on adiponectin levels are not as immediately satisfying as the leptin data in this study, those findings are thought provoking because of the many gender-specific effects of early growth restriction that have been noted.

In contrast to the study by Iniguez et al., in the study by Lopez-Bermejo et al., adiponectin levels were measured, and both insulin resistance and insulin secretion were assessed by using the homeostasis model of assessment (HOMA) in 32 prepubertal SGA children (mean age 5.4 ± 2.9 years) and AGA children (mean age 5.9 ± 3.0 years).[31] Gestational age–adjusted birth weight <10th percentile and >25th percentile defined the SGA and AGA children, respectively. As expected, SGA infants were lighter and shorter but had BMIs similar to those of controls. HOMA analysis of SGA and AGA children >3 years of age demonstrated a tendency toward insulin resistance in the SGA children ($P = 0.046$) after adjustments for gender, age, and BMI SD score. Surprisingly, serum adiponectin levels were significantly higher in the SGA children ($P < 0.0001$), although when the data from the SGA children were broken into BMI quartiles, the findings became more complicated. Compared with lean SGA children, the higher-quartile SGA children had lower serum adiponectin levels ($P = 0.02$). The higher-quartile SGA children also had markedly higher fasting insulin levels ($P = 0.03$), borderline higher HOMA insulin resistance ($P = 0.05$), and higher HOMA beta-cell insulin secretion ($P = 0.01$). Finally, in a multiple regression analysis, HOMA insulin resistance explained 35% of adiponectin variance, and SGA or birth weight status explained an additional 10% or 15% of adiponectin variance.

In general, early malnutrition and subsequent growth restriction appear to affect serum adiponectin levels. Little has been done at this point using specific rodent models to analyze adiponectin biology within the context of growth restriction. As in the case of leptin, we are still at the point of trying to figure out "chicken and egg" type issues. Whether this is a marker for, or cause of, impending morbidity remains to be seen.

Insulin-Like Growth Factor-1

Insulin-like growth factor-1 (IGF-1) is a polypeptide, whose homology resembles proinsulin. The bioavailability and subsequent actions of IGF-1 are regulated by binding proteins, which generally moderate the actions of IGF-1 by competing with IGF-1 receptors. Most tissues synthesize IGF-1, and IGF-1 homeostasis appears to have both systemic and paracrine implications, of which the latter are probably unappreciated. In general, IGF-1 levels in human fetuses increase from 18 to 40 weeks of gestation. IGF-1 and IGF-binding protein-3 (IGFBP-3) serum levels slowly increase before adolescence, steeply increase during puberty, and decrease thereafter. In contrast, IGFBP-1 serum levels gradually decline before adolescence such that the lowest levels are found in puberty.

IGF-1 and its associated binding proteins are intriguing players in the mechanisms relating early malnutrition to adult disease for several reasons. First, IGF-1 plays a key role in fetoplacental growth throughout gestation. Null mutations of IGF-1 in mice reduce fetal size by approximately 40%.[32] In humans, *IGF-1* gene deletion results in severe prenatal growth failure.[33] Second, IGF-1 and IGFBP-3 mediate many of the anabolic and mitogenic actions of growth hormone in postnatal life. Short children have lower IGF-1 and IGFBP-3 levels compared with tall children. Third, a recent nested case-control study found that low IGF-1 and high IGFBP-3 levels in adulthood predicted increased risk for developing ischemic heart disease.[34] Finally, IGF-1 regulates or moderates insulin sensitivity in adulthood. Hepatic IGF-1 is of vital importance for normal carbohydrate metabolism in both mice and humans. In mice, elimination of hepatic IGF-1 production increases serum levels of insulin without significantly affecting glucose elimination.[35] In humans, recombinant IGF-1 is approximately 6% as potent as insulin in the production of hypoglycemia.[36] Severe IGF-1 deficiency leads to insulin resistance, which can be reversed with recombinant IGF-1.[37]

Although not as widely recognized, IGF-1 biology also affects glucose homeostasis before adulthood. Moran et al. hypothesized that the normal increase in insulin resistance that occurs concomitantly with puberty will be associated with changes in IGF-1, IGFBP-1, and IGFBP-3 levels.[38] Studies were performed on 357 adolescents (mean age 13 ± 1.2 years). IGF-1 levels significantly correlated with insulin sensitivity in both boys ($P = 0.0006$) and girls ($P = 0.02$), although IGF-1 correlated significantly with fasting insulin levels only in girls. IGFBP-1 was negatively associated with insulin resistance in both genders, whereas IGFBP-3 was positively associated with insulin resistance only in boys. The findings of this study are provocative in that they can be interpreted to suggest that the IGF-1 axis either contributes or responds to the insulin resistance of puberty. Considering the data on adults, the latter appears to be more likely.

Multiple investigators have found that infants with IUGR or SGA status have lower fetal or cord IGF-1 concentrations compared with AGA infants. In the fetus, both genetic and environmental factors regulate fetal IGF-1 levels.[39] The importance of the latter factor is supported by the observation that serum IGF-1 levels are similar in discordant monochorionic twins but significantly different in discordant dichorionic twins. This suggests that placental function and subsequent in utero substrate delivery may override genetic determinants of IGF-1 production. Furthermore, placental IGF-1 signaling appears altered in association with poor in utero fetal growth. In a recent study of 14 control and IUGR pregnancies, IUGR was found to reduce both IGF-1 receptor protein levels and IGF-1 signal transduction.[40] In contrast, no differences were found in insulin receptor protein levels. The simple conclusion is that IGF-1 homeostasis is altered in both the fetus and the placenta in pregnancies complicated by poor fetal growth. The key question will be which comes first, the poor growth or the altered homeostasis, and the likely answer is that both are possible along the spectrum of the human environmental continuum.

The trend in altered IGF-1 homeostasis continues to be evident in the postnatal period. When comparing IUGR and AGA infants from birth through age 6 to 9 months, Ozkan et al. found that IUGR decreased IGF-1 serum levels and increased serum IGFBP-1, relative to the control infants.[41] When IUGR babies were subdivided into those with catch-up growth and those without, the infants without catch-up growth had the lowest IGF-1 values ($P < 0.05$). Finally, birth weight, postnatal weight, and postnatal height correlated directly with IGF-1 and IGFBP-3 levels, but not IGFBP-1 levels. Similarly, when Fattal-Valavski et al. determined IGF-1 levels in preadolescent IUGR children (mean age 6.5 ± 2.1 years; n = 57) versus control children (7.6 ± 2.8 years; n = 30), IGF-1 serum levels were found to be significantly decreased only in the non–catch-up IUGR group.[42] Again, significant correlations between IGF-1 serum levels and both height and weight percentiles were observed in this study.

The interaction between birth weight and IGF homeostasis continues into early adolescence. Tenhola et al. investigated the relationship between serum IGF-1 and insulin sensitivity in 55 SGA and AGA age-matched children.[43] SGA was defined in this study as birth weight, length, or ponderal index >2 SD below the respective mean for gestational age. Insulin sensitivity was determined by using HOMA. After adjusting for BMI, gender, and puberty, SGA increased serum IGF-1 concentrations ($P = 0.006$). In multiple logistic regression analyses, HOMA insulin resistance predicted high serum IGF-1 levels in SGA children, but not in the AGA control group. Furthermore, SGA children in the highest IGF-1 quartile had higher BMIs ($P = 0.021$), weight ($P = 0.038$), and weight for height ($P = 0.040$), and well as lower birth weights ($P = 0.077$) versus SGA children in the lower IGF-1 quartiles.

In adulthood, the relationship becomes even more complicated, and again, genetic and environmental diversities enter the picture, as does the impact of puberty. Kajantie et al. investigated 421 subjects, who were singleton births between 1924 and 1933 at the Helsinki University Central Hospital.[44] Detailed birth records were available for these subjects, including birth weight, length, head circumference, and gestational age, as well as measurements of height and weight between ages 7 and 15 years. The average birth weight of these subjects was 3504 ± 422 g (males) and 3342 ± 406 g (females). Fourteen of the subjects were classified as SGA and were >2 SD below the norm. When adjusted for gender, current age, and BMI, IGF-1 concentrations did not correlate with any of the measures obtained at birth. However, IGFBP-1 did positively correlate with birth weight ($P = 0.03$) and ponderal index at birth ($P = 0.01$). A positive correlation also existed between adult IGFBP-1 concentration and BMI at age 7 years. Furthermore, serum IGF-1 concentrations were positively associated with adult fasting glucose levels and both systolic and diastolic blood pressures.

Childhood malnutrition also appears to affect adult IGF-1 biology. Elias et al. utilized a group of 87 postmenopausal women who were exposed to the Dutch famine between ages 2 and 20 years.[45] These women were divided into moderately exposed and severely exposed groups on the basis of weight loss, and 163 unexposed women of similar ages were used as controls. After adjusting for characteristics, such as BMI, waist/hip ratio, and cigarette-smoking habit, exposure to famine resulted in a significant increase in IGF-1 ($P = 0.038$) and IGFBP-3 ($P = 0.045$) serum levels.

The relationship between postnatal IUGR and IGF-1 levels is intriguing, although not completely clear, and if one looks at the trend in the studies by age, IGF-1 appears to gradually increase from the initial low levels in the SGA groups relative to the control groups. This may represent an overcompensation that permits catch-up growth, which is a good thing that helps cope with life as an adolescent, but the higher IGF-1 levels may have an as-yet-undefined pathologic or physiologic effect later in life.

Not all of these effects are necessarily bad, however. Early life events have been shown to affect hippocampal neurogenesis and increase age-related learning impairments in the rat. Interestingly, IGF-1 regulates the neurotropic response to aging through multiple mechanisms, including increasing mRNA levels of brain-derived neurotropic fats and stimulating hippocampal neurogenesis. Moreover, a recent study by Gunnell et al. on 547 white singleton boys and girls found that IGF-1 levels positively correlated with intelligence: For every 100 ng/mL increase in IGF-1, the intelligence quotient (IQ) increased by 3.18 points.[46]

Furthermore, aging also leads to decreased brain levels of IGF-1. Although the study by Darnaudery et al. used rats, the findings of the study are worth noting. These authors exposed pregnant dams from day 14 of pregnancy until term (approximately 21.5 days) to confinement as well as exposure to bright light three times a day.[47] After weaning at 21 days, the offspring of stressed and nonstressed dams were housed under identical conditions. At age 24 months, the progeny of the stressed dams were further divided into two groups: one group received vehicle (sodium chloride [NaCl]) into the right lateral ventricle for 21 days, the other group received IGF-1 for the same amount of time. Both groups were then exposed to a water maze task. Females whose dams had been stressed during pregnancy exhibited learning impairment in the water maze task. IGF-1 infusion restored the performance of spatial learning in the water maze such that it approximated that of control animals. One of the debates in the field is whether the adult consequences of early life events are a nonspecific response to early injury or is, in some way, teleologically protective, an evolutionary response, if you will. Such experiments suggest that the latter may be true, at least in some cases. There is a possibility that the benefits of early programming have not been appreciated, but the cost is evident, particularly as humans, as a species, have become more sedentary.

Investigators have used maternal malnutrition in the rat or bilateral uterine artery ligation of the pregnant rat to define this toll. This latter model is attractive in that it produces asymmetric IUGR through fetal hypoxia, acidosis, hypoglycemia, and decreased levels of branched-chain amino acids,[48,49] characteristics shared with human infants suffering from uteroplacental insufficiency.[50,51] IUGR rat pups in this model are 20% to 25% lighter than control pups, and birth weights are normally distributed within and between litters. Furthermore, litter size does not significantly differ between the control and IUGR groups. IUGR pups in this model develop early adipose dysregulation, insulin resistance, and adult-onset diabetes.[52-54]

A variation of this model is unilateral uterine artery ligation, with pups from the unligated side acting as controls. Vileisis and D'Ercole used this model and found that fetal weight correlated with serum glucose ($P < 0.001$), liver IGF-1 protein ($P < 0.001$), and serum IGF-1 protein ($P < 0.001$) levels.[55] No correlation was evident for either serum insulin or lung IGF-1 protein. Interestingly, serum fetal glucose concentrations correlated positively with liver ($P < 0.001$) and serum ($P < 0.002$) IGF-1 protein levels, implicating fetal glucose delivery in the regulation of IGF-1 hepatic synthesis.

Using bilateral uterine artery ligation at day 17 of gestation, Houdijk et al. found that neither male nor female animals exhibited catch-up growth in terms of body weight as they reached adulthood, although the female IUGR rats did catch up to controls in terms of nose-anus length.[56] As one might expect from the data on human children who do not exhibit significant catch-up growth, no differences were noted between control and IUGR IGF-1 levels at 100 days, regardless of gender. Interestingly, baseline growth hormone levels were significantly decreased ($P < 0.05$), suggesting that IUGR in this model may impact tissue, particularly liver, responsiveness to growth hormones.

When maternal malnutrition is utilized, IGF-1 biology is also affected. In 1991 Bernstein et al.[56a] noted that 72 hours of maternal fasting decreased serum IGF-1 levels in term rat pups. Similarly, Woodall et al.[57] investigated the effects of both protein and caloric malnutrition by restricting pregnant rat intake to 30% of an ad libitum control group. As expected, mean body weights were significantly decreased in the term IUGR fetuses versus controls, and this trend continued through the first 90 days of life. Furthermore, plasma IGF-1 levels were significantly decreased in the IUGR group from the end of gestation ($P < 0.01$) through the first 9 days of life ($P < 0.05$).[57] The effects of IUGR on IGF-1 biology have also been well described in the bilateral uterine artery ligation model of IUGR. Growth-restricted pups have decreased serum IGF-1 at birth and in adolescence, at 21 days of life.[58] Fu et al.[58] also measured levels of the various IGF-1 mRNA transcripts in the liver. IGF-1 mRNA processing involves two different start sites involving exon 1 and exon 2, respectively, as well as different 3' processing resulting in *Ea* and *Eb* variants. At birth, all mRNA transcripts were significantly reduced in both male and female IUGR pups relative to their gender-matched controls. By day 21 of life, after some catch-up growth, hepatic mRNA levels of transcripts produced from promoter 2, as well as the *Eb* variant, were still reduced in male and female rat pups compared with their gender-matched controls.[58] An important component of the studies mentioned previously involves analysis of the epigenetic code of the *IGF-1* gene and the effects of in utero nutritional stress on that epigenetic code. Fu et al. have begun to elucidate the role of epigenetics as a mechanism contributing to the complex relationship between in utero nutrition and IGF-1 biology.

Another potential mechanism through which IUGR may alter IGF-1 levels is zinc deficiency. Zinc is one of the most abundant divalent ions in living organisms and performs multiple functions secondary to its unique physiochemical properties. Two of zinc's most important properties include (1) the ability to assume multiple coordination numbers and geometries, which make this ion stereochemically adaptable; and (2) its resistance to oxidation and reduction under physiologic conditions.[59,60]

Zinc deficiency is a worldwide problem, and it is the second most important deficiency in infants.[61] In Western societies, zinc deficiency is often associated with a low socioeconomic status.[62] The effect of prenatal zinc deficiency is IUGR.[63-65] The specificity of this effect is suggested by a double-blind study, which found that zinc supplementation significantly reduced the incidence of IUGR and improved most measured indices of fetal health.[66] Zinc also plays a significant role in determining postnatal growth.[67]

Interestingly, dietary intake of zinc significantly contributes to the regulation of IGF-1 levels in both humans and animals, and the liver is considered to be the major source of circulating IGF-1.[68-70] Devine et al. found that zinc was the major determinant of IGF-1 concentrations ($P < 0.033$) in postmenopausal women after 2 years of nutritional supplementation.[71] Because of this study's careful design, the authors were able to suggest that zinc intake influences IGF-1 concentrations, even in the face of adequate energy and protein intake. Similarly, although less well controlled because of the ages of the study subjects, several groups have found that zinc supplementation increases serum IGF-1 levels in children.[72,73] Unfortunately, in the literature, human studies correlating zinc deprivation to depressed IGF-1 levels are lacking because of the multiple confounding factors, such as low protein and caloric intake, which complicate these studies. As a result, the animal literature is necessary to provide further insight.

A controversy exists in the zinc–IGF-1 literature on whether the effect of zinc deficiency upon IGF-1 hepatic expression is caused by dysregulation of growth hormone receptor pathway or the direct action of zinc on IGF-1. Two studies have investigated this controversy. The first study supplemented mice with zinc and found that although serum and hepatic IGF-1 mRNA levels increased in these animals, serum and hepatic growth hormone receptor mRNA levels remained unchanged.[70] The second study demonstrated that hepatic IGF-1 synthesis requires zinc and that lack of the growth-promoting action of growth hormone in zinc-deficient animals resulted from a defect beyond growth hormone binding to its liver receptors.[74] In other words, although growth hormone biology certainly plays a role in the regulation of hepatic IGF-1 expression, nutritional zinc also contributes in a fashion independent of the GH pathway. This is particularly true in the developing animal for the following reasons: (1) Neither growth hormone receptor mRNA nor specific GH binding is detectable in rat liver until 14 to 20 days of age[75,76]; (2) hepatic IGF-1 mRNA levels are not elevated until age 3 weeks in transgenic mice that are characterized by elevated levels of circulating GH[76]; and (3) liver-specific deletion of IGF-1 in mice reveals that IGF-1 regulates pituitary expression of growth hormone releasing factor, receptor, and secretagogue.[77]

Although the above studies demonstrated causal links between zinc nutrition, IGF-1 biology, and growth, conflicting reports exist. Doherty et al. performed a double-blind, randomized intervention study of 141 children, ages 6 months to 3 years, from the Dhaka Shishu Children's hospital in Bangladesh.[72] Their weight for age was <60% of the National Centre for Health Statistics value. On the basis of the type of malnutrition (marasmus versus kwashiorkor), the presence of diarrhea, and the numbers of days after recruitment, each child was placed in a standardized feeding regimen, which included vitamin supplementation. Randomization further placed the children into one of three regimens: (1) 1.5 mg/kg elemental zinc for 15 days; (2) 6 mg/kg elemental zinc for 15 days; and (3) 6 mg/kg elemental zinc for 30 days. The diet increased ponderal catch-up growth rapidly, although linear growth was only moderately improved. At baseline, IGF-1 and IGFBP-3 were significantly lower than standard values for healthy, well-nourished European children. During the feeding protocol, IGF-1 and IGFBP-3 increased, reaching a plateau by 15 days. The only difference between the regimens was that IGF-1 was higher in the zinc regimen 1 at day 15 ($P = 0.04$). As markers, IGF-1 and IGFBP-3 correlated best with ponderal growth at day 15 and with linear growth at day 90. The authors of this study noted that their inability to demonstrate a clearer effect of zinc in this particular study may be secondary to (1) the lower supplementation providing sufficient zinc or (2) the full nutritional supplementation masking the effects of the higher zinc dosing. The bottom line is that both prenatal and postnatal nutrition affects IGF-1 biology and alters postnatal phenotypic characteristics. On all levels—molecular, endocrinologic, and physiologic—there is a lot of information that has yet to be elicited (Table 11.3). One of the more intriguing factors is the relationship between IGF-1 and early growth, particularly in how that relates to adult phenotype. Issues that need to be addressed include the effects of different macro- and micronutrients on both IGF-1 levels and sensitivity.

Table 11.3 SUMMARY-RELATIONSHIP BETWEEN PURPORTED HORMONES AND NUTRITIONAL SUBSTRATE TO ADULT MORBIDITIES DISCUSSED IN THIS CHAPTER

Hormone/Nutritional Substrate	Relation to Adult Morbidities
Leptin–leptin resistance	Leptin levels correlate with postnatal growth, which may be associated with insulin resistance
Adiponectin	Lower adiponectin levels may be a marker for infants at risk for adult morbidities
Insulin-like growth factor (IGF)-1	Low IGF-1 levels early in life are associated with poor fetal growth; high IGF-1 levels may be associated with the systemic morbidities associated with rapid catch-up growth
Zinc	Prenatal zinc deficiency is associated with poor fetal growth; furthermore, dietary zinc contributes to the regulation of hepatic IGF-1 regulation

Cardiovascular

Poor early nutrition and associated decreased growth are strongly associated with cardiovascular disease, with the three historical cohorts mentioned earlier providing ample evidence. Multiple mechanisms probably play a role with this grouping of morbidity, so the mechanisms that we have focused on are neither exclusive nor exhaustive. The two mechanisms discussed here, renal morphogenesis and endothelial dysfunction, are based on emerging evidence in both human and animal research.

Renal Morphogenesis

Several studies have demonstrated that IUGR predisposes the affected neonate toward impaired renal function as well as an increased risk of adult-onset hypertension. Nephrogenesis increases markedly during the third trimester, and is completed by 34 to 36 weeks, with 60% of the normal complement of nephrons in the human kidney formed during the third trimester. As a result, the kidney is particularly vulnerable to nutritional insults during this period. Subsequently, human and animal studies have shown that IUGR results in smaller kidneys with decreased nephron numbers. For example, Hinchliffe et al. have examined postmortem human kidneys and have remarked upon the decrease in nephron number in IUGR infants.[78,79]

Manalich et al. studied kidneys from SGA and AGA infants who died within 2 weeks of birth as a result of respiratory distress syndrome, infectious complications, cerebral hemorrhage, or perinatal hypoxia–ischemia.[80] The gestational ages of these children were 37 ± 1.05 weeks and 38.9 ± 1.29 weeks, respectively. Gender and race distributions were equal between the two groups. A maternal history of essential hypertension and smoking existed in a significantly higher number of the SGA infants compared with the AGA infants. Histomorphometric analysis was performed by a renal pathologist, who was blinded to the origin of the biopsy. Glomerular number, glomerular volume, and area occupied by glomeruli were measured. A significant positive correlation existed between birth weight and glomeruli number (r = 0.87; $P < 0.0001$) and area occupied by glomeruli (r = 0.935; $P < 0.0001$), whereas a significant negative correlation existed between birth weight and glomerular volume (r = 0.84; $P < 0.001$). These findings appear relevant when considering the findings of relative hypertension in SGA children early in life. For example, Horta et al. studied a cohort of 749 adolescents from Pelotas, in southern Brazil.[81] Approximately 5% of these subjects were marked by birth weights of <2.5 kg, and SGA was defined as birth weight <10th percentile for gestational age. Investigators gathered anthropometric information on these individuals at birth, 20 months, 42 months, and 15 years. After controlling for confounding variables, birth weight was found to be negatively associated with systolic blood pressure. Furthermore, early and late catch-up growth was found to be positively associated with systolic blood pressure in adolescence. As a side note, a separate analysis of this Brazilian cohort noted that catch-up growth in early infancy appeared to provide short-term benefits in that those SGA children who experienced the greatest catch-up growth experienced fewer hospital admissions and lower mortality between 20 and 42 months. This is consistent with this chapter's theme that much of the SGA or IUGR phenotype is an early adaptation that provides initial benefits but that it comes at the cost of later morbidities.

Law et al. used the Brompton study cohort to determine the relative effects of SGA and catch-up growth.[82] This cohort consisted of 1867 individuals from whom data were collected at birth, 6 months, childhood (2-6 years), and young adulthood (22 years of life). Of note, only 12 of these individuals weighed <2.5 kg at birth. In this cohort, a 1-kg decrease in birth weight resulted in an increase of 2.7 mm Hg (95% confidence interval [CI] 0.4-5.0) and 1.6 mm Hg (95% CI 0.1-3.2) of the young adult systolic and diastolic blood pressures, respectively. Although greater weight gain between 1 and 5 years of life correlated with higher adult systolic blood pressures, weight gain during infancy did not. This latter finding may be attributed to the association between childhood BMI and adult BMI. The consequence of the reduced nephron number is more than an amorphous risk factor for hypertension.

In Singapore, a nationwide screening program evaluated the effect of low birth weight on proteinuria and found an eightfold increased risk of proteinuria in the low–birth weight population.[83] Furthermore, SGA children with minimal change disease are more likely to relapse, and SGA children afflicted with IgA nephropathy suffer from an increased incidence of arterial hypertension. Pham et al. used bilateral uterine artery ligation in the Sprague-Dawley rat and found that IUGR decreased glomeruli number by approximately one third both at term and at 21 days of life ($P < 0.01$ for both).[84] This group also demonstrated that the compensatory glomerular hypertrophy was greater in male rats compared with female rats.[85] Interestingly, these investigators also measured IGF-1 mRNA levels and found them to be decreased to 38% of control values ($P < 0.01$). Finally, Merlet-Benichou et al. used partial unilateral artery ligation in the rat to induce IUGR, which reduced nephron number by 37% and glomerular filtration rate by 50%.[86] Among the groups that used maternal malnutrition, Welham et al. and Vehaskari et al. used low-protein diets to induce IUGR and decrease glomeruli number in IUGR rat kidneys.[87,88]

In summary, both human observations and animal studies have demonstrated that the kidney is vulnerable to early nutritional insults. One point of vulnerability may be the dependence of nephrogenesis on apoptosis. Apoptosis, or programmed cell death, is regulated by nutritional and growth factor signals, which are altered in the growth-restricted fetus. Moderation of renal apoptosis is one arena that may be a fruitful intervention in which to minimize the effects of IUGR. However, apoptosis may also be a "safety valve" through which cells minimize the total amount of necrosis. As with many things in this field, future studies are necessary to determine whether apoptosis is truly undesirable or an immediate adaptation that comes with a later cost.

Endothelial Dysfunction

Although reductions in nephron number probably contribute to the hypertensive and cardiovascular complications associated with low birth weight and SGA, other factors are likely to play a role. Biologically and philosophically, this makes sense. Biologically, there is always a reaction or reactions to any particular action. Philosophically, if the adaptations of IUGR are an attempt to increase survival odds, biologic regulation is unlikely to leave the adaptation to a sole event. In fact, evidence is emerging in both human and animal studies suggesting that endothelial function is altered in SGA infants.

Vascular endothelial dysfunction has been linked to both hypertension and coronary artery disease. Leeson et al. investigated 333 British children ages 9 to 11 years.[89] To determine endothelial function, a noninvasive ultrasound technique was used to assess the ability of the brachial artery to dilate in response to increased blood flow, which was induced by forearm cuff occlusion and release. The study group consisted of 165 girls and 168 boys. As expected, birth weight showed a graded positive relationship with flow-mediated dilatation (0.027 mm/kg; 95% CI 0.003-0.051 mm/kg; $P = 0.02$). This relationship was independent of social class, region, ethnic group, and maternal smoking. Furthermore, cardiovascular risk factors, such as blood pressure, total and LDL cholesterol, and salivary carnitine levels, showed no correlation with flow-mediated dilatation, although HDL cholesterol appeared to be inversely related ($P = 0.05$).

This same group studied 165 women and 150 men to determine endothelium-dependent and -independent vascular responses of the brachial artery.[90] The use of a sublingual nitroglycerin spray was used to induce an endothelium-independent dilatation. These subjects were 20 to 28 years of age, and the mean birth weight was 3.27 kg. Again, a significant positive correlation existed between birth weight and flow-mediated dilatation ($P = 0.04$), but not with nitroglycerin-induced dilatation. Birth length, ponderal index at birth, and the ratio of placental weight to birth weight were not related to the measures of vascular function, nor did a relationship exist between vascular function and weight at age 1 year. Because the correlation between birth weight and flow-mediated dilatation was dampened by increasing levels of acquired risk factors, such as smoking, the effect of birth weight appears to be most relevant in those with traditionally lower risk profiles.

One question that typically arises from these types of studies is the extent to which genetics either amplifies or dampens the effects of low birth weight. The best cohort studies deal with this issue statistically, and another option is discordant twin studies. These latter studies have been applied to essentially every aspect of the fetal origins of adult disease paradigm. In the area of vascular endothelial dysfunction, Halvorsen et al. studied 31 twin pairs, of which 21 were monozygotic and nine were dizygotic.[91] Of the monozygotic twins, the gestation of nine pairs was complicated by twin–twin transfusion syndrome. The mean age for the three groups was approximately 8 years. Eight of the 62 twin subjects had a systolic blood pressure above the 90th percentile, and of these eight, seven were from the monozygotic group with a history of poor fetal growth and twin–twin transfusion syndrome. In the monozygotic twin pairs without twin–twin transfusion syndrome, systolic blood pressure was higher and endothelial function more likely to be impaired in the lighter twin. In terms of the mechanism through which endothelial function is likely to occur, multiple factors are likely to be involved. Two factors for which evidence exist are impaired acetylcholine-induced vascular relaxation and impaired angiotensin-converting enzyme (ACE) activity. For the former, Martin et al. investigated 40 newborn infants and their mothers 3 days after delivery, as well as 10 healthy age-matched control women.[92] These investigators induced peripheral vasodilatation through either local application of acetylcholine or local heating, and perfusion differences were assessed by laser Doppler. In response to acetylcholine, SGA infants responded with only a moderate increase in perfusion ($240 \pm 125\%$), whereas AGA infants responded robustly ($650 \pm 250\%$) ($P < 0.01$). Furthermore, when the SGA group was further divided, the lean SGA infants were characterized by a smaller increase in perfusion ($189 \pm 40\%$) versus the symmetrically small SGA infants ($338 \pm 170\%$) ($P < 0.01$). Interestingly, the presence of a family history of cardiovascular disease did not result in changes in perfusion. Furthermore, when comparing either absolute or relative perfusion responses to local heating, no differences were noted between SGA and AGA infants. Because acetylcholine vasodilatation is endothelium dependent and vasodilatation in response to local heat is dependent on smooth muscle, these findings suggest that acetylcholine endothelial dysfunction is present even at birth.

Another mechanism through which endothelial function dysfunction and cardiovascular morbidity may occur is through the altered function of the angiotensin pathways. ACE plays a key role in the regulation of peripheral blood pressure, and the evidence implicating this pathway derives from both human observation and animal studies. In humans, Forsyth et al. performed a prospective study of full-term infants and measured ACE levels at ages 1 and 3 months.[93] Mean birth weight was 3498 ± 506 g. They found a significant negative correlation between ACE activity at both 1 and 3 months and birth weight, $P < 0.001$ and < 0.03, respectively. In rats, Riviere et al. used a 70% caloric restricted model of maternal nutrition to study the effect on offspring angiotensin II serum levels, ACE and ACE2 mRNA levels, and ACE activities in multiple tissues.[94] ACE2 is a newly described member of the angiotensin pathways that competes with ACE for angiotensin peptide hydrolysis. In Riviere et al.'s study, not only was blood pressure moderately increased, but ACE and ACE2 activities were significantly increased in the lung ($P < 0.05$). These authors speculated that increased activity of these enzymes may contribute to the hypertension observed in these animals.

In sheep, several studies have emphasized the potential of the angiotensin pathway in mediating cardiovascular disease. Included among these studies is the work of Roghair et al., who used the programming model of antenatal steroid administration in the preterm sheep.[95] In this model, a catheterized late-gestation fetus receives betamethasone (10 mg/h) over 48 hours, and a control twin receives an identical volume of the 0.9% NaCl vehicle control. Contractile responses of circumflex coronary artery segments were assessed in response to angiotensin, sodium nitroprusside, 8-bromo-cyclic guanosine monophosphate (cGMP), isoproterenol, and forskolin. The betamethasone-treated twins exhibited a significant increase in angiotensin II coronary artery contractility versus the vehicle-treated controls ($P < 0.05$), but no significant difference to the other vasoactive compounds. Interestingly, the mesenteric arteries did not demonstrate the same differential reactivity. Furthermore, increased coronary artery levels of the angiotensin type I receptor differentiated betamethasone-treated and vehicle-treated fetuses ($P < 0.05$).

Multiple other mechanisms may be involved in the dysregulation of endothelial function. These studies, along with those involving the kidney, emphasize the complexity of the adaptations that occur in response to early malnutrition. The questions that need to be asked are how vital these adaptations to fetal survival are and what the costs of moderating them to minimize the effects on adult health are. The changes in blood pressure regulation may very well ensure the survival of the fetus and cost the adult later. As a result, interventions to reverse or change the programming must not be flippantly instituted.

Neuroendocrine Reprogramming

Although these above issues are important, what makes us human is our brain. As a result, the second question parents and physicians ask when looking into a child's future is what the neurologic outcome will be. There are data on humans demonstrating that early malnutrition significantly impacts the brain, and animal models are being used to understand some of the mechanisms that may be involved. This section will discuss the effects on neuroendocrine reprogramming, particularly within the context of the hypothalamic–pituitary–adrenal axis (HPA).

There is hope that changes in HPA may unify many of the phenotypic effects seen in multiple organ systems. Indeed, as with the other systems and organs discussed, a significant amount of effort will be necessary to separate the effects of the reprogrammed HPA axis on the peripheral tissues from the effects of the reprogrammed peripheral tissues on the HPA axis. The associations made by multiple groups suggesting that early exposure to high levels of glucocorticoids may trigger many of the events that we see have complicated the issue, so again, the distinction between cause and effect is blurred.

The place to start is the Dutch famine studies. Bleker et al. investigated survivors who were born term singletons at the Wilhelmina Gasthuis in Amsterdam between November 1943 and February 1947.[96] Sixty normoglycemic men and women from this cohort participated in dexamethasone suppression and adrenocorticotropic hormone-1 (ACTH1)–24-stimulation tests, as well as undergoing clinical and anthropometric assessments. Ten men and 10 women who were born before the famine, during the famine (defined by any 13 weeks of gestation during which the maternal diet consisted of <1000 kcal), and after the famine were tested. In general, higher cortisol levels after dexamethasone suppression and a lower cortisol increment after ACTH1–24 stimulation characterized the men, compared with the women. As expected, a positive correlation between cortisol levels and waist/hip ratios, 2-hour glucose levels, and 2-hour insulin concentrations existed.

When comparing cortisol concentration between those who were exposed to famine and those who were not affected, the authors report that no significant differences were found after dexamethasone suppression and ACTH1–24 stimulation, including peak cortisol levels, incremental rise, and area under the curve. Adjusting for maternal age, maternal weight gain, birth weight, smoking, and socioeconomic status did not alter the results. In their wisdom, the authors of this study pointed out that the study sample was small and the variations in cortisol concentration make it difficult to detect differences. Furthermore, these authors noted that HPA reprogramming may be more evident in those with insulin resistance, as opposed to the normoglycemic population. Finally, the dexamethasone/ACTH1–24 stimulation tests assess the adrenal level of the HPA axis, but not the CNS component. As a result, their studies do not exclude the possibility of CNS HPA reprogramming. When looking at the data from this study closely, it is intriguing that trends suggest an incremental rise in postdexamethasone cortisol and peak cortisol post ACTH1–24 stimulation, as well as an incremental decrease in cortisol increment after ACTH1–24 stimulation when comparing exposure to famine in late gestation, mid-gestation, and early gestation.

The theme of gender-specific HPA reprogramming continues to be discussed in multiple publications. Among the most intriguing is a study by Kajantie et al., which used a cohort of 7086 singleton individuals who were born between 1924 and 1933 at the Helsinki University Hospital to sample for evidence of HPA reprogramming.[97] From the original cohort, 421 individuals underwent measurement of fasting plasma cortisol and corticosteroid binding globulin levels, as well as blood pressure measurement, oral glucose tolerance tests, and body anthropometric assessment.

Similar to the previously discussed study, general gender differences were noted, including higher corticosteroid binding globulin levels in the women ($P < 0.0001$) and higher free cortisol levels in the men ($P < 0.0001$). Furthermore, positive associations between total cortisol and both current BMI ($P = 0.003$) and waist circumference ($P = 0.01$) were also noted, and a positive association between free cortisol index and both diastolic blood pressure ($P = 0.01$) and fasting glucose ($P = 0.02$) were similarly observed. A significant positive association between ponderal index in both genders and free cortisol index was observed.

A unique and important finding in this study is that the associations differed based on gestation age when subgroup analysis was performed. In infants born before 39 weeks of gestation, both total and free cortisol negatively correlated with birth weight and length. In infants born after 40 weeks of gestation, both total and free cortisol positively correlated with birth weight and ponderal index. Multiple logistic regression analysis was used to test this interaction, which revealed that the interaction between birth weight and gestational age was statistically significant for free cortisol. In other words, this study suggests that either adult hyper- or hypocortisolism may occur secondary to fetal reprogramming, based on the infant's biologic maturity at birth. The meaning of these findings supports the neonatologist's mantra that premature infants are different from full-term infants and places further legitimacy on the neonatal community's concern over the reprogramming that probably occurs in the neonatal intensive care unit (NICU).

The animal studies, to date, have focused upon the phenomenon of a fetal overexposure to glucocorticoids, with the general belief that this event programs the newborn to persistent increases in glucocorticoid hormone action. Many of the initial investigations administered dexamethasone to the pregnant animal (rat and sheep), and observed postnatal morbidities in the offspring of these pregnancies. Two of the classic studies were performed by Seckl, one of the pioneers in the field, in the Edinburgh laboratories. In the first study, pregnant female Wistar rats were given dexamethasone in week 1, week 2, or week 3 of pregnancy.[98] Dexamethasone administration during week 3 of pregnancy reduced offspring birth weight ($P = 0.004$) and induced fasting hyperglycemia and hyperinsulinemia ($P = 0.03$). Interestingly, administration of dexamethasone during either week 1 or week 2 did not significantly affect either birth weight or postnatal glucose homeostasis.

Two families of molecules play key roles in determining glucocorticoid hormone action. The first family of molecules is the glucocorticoid receptors. Although the product of one gene, multiple receptor subtypes exist, based on multiple promoter and exon variants, and this variation occurs to some extent in humans, mice, and rats.[99,100] Although not proven definitively, studies have suggested that the teleologic reason for this diversity appears to be allowance for tissue specificity and activity in response to stress. The second family of molecules is the 11b-hydroxysteroid dehydrogenases (11bHSD). 11bHSD1 functions as an 11-oxoreductase and therefore activates cortisone by converting it to cortisol. 11bHSD2 functions as an 11-dehydrogenase and thereby deactivates cortisol. As a result, 11bHSD2 maintains aldosterone receptor specificity, particularly in the kidney.

Expression of these genes is altered in the two rat models of growth restriction that was previously discussed. In the model of growth restriction induced by bilateral uterine artery ligation, Baserga et al. demonstrated that uteroplacental insufficiency and subsequent IUGR increases fetal serum corticosterone levels, as well as gene expression and activation of the hepatic glucocorticoid receptor.[101,102] Conversely, in this model, IUGR significantly decreased hepatic mRNA levels of 11bHSD1 ($P < 0.05$). Similarly, models of maternal malnutrition demonstrate that maternal diet affects the expression of these two gene families. For example, Bertram et al. provided pregnant Wistar dams with either a control diet of 18% casein or a low-protein diet composed of 9% casein throughout the pregnancy.[103] As expected, the offspring of the low-protein diet dams were characterized by reduced birth weight and elevated postnatal blood pressure. In terms of the glucocorticoid receptor, mRNA and protein levels of the gene were increased in the kidney at age 12 weeks. Furthermore, the offspring of the low-protein diet dams were further characterized by significantly decreased renal mRNA levels of 11bHSD2 at age 12 weeks.

What the human and animal studies teach us is that we have a great deal still to learn, but it is reasonable to deduce that glucocorticoid action plays a role in fetal programming, as well as being a target of fetal programming. Glucocorticoid action can be regulated centrally through the HPA axis, peripherally through the degradation of the steroids through aromatases, and locally through the expression of glucocorticoid receptors and the 11bHSD family of genes. This makes sense because it not only allows for a great deal of specificity in the action of these powerful hormones but also adds to the level of difficulty in understanding whether the observed programming is teleologically coordinated.

Postnatal Nutrition, Particularly with the Preterm Infant, and Possible Interventions

The studies linking IUGR with postnatal morbidities and changes in phenotype have increased concern in the neonatal community about the impact of the NICU experience on the preterm infant, particularly in terms of nutrition. Poor nutrition in human preterm infants occurs secondary to clinically indicated feeding volume restriction and/or infant feeding intolerance. Poor nutrition may also take the form of reduced total caloric intake or deficiencies in specific macro- or micronutrients. Despite recommendations for aggressive nutritional management of preterm infants, application of optimal nutritional regimes is difficult because of complex physiologic and management limitations.[104-107] When most preterm infants are discharged home, they are typically growth restricted. In a study with a large cohort of preterm infants, Lucas et al. found that at discharge, three out of four infants weighed <10th percentile of the population's distributions of birth weights by gestation.[108] Similarly, in a multicenter study of more than 24,000 preterm infants from 124 NICUs in North America, between 1998 and 2000, the prevalence of extrauterine growth restriction at hospital discharge (<10th percentile) was 28% for weight, 34% for length, and 16% for head circumference.[109] Poor postnatal growth in preterm humans is associated with an increased risk of neurodevelopmental impairment in later childhood, as well as with less than optimal cognitive and educational outcomes.[110]

Prematurity is associated with many of the issues associated with IUGR, including insulin resistance. In a carefully designed study by Hofman et al., insulin sensitivity was measured using glucose-tolerance tests in 72 healthy children ages 4 to 10 years.[111] Fifty of these children were born at age <32 weeks but were of appropriate size; 12 of these children were both premature and had IUGR. Twenty-two term control and 13 term IUGR infants were also included in the study. The insulin sensitivity for the four groups was as follows (10^{-4} /min/mU/liter): term control = 21.6; term IUGR = 15.1; premature AGA = 14.2 ($P = 0.004$ versus term controls); and term IUGR = 12.9 ($P = 0.009$). Similarly, Bonamy et al. have observed that prematurity is associated with higher brachial and aortic blood pressures in adolescent girls.[112]

In terms of the impact of postnatal nutrition on postnatal metabolic phenotype of the infant discharged from the NICU, a few studies provide some insight. For example, Singhal et al. determined fasting 32 to 33 split proinsulin concentrations (a measure of insulin resistance) in 13- to 16-year-olds who were former preterm infants who had been assigned to either a preterm formula (enriched) or banked breast milk/term formula (nonenriched).[113] They found that the teenagers originally fed nonenriched diets had significantly lower fasting 32 to 33 split proinsulin levels. Furthermore, the fasting 32 to 33 proinsulin levels were associated with greater weight gain in the first 2 weeks of life ($P = 0.001$). Similarly, using the same cohort,

Singhal et al. observed that feeding with banked breast milk results in lower blood pressure ($P = 0.001$), a lower LDL/HDL ratio ($P = 0.03$), and a higher leptin to fat mass ratio ($P = 0.007$).[114-116] Adipose tissue accretion is also influenced by early feeding regimens in preterm infants. Use of these supplemented feedings has been associated with accretion of greater body fat relative to weight at term corrected age,[117,118] as well as increased deposition of visceral adipose.[119] Furthermore, preterm male infants gain weight more rapidly compared with female infants and thus may be at higher risk.[120]

The bottom line is that we are slowly becoming aware that our preterm infants are at risk of many of the same issues that the IUGR infants face. The impact from prematurity has been harder to appreciate because of confounding factors and the relatively young field of neonatology. A pursuit that is going to gain greater importance in the next several years is understanding how nutrition may modulate long-term morbidities and whether we can individualize the nutritional approach based on infants' specific risk factors.

Conclusion

The consequences of altered perinatal environments and poor in utero growth are relatively constant and involve deficits throughout life in many systems, including the cardiovascular and neuroendocrine systems. Although the details may vary, depending on the timing and severity of growth restriction, the overall mechanisms implicated are similar. Primary molecular mediators of growth, cellular function, metabolism and development are disrupted by alterations in perinatal conditions. A caveat is that nutrition in the postnatal period is an important component with the potential to modulate outcomes in the preterm infant. Studies in animal models using postnatal dietary manipulation is an important factor for the identification of dietary and pharmaceutical approaches that can be applied in the preterm human infant during the postnatal period. The goal of this endeavor will be to temper the adult consequences faced by preterm and growth-restricted infants.

REFERENCES

1. Painter RC, Roseboom TJ, Bleker OP. Prenatal exposure to the Dutch famine and disease in later life: an overview. *Reprod Toxicol.* 2005;20(3):345–352.
2. Roseboom TJ, van der Meulen JH, Ravelli AC, Osmond C, Barker DJ, Bleker OP. Effects of prenatal exposure to the Dutch famine on adult disease in later life: an overview. *Twin Res.* 2001;4(5):293–298.
3. de Rooij SR, Painter RC, Phillips DI, Osmond C, Michels RP, Bossuyt PM, et al. Hypothalamic-pituitary-adrenal axis activity in adults who were prenatally exposed to the Dutch famine. *Eur J Endocrinol.* 2006;155(1):153–160.
4. de Rooij SR, Roseboom TJ. The developmental origins of ageing: study protocol for the Dutch famine birth cohort study on ageing. *BMJ open.* 2013;3(6):1–8.
5. Roseboom TJ, Van Der Meulen JH, Ravelli AC, Osmond C, Barker DJ, Bleker OP. Perceived health of adults after prenatal exposure to the Dutch famine. *Paediatr Perinat Epidemiol.* 2003;17(4):391–397.
6. Lakatos HF, Thatcher TH, Kottmann RM, Garcia TM, Phipps RP, Sime PJ. The Role of PPARs in lung fibrosis. *PPAR Res.* 2007;2007:71323.
7. Lopuhaa CE, Roseboom TJ, Osmond C, Barker DJ, Ravelli AC, Bleker OP, et al. Atopy, lung function, and obstructive airways disease after prenatal exposure to famine. *Thorax.* 2000;55(7):555–561.
8. Li J, Liu S, Li S, Feng R, Na L, Chu X, et al. Prenatal exposure to famine and the development of hyperglycemia and type 2 diabetes in adulthood across consecutive generations: a population-based cohort study of families in Suihua, China. *Am J Clin Nutr.* 2017;105(1):221–227.
9. Ravelli GP, Stein ZA, Susser MW. Obesity in young men after famine exposure in utero and early infancy. *N Engl J Med.* 1976;295(7):349–353.
10. Susser E, Neugebauer R, Hoek HW, Brown AS, Lin S, Labovitz D, et al. Schizophrenia after prenatal famine. Further evidence. *Arch Gen Psychiatry.* 1996;53(1):25–31.
11. Roseboom TJ, van der Meulen JH, Osmond C, Barker DJ, Ravelli AC, Bleker OP. Adult survival after prenatal exposure to the Dutch famine 1944–45. *Paediatr Perinat Epidemiol.* 2001;15(3):220–225.
12. Barker DJ, Osmond C. Infant mortality, childhood nutrition, and ischaemic heart disease in England and Wales. *Lancet.* 1986;1(8489):1077–1081.
13. Barker DJ, Winter PD, Osmond C, Margetts B, Simmonds SJ. Weight in infancy and death from ischaemic heart disease. *Lancet.* 1989;2(8663):577–580.
14. Hales CN, Barker DJ, Clark PM, Cox LJ, Fall C, Osmond C, et al. Fetal and infant growth and impaired glucose tolerance at age 64. *BMJ.* 1991;303(6809):1019–1022.

15. Syddall HE, Sayer AA, Simmonds SJ, Osmond C, Cox V, Dennison EM, et al. Birth weight, infant weight gain, and cause-specific mortality: the Hertfordshire Cohort Study. *Am J Epidemiol.* 2005;161(11):1074–1080.

16. Stampfer MJ, Colditz GA, Willett WC, Manson JE, Arky RA, Hennekens CH, et al. A prospective study of moderate alcohol drinking and risk of diabetes in women. *Am J Epidemiol.* 1988;128(3):549–558.

17. Rich-Edwards JW, Colditz GA, Stampfer MJ, Willett WC, Gillman MW, Hennekens CH, et al. Birthweight and the risk for type 2 diabetes mellitus in adult women. *Ann Intern Med.* 1999;130(4 Pt 1):278–284.

18. Troy LM, Michels KB, Hunter DJ, Spiegelman D, Manson JE, Colditz GA, et al. Self-reported birthweight and history of having been breastfed among younger women: an assessment of validity. *Int J Epidemiol.* 1996;25(1):122–127.

19. Rich-Edwards JW, Stampfer MJ, Manson JE, Rosner B, Hankinson SE, Colditz GA, et al. Birth weight and risk of cardiovascular disease in a cohort of women followed up since 1976. *BMJ.* 1997;315(7105):396–400.

20. Mericq V, Ong KK, Bazaes R, Pena V, Avila A, Salazar T, et al. Longitudinal changes in insulin sensitivity and secretion from birth to age three years in small- and appropriate-for-gestational-age children. *Diabetologia.* 2005;48(12):2609–2614.

21. Chessex P, Reichman B, Verellen G, Putet G, Smith JM, Heim T, et al. Metabolic consequences of intrauterine growth retardation in very low birthweight infants. *Pediatr Res.* 1984;18(8):709–713.

22. Jornayvaz FR, Selz R, Tappy L, Theintz GE. Metabolism of oral glucose in children born small for gestational age: evidence for an impaired whole body glucose oxidation. *Metabolism.* 2004;53(7):847–851.

22a. Arends NJ, Boonstra VH, Duivenvoorden HJ, Hofman PL, Cutfield WS, Hokken-Koelega AC. Reduced insulin sensitivity and the presence of cardiovascular risk factors in short prepubertal children born small for gestational age (SGA). *Clin Endocrinol (Oxf).* 2005;62(1):44–50.

23. Soto N, Bazaes RA, Pena V, Salazar T, Avila A, Iniguez G, et al. Insulin sensitivity and secretion are related to catch-up growth in small-for-gestational-age infants at age 1 year: results from a prospective cohort. *J Clin Endocrinol Metab.* 2003;88(8):3645–3650.

24. Zhang Y, Proenca R, Maffei M, Barone M, Leopold L, Friedman JM. Positional cloning of the mouse obese gene and its human homologue. *Nature.* 1994;372(6505):425–432.

25. Pighetti M, Tommaselli GA, D'Elia A, Di Carlo C, Mariano A, Di Carlo A, et al. Maternal serum and umbilical cord blood leptin concentrations with fetal growth restriction. *Obstet Gynecol.* 2003;102(3):535–543.

26. Fernandez-Twinn DS, Ozanne SE, Ekizoglou S, Doherty C, James L, Gusterson B, et al. The maternal endocrine environment in the low-protein model of intra-uterine growth restriction. *Br J Nutr.* 2003;90(4):815–822.

27. Krechowec SO, Vickers M, Gertler A, Breier BH. Prenatal influences on leptin sensitivity and susceptibility to diet-induced obesity. *J Endocrinol.* 2006;189(2):355–363.

28. Yamauchi T, Iwabu M, Okada-Iwabu M, Kadowaki T. Adiponectin receptors: a review of their structure, function and how they work. *Best Pract Res Clin Endocrinol Metab.* 2014;28(1):15–23.

29. Maeda K, Okubo K, Shimomura I, Funahashi T, Matsuzawa Y, Matsubara K. cDNA cloning and expression of a novel adipose specific collagen-like factor, apM1 (AdiPose Most abundant Gene transcript 1). *Biochem Biophys Res Commun.* 1996;221(2):286–289.

30. Iniguez G, Soto N, Avila A, Salazar T, Ong K, Dunger D, et al. Adiponectin levels in the first two years of life in a prospective cohort: relations with weight gain, leptin levels and insulin sensitivity. *J Clin Endocrinol Metab.* 2004;89(11):5500–5503.

31. Lopez-Bermejo A, Casano-Sancho P, Fernandez-Real JM, Kihara S, Funahashi T, Rodriguez-Hierro F, et al. Both intrauterine growth restriction and postnatal growth influence childhood serum concentrations of adiponectin. *Clin Endocrinol (Oxf).* 2004;61(3):339–346.

32. Rajkumar K, Barron D, Lewitt MS, Murphy LJ. Growth retardation and hyperglycemia in insulin-like growth factor binding protein-1 transgenic mice. *Endocrinology.* 1995;136(9):4029–4034.

33. Woods KA, Camacho-Hubner C, Savage MO, Clark AJ. Intrauterine growth retardation and postnatal growth failure associated with deletion of the insulin-like growth factor I gene. *N Engl J Med.* 1996;335(18):1363–1367.

34. Juul A, Scheike T, Davidsen M, Gyllenborg J, Jorgensen T. Low serum insulin-like growth factor I is associated with increased risk of ischemic heart disease: a population-based case-control study. *Circulation.* 2002;106(8):939–944.

35. Isaksson OG, Jansson JO, Sjogren K, Ohlsson C. Metabolic functions of liver-derived (endocrine) insulin-like growth factor I. *Horm Res.* 2001;55(suppl 2):18–21.

36. Guler HP, Zapf J, Froesch ER. Short-term metabolic effects of recombinant human insulin-like growth factor I in healthy adults. *N Engl J Med.* 1987;317(3):137–140.

37. Woods KA, Camacho-Hubner C, Bergman RN, Barter D, Clark AJ, Savage MO. Effects of insulin-like growth factor I (IGF-I) therapy on body composition and insulin resistance in IGF-I gene deletion. *J Clin Endocrinol Metab.* 2000;85(4):1407–1411.

38. Moran A, Jacobs Jr DR, Steinberger J, Cohen P, Hong CP, Prineas R, et al. Association between the insulin resistance of puberty and the insulin-like growth factor-I/growth hormone axis. *J Clin Endocrinol Metab.* 2002;87(10):4817–4820.

39. Corcoran JJ, Charnock JC, Martin J, Taggart MJ, Westwood M. Differential effect of insulin like growth factor-I on constriction of human uterine and placental arteries. *J Clin Endocrinol Metab.* 2012;97(11):E2098–E2104.

40. Laviola L, Perrini S, Belsanti G, Natalicchio A, Montrone C, Leonardini A, et al. Intrauterine growth restriction in humans is associated with abnormalities in placental insulin-like growth factor signaling. *Endocrinology*. 2005;146(3):1498–1505.

41. Ozkan H, Aydin A, Demir N, Erci T, Buyukgebiz A. Associations of IGF-I, IGFBP-1 and IGFBP-3 on intrauterine growth and early catch-up growth. *Biol Neonate*. 1999;76(5):274–282.

42. Fattal-Valevski A, Toledano-Alhadef H, Golander A, Leitner Y, Harel S. Endocrine profile of children with intrauterine growth retardation. *J Pediatr Endocrinol Metab*. 2005;18(7):671–676.

43. Tenhola S, Halonen P, Jaaskelainen J, Voutilainen R. Serum markers of GH and insulin action in 12-year-old children born small for gestational age. *Eur J Endocrinol*. 2005;152(3):335–340.

44. Kajantie E, Fall CH, Seppala M, Koistinen R, Dunkel L, Yliharsila H, et al. Serum insulin-like growth factor (IGF)-I and IGF-binding protein-1 in elderly people: relationships with cardiovascular risk factors, body composition, size at birth, and childhood growth. *J Clin Endocrinol Metab*. 2003;88(3):1059–1065.

45. Elias SG, Keinan-Boker L, Peeters PH, Van Gils CH, Kaaks R, Grobbee DE, et al. Long term consequences of the 1944-1945 Dutch famine on the insulin-like growth factor axis. *Int J Cancer*. 2004;108(4):628–630.

46. Gunnell D, Miller LL, Rogers I, Holly JM. Association of insulin-like growth factor I and insulin-like growth factor-binding protein-3 with intelligence quotient among 8- to 9-year-old children in the Avon Longitudinal Study of Parents and Children. *Pediatrics*. 2005;116(5):e681–e686.

47. Darnaudery M, Perez-Martin M, Belizaire G, Maccari S, Garcia-Segura LM. Insulin-like growth factor 1 reduces age-related disorders induced by prenatal stress in female rats. *Neurobiol Aging*. 2006;27(1):119–127.

48. Ogata ES, Bussey ME, Finley S. Altered gas exchange, limited glucose and branched chain amino acids, and hypoinsulinism retard fetal growth in the rat. *Metabolism*. 1986;35(10):970–977.

49. Ogata ES, Bussey ME, LaBarbera A, Finley S. Altered growth, hypoglycemia, hypoalaninemia, and ketonemia in the young rat: postnatal consequences of intrauterine growth retardation. *Pediatr Res*. 1985;19(1):32–37.

50. Economides DL, Nicolaides KH, Campbell S. Metabolic and endocrine findings in appropriate and small for gestational age fetuses. *J Neonatal Perinatal Med*. 1991;19(1-2):97–105.

51. Economides DL, Nicolaides KH, Gahl WA, Bernardini I, Evans MI. Plasma amino acids in appropriate- and small-for-gestational-age fetuses. *Am J Obstet Gynecol*. 1989;161(5):1219–1227.

52. Joss-Moore LA, Wang Y, Campbell MS, Moore B, Yu X, Callaway CW, et al. Uteroplacental insufficiency increases visceral adiposity and visceral adipose PPARgamma2 expression in male rat offspring prior to the onset of obesity. *Early Hum Dev*. 2010;86(3):179–185.

53. Simmons RA, Templeton LJ, Gertz SJ. Intrauterine growth retardation leads to the development of type 2 diabetes in the rat. *Diabetes*. 2001;50(10):2279–2286.

54. Tsirka AE, Gruetzmacher EM, Kelley DE, Ritov VH, Devaskar SU, Lane RH. Myocardial gene expression of glucose transporter 1 and glucose transporter 4 in response to uteroplacental insufficiency in the rat. *J Endocrinol*. 2001;169(2):373–380.

55. Vileisis RA, D'Ercole AJ. Tissue and serum concentrations of somatomedin-C/insulin-like growth factor I in fetal rats made growth retarded by uterine artery ligation. *Pediatr Res*. 1986;20(2):126–130.

56. Houdijk EC, Engelbregt MJ, Popp-Snijders C, Delemarre-Vd Waal HA. Endocrine regulation and extended follow up of longitudinal growth in intrauterine growth-retarded rats. *J Endocrinol*. 2000;166(3):599–608.

56a. Bernstein IM, DeSouza MM, Copeland KC. Insulin-like growth factor I in substrate-deprived, growth-retarded fetal rats. *Pediatr Res*. 1991;30(2):154–157.

57. Woodall SM, Breier BH, Johnston BM, Gluckman PD. A model of intrauterine growth retardation caused by chronic maternal undernutrition in the rat: effects on the somatotrophic axis and postnatal growth. *J Endocrinol*. 1996;150(2):231–242.

58. Fu Q, Yu X, Callaway CW, Lane RH, McKnight RA. Epigenetics: intrauterine growth retardation (IUGR) modifies the histone code along the rat hepatic IGF-1 gene. *FASEB J*. 2009;23(8):2438–2449.

59. Dudev T, Lim C. Principles governing Mg, Ca, and Zn binding and selectivity in proteins. *Chem Rev*. 2003;103(3):773–788.

60. Vallee BL, Falchuk KH. The biochemical basis of zinc physiology. *Physiol Rev*. 1993;73(1):79–118.

61. Hess SY. National risk of zinc deficiency as estimated by national surveys [published online Jan 1, 2017]. *Food Nutr Bull*. https://doi.org/10.1177/0379572116689000.

62. Simmer K, Thompson RP. Zinc in the fetus and newborn. *Acta Paediatr Scand Suppl*. 1985;319:158–163.

63. Higashi A, Tajiri A, Matsukura M, Matsuda I. A prospective survey of serial maternal serum zinc levels and pregnancy outcome. *J Pediatr Gastroenterol Nutr*. 1988;7(3):430–433.

64. Neggers YH, Cutter GR, Acton RT, Alvarez JO, Bonner JL, Goldenberg RL, et al. A positive association between maternal serum zinc concentration and birth weight. *Am J Clin Nutr*. 1990;51(4):678–684.

65. Simmer K, Thompson RP. Maternal zinc and intrauterine growth retardation. *Clin Sci (Lond)*. 1985;68(4):395–399.

66. Simmer K, Lort-Phillips L, James C, Thompson RP. A double-blind trial of zinc supplementation in pregnancy. *Eur J Clin Nutr*. 1991;45(3):139–144.

67. King JC, Brown KH, Gibson RS, Krebs NF, Lowe NM, Siekmann JH, et al. Biomarkers of nutrition for development (BOND)-zinc review. *J Nutr*. 2016;146(4):S858–S885.

68. D'Ercole AJ, Stiles AD, Underwood LE. Tissue concentrations of somatomedin C: further evidence for multiple sites of synthesis and paracrine or autocrine mechanisms of action. *Proc Natl Acad Sci USA*. 1984;81(3):935–939.

69. Murphy LJ, Bell GI, Friesen HG. Tissue distribution of insulin-like growth factor I and II messenger ribonucleic acid in the adult rat. *Endocrinology*. 1987;120(4):1279–1282.

70. Yu ZP, Le GW, Shi YH. Effect of zinc sulphate and zinc methionine on growth, plasma growth hormone concentration, growth hormone receptor and insulin-like growth factor-I gene expression in mice. *Clin Exp Pharmacol Physiol*. 2005;32(4):273–278.

71. Devine A, Rosen C, Mohan S, Baylink D, Prince RL. Effects of zinc and other nutritional factors on insulin-like growth factor I and insulin-like growth factor binding proteins in postmenopausal women. *Am J Clin Nutr*. 1998;68(1):200–206.

72. Doherty CP, Crofton PM, Sarkar MA, Shakur MS, Wade JC, Kelnar CJ, et al. Malnutrition, zinc supplementation and catch-up growth: changes in insulin-like growth factor I, its binding proteins, bone formation and collagen turnover. *Clin Endocrinol (Oxf)*. 2002;57(3):391–399.

73. Ng HH, Bird A. DNA methylation and chromatin modification. *Curr Opin Genet Dev*. 1999; 9(2):158–163.

74. Ninh NX, Maiter D, Lause P, Chrzanowska B, Underwood LE, Ketelslegers JM, et al. Continuous administration of growth hormone does not prevent the decrease of IGF-I gene expression in zinc-deprived rats despite normalization of liver GH binding. *Growth Horm IGF Res*. 1998;8(6):465–472.

75. Mathews LS, Enberg B, Norstedt G. Regulation of rat growth hormone receptor gene expression. *J Biol Chem*. 1989;264(17):9905–9910.

76. Tiong TS, Herington AC. Ontogeny of messenger RNA for the rat growth hormone receptor and serum binding protein. *Mol Cell Endocrinol*. 1992;83(2-3):133–141.

77. Wallenius K, Sjogren K, Peng XD, Park S, Wallenius V, Liu JL, et al. Liver-derived IGF-I regulates GH secretion at the pituitary level in mice. *Endocrinology*. 2001;142(11):4762–4770.

78. Hinchliffe SA, Lynch MR, Sargent PH, Howard CV, Van Velzen D. The effect of intrauterine growth retardation on the development of renal nephrons. *Br J Obstet Gynaecol*. 1992;99(4):296–301.

79. Hinchliffe SA, Sargent PH, Howard CV, Chan YF, van Velzen D. Human intrauterine renal growth expressed in absolute number of glomeruli assessed by the disector method and Cavalieri principle. *Lab Invest*. 1991;64(6):777–784.

80. Manalich R, Reyes L, Herrera M, Melendi C, Fundora I. Relationship between weight at birth and the number and size of renal glomeruli in humans: a histomorphometric study. *Kidney Int*. 2000;58(2):770–773.

81. Horta BL, Barros FC, Victora CG, Cole TJ. Early and late growth and blood pressure in adolescence. *J Epidemiol Community Health*. 2003;57(3):226–230.

82. Law CM, Shiell AW, Newsome CA, Syddall HE, Shinebourne EA, Fayers PM, et al. Fetal, infant, and childhood growth and adult blood pressure: a longitudinal study from birth to 22 years of age. *Circulation*. 2002;105(9):1088–1092.

83. Ramirez SP, Hsu SI, McClellan W. Low body weight is a risk factor for proteinuria in multiracial Southeast Asian pediatric population. *Am J Kidney Dis*. 2001;38(5):1045–1054.

84. Pham TD, MacLennan NK, Chiu CT, Laksana GS, Hsu JL, Lane RH. Uteroplacental insufficiency increases apoptosis and alters p53 gene methylation in the full-term IUGR rat kidney. *Am J Physiol Regul Integr Comp Physiol*. 2003;285(5):R962–R970.

85. Baserga M, Bares AL, Hale MA, Callaway CW, McKnight RA, Lane PH, et al. Uteroplacental insufficiency affects kidney VEGF expression in a model of IUGR with compensatory glomerular hypertrophy and hypertension. *Early Hum Dev*. 2009;85(6):361–367.

86. Merlet-Benichou C, Gilbert T, Muffat-Joly M, Lelievre-Pegorier M, Leroy B. Intrauterine growth retardation leads to a permanent nephron deficit in the rat. *Pediatr Nephrol*. 1994;8(2):175–180.

87. Vehaskari VM, Aviles DH, Manning J. Prenatal programming of adult hypertension in the rat. *Kidney Int*. 2001;59(1):238–245.

88. Welham SJ, Wade A, Woolf AS. Protein restriction in pregnancy is associated with increased apoptosis of mesenchymal cells at the start of rat metanephrogenesis. *Kidney Int*. 2002;61(4):1231–1242.

89. Leeson CP, Whincup PH, Cook DG, Donald AE, Papacosta O, Lucas A, et al. Flow-mediated dilation in 9- to 11-year-old children: the influence of intrauterine and childhood factors. *Circulation*. 1997;96(7):2233–2238.

90. Leeson CP, Kattenhorn M, Morley R, Lucas A, Deanfield JE. Impact of low birth weight and cardiovascular risk factors on endothelial function in early adult life. *Circulation*. 2001;103(9):1264–1268.

91. Halvorsen CP, Andolf E, Hu J, Pilo C, Winbladh B, Norman M. Discordant twin growth in utero and differences in blood pressure and endothelial function at 8 years of age. *J Intern Med*. 2006;259(2):155–163.

92. Martin H, Gazelius B, Norman M. Impaired acetylcholine-induced vascular relaxation in low birth weight infants: implications for adult hypertension? *Pediatr Res*. 2000;47(4 Pt 1):457–462.

93. Forsyth JS, Reilly J, Fraser CG, Struthers AD. Angiotensin converting enzyme activity in infancy is related to birth weight. *Arch Dis Child Fetal Neonatal Ed*. 2004;89(5):F442–R444.

94. Riviere G, Michaud A, Breton C, VanCamp G, Laborie C, Enache M, et al. Angiotensin-converting enzyme 2 (ACE2) and ACE activities display tissue-specific sensitivity to undernutrition-programmed hypertension in the adult rat. *Hypertension*. 2005;46(5):1169–1174.

95. Roghair RD, Lamb FS, Bedell KA, Smith OM, Scholz TD, Segar JL. Late-gestation betamethasone enhances coronary artery responsiveness to angiotensin II in fetal sheep. *Am J Physiol Regul Integr Comp Physiol*. 2004;286(1):R80–R88.

96. Bleker LS, de Rooij SR, Painter RC, van der Velde N, Roseboom TJ. Prenatal undernutrition and physical function and frailty at the age of 68 years: the Dutch famine birth cohort study. *J Gerontol A Biol Sci Med Sci*. 2016;71(10):1306–1314.

97. Kajantie E, Phillips DI, Andersson S, Barker DJ, Dunkel L, Forsen T, et al. Size at birth, gestational age and cortisol secretion in adult life: foetal programming of both hyper- and hypocortisolism? *Clin Endocrinol (Oxf)*. 2002;57(5):635–641.

98. Nyirenda MJ, Lindsay RS, Kenyon CJ, Burchell A, Seckl JR. Glucocorticoid exposure in late gestation permanently programs rat hepatic phosphoenolpyruvate carboxykinase and gluco-corticoid receptor expression and causes glucose intolerance in adult offspring. *J Clin Invest*. 1998;101(10):2174–2181.

99. Geng CD, Pedersen KB, Nunez BS, Vedeckis WV. Human glucocorticoid receptor alpha transcript splice variants with exon 2 deletions: evidence for tissue- and cell type-specific functions. *Biochemistry*. 2005;44(20):7395–7405.

100. Turner JD, Schote AB, Macedo JA, Pelascini LP, Muller CP. Tissue specific glucocorticoid receptor expression, a role for alternative first exon usage? *Biochem Pharmacol*. 2006;72(11):1529–1537.

101. Baserga M, Hale MA, McKnight RA, Yu X, Callaway CW, Lane RH. Uteroplacental insufficiency alters hepatic expression, phosphorylation, and activity of the glucocorticoid receptor in fetal IUGR rats. *Am J Physiol Regul Integr Comp Physiol*. 2005;289(5):R1348–R1353.

102. Turner JD, Vernocchi S, Schmitz S, Muller CP. Role of the 5'-untranslated regions in post-transcriptional regulation of the human glucocorticoid receptor. *Biochimica et biophysica acta*. 2014;1839(11):1051–1061.

103. Bertram C, Trowern AR, Copin N, Jackson AA, Whorwood CB. The maternal diet during pregnancy programs altered expression of the glucocorticoid receptor and type 2 11beta-hydroxysteroid dehy-drogenase: potential molecular mechanisms underlying the programming of hypertension in utero. *Endocrinology*. 2001;142(7):2841–2853.

104. Ramel SE, Brown LD, Georgieff MK. The impact of neonatal illness on nutritional requirements – one size does not fit all. *Curr Pediatr Rep*. 2014;2(4):248–254.

105. Schulzke SM, Pillow JJ. The management of evolving bronchopulmonary dysplasia. *Paediatr Respir Rev*. 2010;11(3):143–148.

106. Jobe AH. The new bronchopulmonary dysplasia. *Curr Opin Pediatr*. 2011;23(2):167–172.

107. Jobe AH. Let's feed the preterm lung. *J Pediatr (Rio J)*. 2006;82(3):165–166.

108. Lucas A, Gore SM, Cole TJ, Bamford MF, Dossetor JF, Barr I, et al. Multicentre trial on feeding low birthweight infants: effects of diet on early growth. *Arch Dis Child*. 1984;59(8):722–730.

109. Clark RH, Thomas P, Peabody J. Extrauterine growth restriction remains a serious problem in prematurely born neonates. *Pediatrics*. 2003;111(5 Pt 1):986–990.

110. Harmon HM, Taylor HG, Minich N, Wilson-Costello D, Hack M. Early school outcomes for extremely preterm infants with transient neurological abnormalities. *Dev Med Child Neurol*. 2015;57(9):865–871.

111. Hofman PL, Regan F, Jackson WE, Jefferies C, Knight DB, Robinson EM, et al. Premature birth and later insulin resistance. *N Engl J Med*. 2004;351(21):2179–2186.

112. Bonamy AK, Bendito A, Martin H, Andolf E, Sedin G, Norman M. Preterm birth contributes to increased vascular resistance and higher blood pressure in adolescent girls. *Pediatr Res*. 2005;58(5):845–849.

113. Singhal A, Fewtrell M, Cole TJ, Lucas A. Low nutrient intake and early growth for later insulin resistance in adolescents born preterm. *Lancet*. 2003;361(9363):1089–1097.

114. Singhal A, Cole TJ, Fewtrell M, Lucas A. Breastmilk feeding and lipoprotein profile in adolescents born preterm: follow-up of a prospective randomised study. *Lancet*. 2004;363(9421):1571–1578.

115. Singhal A, Cole TJ, Lucas A. Early nutrition in preterm infants and later blood pressure: two cohorts after randomised trials. *Lancet*. 2001;357(9254):413–419.

116. Singhal A, Farooqi IS, O'Rahilly S, Cole TJ, Fewtrell M, Lucas A. Early nutrition and leptin concentrations in later life. *Am J Clin Nutr*. 2002;75(6):993–999.

117. Gianni ML, Roggero P, Taroni F, Liotto N, Piemontese P, Mosca F. Adiposity in small for gestational age preterm infants assessed at term equivalent age. *Arch Dis Child Fetal Neonatal Ed*. 2009;94(5):F368–F372.

118. Roggero P, Gianni ML, Liotto N, Taroni F, Orsi A, Amato O, et al. Rapid recovery of fat mass in small for gestational age preterm infants after term. *PLoS One*. 2011;6(1):e14489.

119. Cooke RJ, Griffin I. Altered body composition in preterm infants at hospital discharge. *Acta paediatrica (Oslo, Norway : 1992)*. 2009;98(8):1269–1273.

120. Rigo J. Body composition during the first year of life. *Nestle Nutr Workshop Ser Pediatr Program*. 2006;58:65–76; discussion 76–78.

CHAPTER 12

What Are the Controversies, and Where Will the Field be Moving in the Future?

Brenda Poindexter, MD, MS, Josef Neu, MD

In this third edition of *Gastroenterology and Nutrition: Neonatology Questions and Controversies*, a number of emerging controversies have been identified by esteemed leaders in the field of neonatal nutrition. Gastroesophageal reflux (GER) and intestinal motility remain extremely important issues in the care of preterm infants. GER, in itself, is a benign physiologic process that only becomes a disease, that is, gastroesophageal reflux disease (GERD), if it causes clinical symptoms or complications. These include worsening of lung disease, irritability, feeding intolerance, failure to thrive, and stridor. Considerable attention has also been paid to respiratory instabilities, such as apnea and bradycardia, but most recent studies have suggested that the relationship among GER, apnea, and bradycardia is weak and that in most cases, GER is not a cause of apnea and/or bradycardia. Therapeutic interventions used routinely in the past for the prevention of apnea and bradycardia, such as histamine 2 blockers, are not warranted, and nonpharmacologic expectant management should be the mainstay of treatment for most infants with suspected apnea and bradycardia. The exact nature of these treatments and strategies requires further study.

Feeding intolerance is a major problem in many preterm infants and has a multifactorial etiology that is primarily rooted in various immaturities of the developing intestinal tract. Gastrointestinal motility, in many cases, may not be of sufficient maturity to allow rapid advancement to full feedings in preterm infants. This is often complicated by comorbidities, such as hypoxia, sepsis, and inflammation. Management of these motility issues should be tailored to the functional maturity level in an individual infant, rather than based on birth, gestation, or postmenstrual age. A combination of systemic signs and symptoms needs to be considered when interpreting feeding readiness in a preterm infant. Of crucial importance is that enteral feedings accelerate gut motility patterns and that even small quantities may be capable of inducing maturation. Thus prolonged periods of *nulla per os* (NPO) should be unacceptable in these infants. Gastric capacity is small in most of these infants and emptying delayed because of immaturity. Smaller more frequent feedings may be very helpful in such infants. Drug therapy with erythromycin as a prokinetic agent that induces migrating motor complexes may be beneficial, but its safety and efficacy remain inadequately defined. Its use should be limited to rescue treatment of severe persistent feeding intolerance. New technologies that may provide the clinician with tools beyond clinical examination are being developed to aid in deciding how to best proceed with feeding advancement in these infants.

The composition of nutrients provided to preterm infants remains of major importance. For preterm infants, the quantity, timing, and composition of lipids, provided both parenterally and enterally, have been subject to controversy. Too much lipid, especially when provided intravenously in a preparation that may not be physiologic for the preterm infant, can result in liver damage, cholestasis, and lung disease. Newer preparations with different blends of lipids have been developed and are under scrutiny in their effectiveness and safety for the preterm infant. Although human milk lipids are thought to provide the greatest benefit for preterm infants, their delivery in donor human milk that does not contain active lipases may be limiting.

Infants undergoing surgical procedures, especially those related to the intestinal tract for congenital disorders, such as gastroschisis, or acquired disorders, such as necrotizing enterocolitis (NEC), go through prolonged periods of not being able to feed using the gastrointestinal tract. These infants represent a group that is in high need for specialized formulations of parenteral nutritional products, especially essential lipids that provide for optimal growth and neurodevelopment and that do not cause harm. We have the capability to evaluate and develop such products, and it will take a concerted effort by the scientific community, industry, and the regulatory agencies to move forward in this very critical field.

Human milk provides the best form of enteral nutrition for both term and pre-term neonates. However, the rapid growth of extremely low–birth weight infants as well as mitigating factors related to intestinal immaturities often necessitates addition of proteins, minerals, and other fortifiers that will help meet their needs for growth and development. Human milk lipids, microbes, and oligosaccharides are difficult to duplicate in commercial preparations, but studies are suggesting that these are valuable components that may be personalized for each infant. The American Academy of Pediatrics and Canadian Pediatric Society have recommended that all babies of a very low gestational age in neonatal intensive care units (NICUs) be provided with either their own mothers' milk or banked donor milk. Donor milk is pasteurized, and thus microbial components as well as enzymes, cells and other bioactive molecules lose activity and do not provide the same potential value as the baby's own mother's milk. There is a need for studies that will enhance provision of the baby's own mother's milk and/or provide a human milk substitute that is as effective nutritionally and immunologically as the baby's own mother's milk.

NEC is a devastating disease that represents one of the major causes of mortality and morbidity in NICUs. Despite this, even the definition of this disease remains poorly defined and there are multiple pathways to reach intestinal necrosis. Thus what is being termed "NEC" likely represents several different diseases. The prevalence of NEC increases with decreasing gestational age and appears to peak between 29 and 32 weeks' corrected gestational age. Several developmental components relate to the development of the classic forms of this disease. These include the innate immune system (e.g., Toll-like receptors), development of the microvasculature (with the developing vascular endothelial growth factor pathways) and the developing microbial ecology of the intestine, which interacts with the developing intestinal immune system, as well as formation of interepithelial tight junctions and inflammatory responses. The microbial ecology of babies who develop NEC differs from those who do not develop this disease, and this fact is leading to intense investigation for microbial therapies that may be utilized to prevent this disease.

Infants with surgical conditions continue to present a major challenge for neonatologists, pediatric surgeons, nutritionists, and others caring for these infants. Surgical infants represent a special population at risk for nutrient deficiencies and growth failure. At this time, the appropriate amino acid and lipid composition for these infants is not defined. Long-term outcomes, such as linear growth, body composition, and neurodevelopment, need to be investigated to help guide the nutritional management of these infants.

Index

Note: Page numbers followed by "f" refer to illustrations; page numbers followed by "t" refer to tables; page numbers followed by "b" refer to boxes.

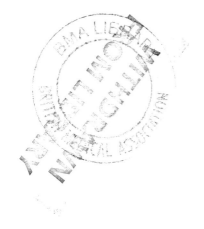